The Healthy School Handbook

Conquering the Sick Building Syndrome and Other Environmental Hazards In and Around Your School

NORMA L. MILLER, ED.D., EDITOR

NEA Professional Library
National Education Association
Washington, D.C.

Printing History
First Printing: June 1995

Note: The opinions expressed in this publication should not be construed as representing the policy or position of the National Education Association. Books published by the NEA Professional Library are intended to be discussion documents for educators who are concerned with specialized interests of the profession.

Printed on acid-free paper

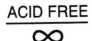

Printed with soy ink

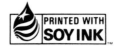

Library of Congress Cataloging-in-Publication Data

The healthy school handbook : conquering the sick building syndrome
 and other environmental hazards in and around your school / Norma L.
 Miller, editor.
          p.   cm.
     Includes Bibliographical References and Index.
     ISBN 0-8106-1863-X
     1. School hygiene—United States—Handbooks, manuals, etc.
2. School children—Health and hygiene—United States—Handbooks. manuals, etc. 3.
School environment—United States—Evaluation—Handbooks, manuals, etc. 4. Sick
building syndrome—United States—Handbooks, manuals, etc. I. Miller, Norma L.
LB3409.U5H42   1995
371.7'7—dc20   95-6345
                           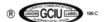   CIP

CONTENTS

Advisory Panel

Faye Chlorie
Substitute paraprofessional
Richmond Public Schools
Richmond, Virginia

M. Elaine Prom
Family Life Science Teacher
John Marshall High School
Rochester, Minnesota

Ellen H. Stein
Kindergarten Teacher
Fort Garrison Elementary
Baltimore, Maryland

Dewey White
Ariz. Ed. Assoc. Board of Directors
ESP-At-Large

PREFACE

The temperature soared to 100 degrees each day during September. Our school was not air-conditioned. We sweltered in 90-degree-plus heat. A few feet outside my elementary school classroom, two large transformers hummed constantly. Inside my classroom, rows of cool white fluorescent lights hung not far above my head.

Each day, about 200 students attended art classes in my classroom. These students came bearing odors of perfume and scented hair preparations. In the hall, custodians used sawdust to help sweep the floors. After one long weekend, we returned to school to see shining desktops that emitted a strong odor of fresh wax. I used a mimeograph machine to make copies of workbook activities. I brought these copies, still wet with ink, into the classroom. The teachers' lounge was hazy with cigarette smoke.

About six weeks after the school year began, I developed a sore throat, hoarseness, and respiratory problems. Somedays, I had difficulty talking. My health continued to deteriorate. A physician told me that my work environment was making me ill. I eventually resigned from my job as an art teacher. I felt very alone.

I continued to be hypersensitive to many chemical fumes. After a time my health improved enough for me to attend graduate school part-time. Because I wanted a better understanding of how the environment could affect the health and the learning ability of students, I chose "The Healthful School Environment" as the topic of my doctoral research at Texas Woman's University. The research data identified the top 10 areas of concern associated with the construction and maintenance of healthful school buildings. I realized that I was not alone.

The idea for this book had been germinating in my mind for some time before I was invited to Chicago to speak at the professional-development program for the 27th Annual Meeting of the American Academy of Environmental Medicine (AAEM) in October 1992. Gary R. Oberg, Annual Meeting Program Director for AAEM, had planned an entire day of sessions on the topic "Environmental Causes of Learning, Behavioral, and Other Health Problems in School Children." If each of the speakers, I thought, would write a chapter based on their topic, my idea would blossom into a very valuable handbook. The book would contain chapters covering a wide range of indoor school environment issues and discuss how sick building syndrome affects the health and the learning ability of students.

I contacted Earon Davis, Esq., Executive Director of AAEM. He liked the idea of a comprehensive book about school environmental concerns. He discussed the suggestion with Dr. Oberg who gave me the go-ahead to contact the speakers about the book. Next, I needed a publisher. I spoke with Timothy Crawford, General Manager of the NEA Professional Library----a book publishing group at the National Education Association in Washington, D.C.

Mr. Crawford attended the AAEM meeting in Chicago, and invited the distinguished cadre of environmental scientists, physicians, engineers, psychologists, and educators who presented at the meeting to write chapters for the book. Following the meeting he prepared an outline of proposed contents, that is nearly identical to the table of contents of this handbook. To cover all the topics outlined for the proposed book, I asked several other individuals who had specific expertise to contribute a chapter to the book. Mary Claycomb, a freelance editor, was hired by NEA to copyedit the voluminous manuscript. The result is the handbook you are reading now.

Every generation encounters unique problems unknown to previous generations. Parents, teachers, administrators, and school boards across the country should be concerned about the effect of the indoor environment on teaching and learning. Although there are many factors that can contribute to sick school building syndrome today, two are particularly disturbing to me:

- "cave-like" classrooms that have no windows, and
- the hazards in the computer classroom, where children are often exposed to electromagnetic fields, ozone emissions, and toner dust from laser printers. Pupils may be in that particular classroom for only 30 minutes twice a week, but the teacher is continually exposed to any hazards present in the computer classroom.

Landmark studies have shown that if the workplace environment is improved, the productivity of a worker in that environment can go up as much as 25 percent. Could the same principle be applied in schools? If the *classroom* environment is improved, will learning ability and productivity also increase?

I hope that this handbook will help patients who became sick due to the indoor environment in their school understand that they are not alone, and that it will be a catalyst for change that will alleviate some of the discomfort teachers, students, and other school staff experience because of unhealthy* environmental conditions at school.

Norma L. Miller, Ed.D.

---

* Healthy or healthful? Why does this handbook refer to *healthy* or *unhealthy* schools, when *healthful* is widely viewed as the more grammatically correct adjective to use when referring to inanimate objects like buildings? The answer is that many people experience their school building as being akin to an organic entity that breathes and pulses with the constant vitality of the activities that go on within it. A school building is, thus, capable of developing symptoms and diseases. It can succumb to illness, and it can also be brought back to health by the means described in this handbook. Besides, the term "healthy school" has a lively ring to it that conveys the dynamic nature of a building in which learning takes place.

Part One

Is Your School Sick?

IS THIS YOUR SCHOOL?
One Typical Example

by Doris Rapp, M.D.

In this chapter, Dr. Rapp—an internationally recognized author-ity on environmental medicine—examines a fictional school that typifies many of the "ailments" of sick school buildings. Empha-sizing that a major consideration in any school must be the health of students, teachers, and support personnel, she discusses in detail how environmental problems begin, progress, and, often needlessly, persist. She makes clear that restoring a school build-ing to health requires not only the satisfactory resolution of any existing air-quality problems, but also a sincere attempt on the part of everyone involved in management of the school to main-tain the highest possible air-quality standards at all times. Al-though some buildings may be returned to good health quickly and inexpensively, she writes, in many cases school districts face enormous challenges when they attempt to enhance the health and academic performance of those children and adults who spend their days in a sick school building. This chapter will give teachers, support personnel, administrators, parents, and health-care pro-fessionals valuable answers to many questions about the health of the schools in their communities. Among these questions are:

□ *What is a sick school building?*

□ *How does a sick school building affect teaching and learning?*

□ *How can you tell if your school building is sick?*

□ *How does a school building become sick?*

□ *Is there a cost-effective approach that can make a sick school building "healthy" again?*

□ *What are the long-term benefits of speedy and effective treat-ment of a sick school building?*

Let us look at one typical sick school building, which we will call the *Oldtown School*, and review how teachers, students, parents, administrators, and physicians sometimes approach the same contaminated situation. The Oldtown School does not exist. It is not part of a real school system, but is a composite of many sick schools in many systems around the the United States. The experience of our Oldtown School represents just one example of the way problems can develop in school buildings, how they can progress, and what allows them to persist.

If a school's administration is aware of illness resulting from the school building, the major consideration must be the restoration of good health to the students, teachers, and other staff members as soon as possible. To achieve the goal of ideal health, action that is appropriate, decisive, and forthright must be taken as soon as school officials are aware of the existence of the potentially unhealthful situation. Appropriate action means not only the satisfactory resolution of air-quality problems, but also a sincere attempt to ensure the highest possible air-quality standards in the future. Sometimes the solutions for an individual school can be applied quickly, easily, and inexpensively, but in other situations, it may become extremely challenging to enhance the health and academic performance of those who attend classes in the school.

WHY AND WHEN DO PROBLEMS BEGIN?

In the summer of 1992, the Oldtown School underwent major renovations that included indoor reconstruction, the installation of carpets, replacement of some roof insulation, painting, staining, masonry repair, and other similar operations. Due to unanticipated delays, fresh carpet that was particularly odorous was installed within days after its manufacture. Part of the carpet was installed during the first few weeks of the fall semester. The adhesive used to secure it to the floor required extraordinary ventilation because of its known neurotoxicity. In addition, just after school opened, pesticides were applied in the kitchen area to control ants.

Replacement of the roof insulation required that an isocyanate insulating material be sprayed on the roof when students and teachers were in the building or nearby on the school grounds. Particles of the insulation drifted through the air and settled in the hair and on the clothing of the children.

During the early weeks of the fall session, the school buses had their engines running when they parked to drop off and pick up the students. Each of the 10 buses idled for several minutes while they waited. This routine allowed exhaust fumes to permeate the air, and many students breathed the resulting pollution on a regular basis.

PROGRESSION OF PROBLEMS

About two weeks after school began, there was a sudden rash of obvious medical symptoms at Oldtown School. As the days passed, these symptoms became progressively and alarmingly more apparent in both students and teachers. By early October, about 44% (34 of 78) of the teachers had complaints, and by the end of that month, a survey indicated that 82% (64 of 78) were ill. In addition, an expanding number of students similarly complained about symptoms of the types listed in *Figures 1-1* and *1-2*.

- ☐ Headaches, fatigue, weakness, exhaustion, listlessness
- ☐ Depression, easy crying
- ☐ Moodiness, anger, confusion
- ☐ Excessive talking, explosive speech, stuttering, slurred speech
- ☐ Inattentiveness, disruptive behavior, impulsiveness
- ☐ Nervousness, irritability, agitation
- ☐ A short attention span, inability to concentrate
- ☐ Memory loss, learning problems
- ☐ Numbness and/or tingling of face, hands, arms
- ☐ Dizziness, clumsiness
- ☐ Restless legs, fingertapping, tremors, tics
- ☐ Excessive fatigue and tiredness, nightmares
- ☐ Hyperactivity, wild unrestrained behavior
- ☐ Increased sensitivity to odors, light, sound, temperature, touch and pain

Figure 1-1.
Complaints related to the nervous system.

Nose	stuffiness, watery secretions, sneezing, nose rubbing, nosebleeds, burning or irritation in nose
Chest	congestion of chest or asthma, shortness of breath, difficulty breathing, tight or heavy chest, coughing
Eyes:	irritation, burning, blurred or double vision
Skin	rashes, prickly sensations, ants crawling on skin
Throat	tightness, burning, soreness, sudden hoarseness
Aches	head, back, neck, muscles, or joint aches (e.g., "growing pains"), or aches unrelated to exercise
Intestinal	abdominal pain, nausea, belching, upset stomach, bloating, bad breath, rectal gas, vomiting, diarrhea, constipation, loss of appetite or unusual weight gain
Bladder	wet pants in the daytime or in bed, need to rush to urinate, frequent urination, burning or pain with urination, excessive thirst
Face	pallor; dark eye circles; puffiness below eyes; red cheeks, nose or ears
Glands	swelling of neck lymph node glands
Ear	repeated fluid formation behind eardrums, ear ringing, dizziness
Misc.	excessive perspiration, low-grade fever

Figure 1-2.
Other associated medical problems.

Some parents who complained that their children were ill began to receive threatening phone calls from individuals who refused to identify themselves. The callers told the parents to keep quiet and not discuss any aspect of the school situation with anyone. Teachers also received threatening phone calls from anonymous callers.

In addition, several teachers were warned repeatedly that if they discussed the school situation with anyone they would be "punished for insubordination," so most of them were afraid to tell anyone about the many health problems. Teachers who reported symptoms were frequently told by the school administration that their illnesses were psychological. Although some of the affected teachers applied for transfers to other schools, few transfers were granted. A few teachers became too ill to work. With the help of the teachers' association, some applied for—and received—Workers' Compensation.

The children had no organization to help or represent them. Furthermore, their parents did not know how to arrange for a large meeting to compare their children's medical complaints and express their concerns.

After several months, one parent's informal survey of a number of other parents indicated that about 30% of a total of the nearly 400 students had developed medical symptoms. These symptoms had first appeared during the month after school started. Initially, many parents were not fully aware of the possible pattern of illness or the potential seriousness of certain chemical exposures. Some sought treatment for their sons and daughters because they recognized the possible gravity of the children's complaints. Others recognized the problem, but, having no insurance and little money, they could not afford a neurological or environmental medical evaluation. The necessary immunologic diagnostic blood tests, or brain imaging procedures such as the Single Photo Emission Computerized Tomography (SPECT) test were not available to the children because of the parents' financial condition. Although children became ill whenever they went to school, some parents were still not knowledgeable about the scope of the school problem, even 20 months later.

When some of the sickest children went to the school nurse or health office to complain, a few were allowed to go home. Others, however, were reassured that they were all right and were sent back to their classrooms. Some of the mothers who had repeatedly requested to be notified about their children's symptoms in school, were not called, and their children were forbidden to use the telephone to call home. The parents wondered why this policy was initiated, because the attitude was so atypical of the caring nature that characterizes the Oldtown School.

Initially, the school authorities adamantly refused to transfer the students or teachers who complained of illness to other schools, even though their symptoms appeared to be directly related to the Oldtown School building. The administration continually reassured everyone that the school was safe and that the ill children and teachers merely had infections, prolonged forms of flu, mass hysteria, psychological problems, or preexisting medical conditions. They did state, however, that they had been told that allergy-like reactions that "are not too serious" could develop from materials such as carpets.

THE OLDTOWN SCHOOL ISSUES A REPORT

When the entire ventilation system was inspected and its maintenance and filtration were evaluated, it was found to have been malfunctioning in a number of ways. An examination of the entire school by the county and eventually the state health departments revealed that the ventilation system indeed had a number of defects, and appropriate changes were implemented to remedy the problems.

After the ventilation system malfunction was discovered, school officials made some changes in the system. The maintenance staff also increased the fresh air exchange markedly. Since this caused the school temperature to be about 60 degrees Fahrenheit or lower during the winter, some students and teachers wore their coats and gloves during class to keep warm. The sickest teachers and students routinely sat near open windows so they could put their heads outside from time to time to breathe cleaner air.

In addition, two "very minuscule" natural gas leaks were discovered, but these were said not to alter the indoor air quality significantly. A water heater leaked carbon monoxide sporadically. A newly constructed room had no windows, so that the air circulation there was exceedingly poor; indeed the air in that room was so improperly balanced that it necessitated the use of diffusers and exhaust fans to distribute fresh air more effectively.

Because some of the intake ventilation and exhaust ducts were located at the ceiling level, the *ceiling* was well-ventilated with recirculated air. The floor, however, which was layered with carpet and adhesive chemicals, received less adequate air exchange.

On several occasions, during October and November, 1992, officials closed the school while the building was "baked out"—heated to 85 degrees Fahrenheit—to help eliminate the chemical odors. Intensive heat can outgas chemicals by 400% and reduce chemical levels in homes by 25%. (Green 1991) The building was well-aerated after each baking. Prior to the bakeout, one air-quality evaluation had reported that there were volatile organic chemicals or compounds (VOCs) "just above the detectable limits" in the air. These included trichloroethane, benzene, toluene, and methylene chloride. (See *Figure 1-3*.)

CHEMICAL	WHERE IS IT FOUND?	WHAT DOES IT DO?
TRICHLORO-ETHANE	Art class, duplicating fluid, Vinyl floortile, VOCs, degreaser/solvent, dry cleaning fluid, fumigants, insecticides, insulators, paint, solvents, water.	Cause of cancer. Dizziness, headaches, possible liver damage.
BENZENE	Adhesives, anthraquinone colors, art class, automobile exhaust, cigarette smoke, degreaser/solvent, eggs, fossil fuel, fungicide, gasoline, glue, paint, paint stripper, plastics, room deodorizers, solvents, spot removing products, synthetic fibers, tobacco smoke, VOCs, water, wood finish.	Cause of cancer. Immunotoxic. Anorexia, aplastic anemia, blurred vision, bone marrow and central nervous system depression, chromosomal abnormalities, dermatitis, disorientation, drowsiness, drunken behavior, euphoria, eye, gastrointestinal and respiratory tract irritation, fatigue, headache, leukemia, leukopenia, lightheadedness, loss of appetite, multiple myeloma, pancytopenia, paralysis, polyneuritis, reproductive hazard.
TOLUENE	Adhesives, carpets, classrooms, cleaners, composite wood products, room deodorizers, floor tile, fossil fuel, fuel additive, gasoline, furniture, glue, insulation, lacquer, liquid paper/whiteout, paint, paint thinner and stripper, petroleum products, polyethylene, polyurethane wood finish, printing materials, solvents, tobacco smoke, varnish, wallcoverings, water.	Cause of cancer. Narcotic. Brain malfunction, central nervous system damage, depression, disorientation, eye, lung, nose and skin irritation, fatigue, hoarseness, irritability, kidney, liver and spleen damage, loss of coordination, marrow suppression, reproductive hazard; with prolonged exposure, permanent neurological damage.
METHYLENE CHLORIDE	Adhesives, classrooms, coffee, epoxy, furniture, glue, paint, paint remover, pharmaceuticals, phenolic thermosetting resins, wallcoverings.	Suspected carcinogen. Mutagen. Bronchitis, central nervous system and heart damage, eye, lung and skin irritation, metabolizes to carbon monoxide in blood, pulmonary edema or lung fluid.

Figure 1-3.
Volatile organic compounds (VOCs): what they do; where they are found.

The maintenance staff sprayed the carpets with a water-soluble herbal deodorant and used a liquid bacterial digestive enzyme that caused them to feel slimy. They were then cleaned, and all the carpeting was removed from one room. Water-damaged tiles were also repaired.

While the Oldtown School building was being baked and then aired out, the students and teachers attended a different school. Children and staff members who had been ill from the beginning of school had fewer or no symptoms during their time in the other building, but upon returning to the Oldtown School, they promptly developed symptoms again.

When all the work was completed, the official school reports indicated that the school was safe. Stating that rumors to the contrary were exaggerated and misleading, the school officials urged that such misinformation about the school building not be believed.

THE HEALTH DEPARTMENT

After each of a number of changes to improve the situation, county and state health departments evaluated the improvements, and their reports gave assurances that the school was now safe.

Health departments in such situations have a number of dilemmas. What is to be their gold standard? In their recommendations, the American Society of Heating, Refrigerating, and Air-Conditioning Engineers (ASHRAE), the Environmental Protection Agency (EPA), National Institute for Occupational Safety and Health (NIOSH), and Occupational Safety and Health Administration (OSHA) sometimes set varying standards for "tolerated or safe" levels of different gases and other air pollutants. These standards, which are designed for healthy males in workplaces and not for children in schools, serve only as suggested guidelines. So what should a health department do if, even though the suggested levels are not exceeded, certain children and teachers continue to be ill in a particular school?

The disparity between the health department reports and the continued medical complaints at the Oldtown School suggests that something in the air had not been investigated. There are innumerable potential pollutants in indoor air, and some of them can be present in lower concentrations than the usual methods of analysis can detect. Some pollutants in the Oldtown School might have eluded evaluation because their small quantity suggested they were too negligible to investigate. In addition, some water- or fat-soluble airborne chemicals are never easy to detect.

Even if the health department's thorough evaluation indicated that no problem existed, it is still realistic to think that there must have been a reason why some students and teachers continued to be ill whenever they entered the building. The ultimate challenge for the health department was not so much to confirm that a problem existed as to detect and eliminate the etiologic causative factors of the problem.

Another aspect of the confusion about pollutants is the problem of acceptance of the medical entity called "multiple chemical sensitivity." (Ashford 1991; Green 1991; Levin 1985; Rapp 1995; Rea 1989, 1991, 1992)

The Americans with Disabilities Act (Public Law 101-336, 101st Congress, July 26, 1990) acknowledges multiple chemical sensitivity as a medical illness, so it is recognized by the federal government. The bottom line, then, is not whether a particular chemical is below an "accepted tolerated" level, but rather whether its level is lower than that at which characteristic symptoms are triggered. The level that indicates a chemical sensitivity can be, and usually is, much lower than the amount routinely considered to be "safe." Disagreement arises because individuals who are not chemically sensitive neither smell nor become ill from exceedingly low odor levels. In contrast, chemically-sensitized children and adults not only smell minute levels of an ever-expanding variety of chemicals, but they also become ill from a small amount of exposure. Although the trigger level will vary from student to student and teacher to teacher, in general, the amount that causes symptoms is minuscule. It is also much lower than the level usually recognized as toxic. (Ashford 1991)

One other challenge for health officials who set standards is to designate the point at which acceptable levels should be set. The cut-off point between an acceptable level and a potential problem level can vary surprisingly at different times. From the medical viewpoint, however, a single individual who is ill can represent the warning "canary in the coal mine." That person can alert an entire school system that something may be awry, and his or her symptoms may result in action that will defuse a potentially serious situation. From a practical standpoint, there is a tendency to discount the complaints of a single individual or a few who are ill from chemical levels that don't bother the majority. This view, however, is acceptable only if you—or a member of your family—do not represent the exception.

When a school's air quality is in question, it is unwise to introduce any additional potentially harmful chemicals into the indoor environment. Unfortunately, in the Oldtown School, new wooden cabinets were purchased, and chemically-laden, vinyl folding partitions were installed in some areas of the building during the Christmas vacation. Both outgassed formaldehyde and other chemicals. By early January 1993, a new rash of complaints rapidly developed when the youngsters and teachers returned to school. The sickest teachers were often those who taught in the refurbished rooms in which the majority of the affected children also spent most of their time.

In May 1993, to evaluate the indoor air quality more completely, the state health department decreased the school's ventilation to 15% and kept the windows closed. During that period, the school was purposely kept in session so observers could gauge more accurately the typical air quality in the school. Unfortunately, the children with the more severe symptoms remained in school on that day, and at least one child became so ill from this exposure that her parents later stated "she has never been the same." On the day of the evaluation, this student became pale and nauseated, felt faint, and developed weak arms and a headache a few minutes after entering one of the most problematic classrooms. Since that time, her sensitivity to chemical odors has increased dramatically, and she has had daily headaches and fatigue.

MEDICAL ASPECTS OF THE PROBLEM

The vast majority of the school personnel and students who sought care from environmental medical specialists because of obvious school-related illnesses were found to have classical allergies and/or "allergy relatives" such as asthma and hay fever. The major complaints of both the students and the teachers were similar, as indicated in *Figures 1-1* and *1-2*. Most had the following complaints in varying numbers and degrees: headaches, recurrent flu-like infections, muscle aches, burning of the eyes and throat, loss of appetite, nausea, abdominal cramps, coughing, difficulty breathing, easy crying, and numbness and tingling of the arms, fingers, or face.

Many reported congestion and worsening of their asthma and hay fever. Some appeared to develop asthma for the first time. Some noted easy bruising or nosebleeds. A few passed out. One boy had burning eyes early in the day and developed blurred or double vision by the late afternoon. Some teachers and children noticed an impaired memory; a few became confused and had difficulty concentrating. A few children could not stay awake and found they repeatedly fell asleep during class, and a frequent complaint was daily fatigue or exhaustion. Some of them routinely required naps or collapsed as soon as they arrived home from school. Some boys were too tired to deliver newspapers. A few were in tears because they were too exhausted to play ball. Behavior problems, irritability, negativity, and mood changes became evident, and the grades of a few of the children dropped suddenly. Some girls and teachers had problems with their menses.

Many of the complaints became evident within an hour after the students entered the Oldtown School each day. The symptoms gradually worsened, becoming more severe by the time the school day ended. At first, most children and teachers were better within one to four hours after they left the school building. In time, however, the more seriously ill found that their symptoms did not subside until late Sunday afternoon. As more time passed, a weekend was no longer adequate. They needed a long vacation before they felt better. For a few, total avoidance of the problem school did not relieve their illness, and it still persisted 20 months later.

TWENTY MONTHS LATER

Teachers

Twenty months after the first symptoms appeared, most teachers in the Oldtown School were better. The school administrators, however, consistently refused to allow two of the ill teachers to transfer to other schools. They also refused to place air purifiers in the classrooms, so these two teachers had to force themselves to continue teaching in a polluted school, knowing that their future health could be seriously and perhaps permanently jeopardized. They feared loss of employment.

A few of the teachers continued to be much too ill to return to school. At least six of them remained seriously affected and two had to live a very restricted life, confined mainly to their homes. Some of the sickest had not been able to afford appropriate medical care.

The stress some teachers endured during those 20 months could certainly affect anyone adversely. It is a well-known fact that certain chemicals can alter the nervous system directly, producing changes in activity, behavior, and memory. The lives of some of the teachers exposed to chemicals during the school renovation will never be the same again. Some have been diagnosed as having psychological problems, although they had always coped well before the renovations took place. One was even forced by the expense of medical treatment to move back to her parents' home.

After 20 months, a few staff members who had at first scoffed at the idea of symptoms being caused by a school building found that they too had illnesses that might be related to a chemical exposure in the Oldtown School.

Students

Most of the students who were transferred to other schools had fewer health problems than they had experienced in the Oldtown School. One girl who had had severe headaches, continued to have them each day, but the pain was less severe. One year after treatment, however, and 15 months after the initial exposure, she still could not attend school.

Some students tried more than one substitute school before they found one they could tolerate. One such child continued to have intermittent daily headaches, nausea, and fatigue. These symptoms usually occurred within a few minutes of exposure to unavoidable substances such as perfumes, fingernail polish, and certain common cleaning agents. In addition to intense headaches and fatigue, she would also have a sharp pain in her left ear, pain in her lower right abdomen, nausea, and shakiness. These symptoms could last from two to ten days at a time.

Both Students and Teachers

Twenty months after the initial exposures in the Oldtown School, a few of the affected students and teachers found they could not tolerate the lesser chemical exposures normally present in most other schools. The children remained in home-teaching programs; the teachers also had to remain at home and were unable to work or live in a normal manner. They were forced to weigh carefully the possibility of a sudden exacerbation of their illness whenever they ventured from their homes. What chemicals would they accidentally encounter, and where would they encounter them? A challenge could be as simple as finding a service station where an attendant filled the gas tank so one didn't have to have contact with gasoline, only to be overcome by gasoline fumes when opening the window to pay for the service. Sometimes that exposure alone was enough to trigger illness that could last for hours or even days.

Because most of these students and teachers are still so sensitized, they must limit their exposure to chemicals in foods, in water, and in the air they breathe. Their experience is typical of the "spreading phenomenon" so commonly noted in individuals who have been sensitized by some previous chemical exposure. The odors of malls, restaurants, churches, public lavatories, movies, or any public gathering now can cause a recurrence of their original symptoms. (Ashford 1991; Rapp 1995) The slightest whiff of such diverse substances as perfume, tobacco, scouring powder, a disinfectant, deodorizer, or exhaust fumes now causes illness. Freshly dry-cleaned clothing and other chemically treated articles can also cause symptoms. Several years later some of the most seriously ill children and teachers continue to notice a recurrence of their original complaints within minutes after they enter the Oldtown School where their problems began.

The health of all the children and teachers who received environmental medical care has improved. Some have been treated mainly by avoidance of as many chemicals as possible. Unfortunately, a few of the children did not receive this type of care until 1994, two years after the initial exposure. They are certainly not as well at this time as those children who received comprehensive environmental medical treatment soon after their symptoms first occurred.

The vast majority of the students and teachers who had immunological blood evaluations were found to have changes in their immune systems. A few had elevated levels of chemicals in their blood. Many had antibodies against the myelin or fat covering their nerves. A few had nerve conduction changes.

When a combined total of nine children and teachers had brain image SPECT tests, they all had changes in the blood flow and function in their brains of the type caused by exposure to neurotoxic substances. The remaining 14—both students and teachers seen in late 1992—did not have this test performed.

During single-blinded testing with allergy extracts prepared from the school carpet or the school air or both, many children and teachers had symptoms that were very similar to those noted in the polluted classroom. Many also reacted to such chemicals as formaldehyde, phenol, glycerin, and hydrocarbons, all commonly found in schools.

The school carpet was analyzed by the Anderson Laboratories. During the test, air was blown over a small year-old piece of the carpet into a cage containing four mice. After exposure to this air for a total of four hours, some of the mice developed facial swelling, breathing problems, hemorrhages in their skin, eye problems, and paralysis. One mouse died after the third hour of exposure.

Physicians' Diagnoses

The usual diagnosis for both the children and the teachers was prolonged flu. This is a common diagnosis, because many of the symptoms of a chemical sensitivity are similar to the headaches, joint pains, fatigue, nausea, dizziness, and weakness so typical of flu.

Most general practitioners in the small town in which the Oldtown School is located earnestly continue to believe the children's and teachers' problems are symptoms of a prolonged variety of flu or are emotional in nature. Some of the medical specialists who saw the students and teachers also have attributed the symptoms to flu or psychological causes.

Although many of the children and teachers were seen by a number of environmental medical specialists, some physicians in non-environmental specialty practices refused to see the ill children after they heard a few details of the situation. One stated she did not want to become involved, because there might be endless hours of litigation.

Since vast numbers of individuals presently have multiple chemical sensitivities, however, many physicians are becoming increasingly knowledgeable about and accepting of the concept of illness resulting from chemical sensitivities. The literature discussing chemical sensitivities dates back to the 1940's, and since then innumerable scientific articles and books for physicians and the general public have been published about this medical problem.

FINAL HEALTH DEPARTMENT AND SCHOOL REPORTS

The health department and school officials have issued repeated reports that consistently reassure everyone that the situation has been evaluated, that minor problems have been corrected, and that the Oldtown School is safe for occupancy. Having found no measurable toxic levels of any chemicals, neither the health department nor school officials have explained why some individuals continue to become ill within minutes after they enter the Oldtown School building.

WHAT SHOULD SCHOOLS DO ABOUT ENVIRONMENTAL PROBLEMS?

Implementing some of the following measures will prove to be surprisingly health- and cost-effective for schools in which problems have been discovered or are suspected:

1. If investigation confirms the existence of a suspected problem, it should be faced head on. It is only fair and right that someone other than the parents and school personnel should provide immediate and appropriate diagnostic and therapeutic medical help to seriously affected youngsters and teachers.

2. A random check of any available school health records should reveal if and when the number of medical complaints has suddenly risen. If these records reflect a significant deviation from normal, the data can be correlated with information about changes that have occurred inside the school building immediately prior to the rise in health problems. Such a correlation, however, will help environmental planning only if a large number of individuals are affected. Isolated cases of adverse effects from localized exposures would have to be evaluated on an individual basis.

3. In an effort to prevent future air-quality problems, all renovations should begin as early as possible after school is out of session so there is adequate time for any chemical odors to dissipate before classes are resumed.

4. School administrators should pinpoint the most probable causes of their school's health problem, and then take corrective steps that will be quick, easy, practical and inexpensive. (See *Figure 1-4*.)

5. Schools must eliminate such recognized sources of problems as those shown in *Figure 1-5* in an expeditious manner, making any adjustments necessary to correct unhealthy conditions:

   □ If a problem is related to the ventilation system, a heating/ventilation/air-conditioning (HVAC) engineer or specialist should

TO HELP THE MAJORITY RIGHT AWAY

☐   Have the school's ventilation system thoroughly evaluated.

☐   The ductwork should be cleaned being certain the insulation is not moldy. Never put chemicals into the duct work.

☐   Be sure filters are maintained properly. Be sure they fit and are not dirty or contaminated with molds or bacteria.

☐   Be sure ancillary ventilation hoods and supplementary exhaust systems function well, especially in print areas, chemistry and biology classrooms, lavatories, etc.

☐   Install air purifying machines in each problem classroom for localized illness and/or in the central ventilation system if the scope of the school problem is extensive in nature.

☐   Use only environmentally safe cleaning materials.

☐   Use dehumidifiers and environmentally safe mold retardant cleaning agents. Eliminate water leaks.

☐   Clean more thoroughly and often to reduce the amount of dust. Vacuum highly trafficked areas often.

☐   Check for localized pockets of mold and bacterial contamination.

☐   Stringently reduce the number of chemicals used in any school buildings. Check storage areas for safety. Read Material Safety Data Sheets (MSDS) and have them available for those who are concerned.

☐   Stop buses from running their engines except when they are in motion.

☐   Try to have more pure and less chemically contaminated water and foods available in school cafeterias and for snacks.

☐   Be sure drain traps contain water to decrease sewer gas.

☐   Stop all routine pesticide use and implement an Integrated Pest Control System.

Figure 1-4.
What help is quick, easy, and inexpensive?

INDOOR AIR POLLUTION SOURCES

1. Ventilation
Inadequate fresh air circulation
Cleaning of ductwork
Poor filtration
Molds, bacteria or chemicals in ductwork

2. Chemicals
Pesticides
Cleaning solutions
Printing
Renovation substances:
      paint, varnish, sealants, plywood
      New carpets
      New furniture
      Insulation

3. Asbestos

4. Radon

5. Electromagnetic radiation
Fluorescent lighting
High power wires
Television or radio stations
Computers

Figure 1-5.
The major categories of indoor air pollution.

evaluate the system thoroughly, and it should be corrected according to the specifications of the specialist. (Good 1988, 1980; Bower 1993; Rousseau 1989) It is easy and inexpensive to monitor the level of CO_2 in a building. Duct work and filters should be cleaned. Intakes and outlets should be checked. Circulation should be improved throughout the school with special attention to supplying adequate fresh air to highly polluted areas. Sufficient exhaust vents, hoods, and ducts should be located near copy machines, chemistry and biology labs, cafeterias, locker rooms, swimming pools, etc.

☐ County and state health departments and other environmental evaluation agencies should be consulted for assistance and guidance.

☐ A toxicologist might be contacted to assess the air quality for toxic chemicals and to help determine the source and level of possible pollutants.

☐ After a bake-out at a very high temperature, thorough ventilation of the building would help eliminate any chemicals emitted during the bake-out.

☐ The school's ventilation should not be stringently decreased while the windows are closed during indoor air evaluations unless the most seriously ill students and teachers are not present at that time.

☐ If dust is a major or minor contributing factor to an unhealthy building condition, better and more frequent cleaning, using higher-quality vacuums and room, ceiling, or central air purifiers will help reduce the problem.

☐ If excessive molds are present, sources of moisture should be eliminated. Any damp areas should be cleaned with environmentally safe mold retardants. Drains should be cleaned, leaks fixed, and dehumidifiers should be used.

☐ If formaldehyde is outgassing from pressed wood furniture or paneling, the source should be sealed. (Krohn 1991; Rapp 1995; Small 1985, 1982)

☐ If sewer gas is present, the source should be found and the problem corrected as soon as possible. Adding water to the drain may be all that is needed.

☐ If there is a pesticide problem, an Integrated Pest Management (IMP) program should be implemented. Such a program utilizes mainly nontoxic pest control and stresses education of the faculty and maintenance personnel about how to eliminate pests, as well as control the source of the pest problem. (Forbes 1990, 1991; Mott 1987)

☐ If new carpeting is in question, a mouse bioassay should be undertaken. Anderson Laboratories will do a study to determine whether a piece of a suspect carpet adversely affects the health of test mice. If a carpet is proven to be a significant problem, it should be removed. If a school must have carpets, only those carpets proven to be totally safe should be installed, and only the safest carpet adhesives used.

It took the EPA several years to remove 27,000 square feet of contaminated carpet that reportedly caused illness to their employees. Although they no longer allow any carpet containing 4-PC or phenylcyclohexene to be installed in EPA buildings, it is perplexing that they have not issued similar warnings to protect the public in other buildings. Some carpets do not contain 4-PC, but many *do* contain a plethora of other potentially harmful chemicals.

Every school official should realize that although the purchase, installation, and maintenance of carpeting in a school costs approximately half as much as hard tile, the tile lasts four times longer (33 years) than carpet (eight years).

One must ask if the advantage of noise reduction and less floor cleaning in school buildings is worth the obvious possible health, emotional, and academic risks associated with exposure to some carpets. Infections, allergies, and chemicals that outgas from the carpet or its adhesives can all contribute to environmental illness and learning problems. This creates a benefit/risk ratio that is far less than desirable.

Administrators should bear in mind that consultants for nontoxic and environmentally safe buildings are available. (See Resources in the Reference section at the end of this chapter.)

DIAGNOSING AND HELPING RESOLVE PRESENT PROBLEMS

Many sick children and teachers need an evaluation by an experienced environmental medical specialist who understands chemical sensitivities. The therapeutic program outlined in *Figure 1-6* should help eliminate current problems and prevent other children and teachers from becoming ill.

Specialists can help determine whether an illness is due to an environmental factor or not. The typical symptoms noted in some children and teachers during school sessions often can be easily reproduced using allergy extracts prepared from school air or carpets that are suspected of

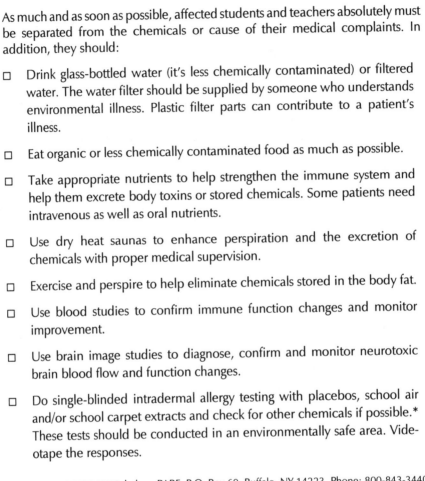

As much and as soon as possible, affected students and teachers absolutely must be separated from the chemicals or cause of their medical complaints. In addition, they should:

☐ Drink glass-bottled water (it's less chemically contaminated) or filtered water. The water filter should be supplied by someone who understands environmental illness. Plastic filter parts can contribute to a patient's illness.

☐ Eat organic or less chemically contaminated food as much as possible.

☐ Take appropriate nutrients to help strengthen the immune system and help them excrete body toxins or stored chemicals. Some patients need intravenous as well as oral nutrients.

☐ Use dry heat saunas to enhance perspiration and the excretion of chemicals with proper medical supervision.

☐ Exercise and perspire to help eliminate chemicals stored in the body fat.

☐ Use blood studies to confirm immune function changes and monitor improvement.

☐ Use brain image studies to diagnose, confirm and monitor neurotoxic brain blood flow and function changes.

☐ Do single-blinded intradermal allergy testing with placebos, school air and/or school carpet extracts and check for other chemicals if possible.* These tests should be conducted in an environmentally safe area. Videotape the responses.

*See MISCELLANEOUS RESOURCES, below: PARF, P.O. Box 60, Buffalo, NY 14223. Phone: 800-843-3440.

Figure 1-6.
What health measures help the chemically sensitized?

contamination. These physicians can either initiate appropriate diagnostic and therapeutic modalities or can refer to an appropriate physician those patients who are ill for reasons unrelated to the school exposures. Some patients may need to be seen by a variety of other medical specialists to have a particular diagnosis confirmed or negated.

Some specialists who might be most helpful include:

- *Pediatricians* and *internists* who can conduct a thorough initial examination.

- *Neurologists* who can evaluate the nervous system thoroughly.

- *Neuropsychologists* and *psychologists* who can help determine how much of a patient's problem is medical, due to a neurological problem, or psychological in nature. Patients who have a chemical sensitivity can act abnormally because of the effect that chemical exposures have upon the brain and nervous system. There is also a secondary psychological aspect to their illnesses. Both the stress caused by the stringent limitations in lifestyle due to chemical sensitivities, and the emotional impact that results from those members of the patient's family (or his or her acquaintances) who deny the presence of this type of illness, take a definite toll.

- *Physiatrists* who measure the time it takes for nerve impulses to travel from a body part to the brain and back.

- *Radiologists* who use high-tech brain imaging techniques including SPECT tests (triple head) to evaluate both the blood flow and function of the brain.

- *Detoxification medical specialists* who are knowledgeable about how to rid the body of stored chemicals or toxins. (See *Figure 1-8*.)

WHAT ARE THE MAJOR, LONG-TERM MEDICAL CONCERNS ABOUT TOXIC EXPOSURES?

There are several important long-term medical concerns that are raised by toxic exposures, including:

- *Will these medical complaints and illnesses subside after appropriate medical therapy?*

We anticipate that children and adults will have less illness if they respond favorably to comprehensive environmental medical care.

Some will improve much more than others. The degree to which patients are helped and the time required for remediation, however, will vary. Roughly 80% should be better in six to twelve months, 15% will remain the same, and 5% might become worse, in spite of therapy. Theoretically, the least ill, less exposed, and youngest, as well as those who have the strongest immune and detoxification systems should do best.

The more comprehensive the therapy, the better the patient should be as a result, and those who are treated only with avoidance are denied critical therapy. If the body's metabolic pathways are not functioning optimally, the chemical stores cannot be adequately detoxified. To enhance detoxification, proper nutrients must be available.

In one group of 19 students and 5 teachers, it was found that 20 months after initial exposure, all but one continued to manifest definite limitations in lifestyle due to the "spreading phenomenon." In general, teachers remained less healthy than most of the students, and some remained too ill to resume a normal lifestyle.

One aspect of the prognosis that appears obvious is that the earlier the correct diagnosis is made and proper comprehensive treatment is implemented, the better chance these affected children and educators have of a complete recovery.

■ *If affected individuals appear to recover completely, will they remain well when they are older?*

Many teachers and students are better to varying degrees the longer the time lapse after initial exposure, but we have no long-term follow up studies. Even if affected individuals appear to be entirely well, will they be more prone to relapse at any time in the future if they are accidentally and unavoidably exposed to some chemical? We can't be entirely sure, but, from experience, this would certainly appear to be a realistic concern.

One child in the Oldtown School who had been feeling well recently complained of a sudden recurrence of his original symptoms shortly after a chemical spill occurred a few blocks from his home. How many years will it take before he can be assured that some accidental chemical exposure won't cause another return of his original symptoms?

We need long-term scientific studies to predict more accurately what can be anticipated. The bottom line will depend upon the integrity of each individual's immune and detoxification system. Will those systems be adequate to compensate for and

cope with the diverse, potentially deleterious exposures facing all of us now and in the future?

■ *Will the abnormalities in the blood, nervous system, and brain
return to normal?*
We don't know how long these changes will last. There is presently definitive evidence that the immune or nervous system
of some children and teachers can be impaired after certain
exposures. It is obvious that appropriate baselines and monitoring are required in relation to the immunological changes
in the blood, the antibodies against an individual's own nervous system, and the changes in the brain flow and function. It
is encouraging that sometimes the brain images return almost
to normal when an individual's only treatment is separation
from the source of the problem. This indicates that the body
can and will, at times, heal itself.

■ *Will chemical exposures alter reproductive capacity in the affected
teachers and in children when they become adults?*

We simply do not know at this time. There are entire medical
texts covering the effect of chemicals on reproduction. (Colborn, et al., 1992; Council on Scientific Affairs 1985) They can
cause mutation or DNA genetic coding problems that result in
infertility or congenitally malformed babies. Some investigators have suggested that hydrocarbons and other chemicals,
for example, can be related to a drop in the male sperm count
from 120 M/ml in 1930 to 20 to 80 M/ml in more recent studies. Sterility has risen from 0.5% to 25% in some college
males. Certain pesticide exposures are known to cause atro-
phy of the testicles and a decreased sperm count in various
animal species. There is even some evidence that the health
of the offspring of parents exposed to toxic chemicals long before a child is conceived can be affected by that exposure. For
example, the children of the Vietnam soldiers exposed to
Agent Orange, appear to have more birth defects than normal
even if they were conceived long after the parent's exposure.
More long-term follow-up studies of students and teachers
are definitely indicated.

WHO IS RESPONSIBLE?

The question of responsibility is complex because:

- *The health departments* will investigate a school and provide guidelines and suggestions. They are reluctant to pass mandates or laws, however. If they do not have the authority, do they have the responsibility to enforce rules about the air quality inside schools? Are they or should they be responsible for the medical diagnosis or care of either the sick youngsters or teachers?

- *The individuals who brought chemicals into the schools* can claim they only did what they were told to do.

- *School administrations, supervisors, and other school district officials* can claim their decisions were approved by their school boards. Is it their responsibility to pay for the diagnosis and treatment of sick teachers and students if the school caused the illness?

- *School boards* are, therefore, the end of the line. Board members often have insurance to protect them from the results of their decisions. The problem is that the key players, the superintendents and board members, will no longer be making the decisions several years down the line when the sequelae from the chemical exposures are more fully understood.

- Why aren't the *medical insurance companies* responsible for reimbursement for appropriate diagnostic and therapeutic medical care? Ironically, though they often pay for medical care that does not help, they also often refuse to pay for the care and therapy that will relieve the illness, and enable some teachers to resume their professional activities. In spite of numerous scientific articles and an immense number of patient successes, some continue to claim that environmental medicine is "experimental and unproven." Do the medical advisors of the insurance companies have vested interests?

- *Social Security benefits* have been denied repeatedly for most of the teachers who have suffered environmental illnesses. Workers' compensation commissions are reviewing 4 to 6 teachers' claims every few months. Where do the teachers turn for help when the decisions of these agencies fail to provide adequate resources for reimbursement and care?

Once again, the answers are not easy. One thing, however, is certain: For occupants of a sick school building to have the best possible chance of recovery, *they must receive the appropriate and comprehensive treatment* that heretofore has been needlessly delayed or denied because no one would accept the responsibility of protecting the health of our children and teachers.

WHAT HAPPENED TO ONE CHILD AND TWO TEACHERS WHO ATTENDED AFFECTED SCHOOLS

Case Study #1: Child AB

AB is a handsome 13-year-old boy who lives in a small town in upper New York State. After having allergies and "allergy relatives," he developed new medical complaints that started shortly after he returned to school in September 1992. Within two weeks he had: nasal symptoms, a tight chest, chest pain, full ears, headaches, flushing, and hives. By October 1992, he was experiencing extreme fatigue, and was too tired to play. He would come home and collapse on the floor. He also had mood swings, a weak voice, an unpleasant taste in his mouth, itchy skin, muscle aches, and daily severe abdominal cramps with nausea, diarrhea, and a poor appetite.

At first these symptoms routinely subsided within one to four hours after he left school or when he was on vacation. During the next few months his symptoms promptly recurred within 15 minutes after he entered the school building, despite efforts on the part of the school to correct the environmental problems school officials acknowledged.

AB's complaints lessened when the school was closed in November, but worsened again when he returned a month later. During the Christmas vacation he improved. With his return to school in January 1993, his medical problems also returned. By then he had developed additional symptoms—numbness and tingling in his arms and fingers. Because of his persistent and worsening symptoms, his parents obtained permission for him attend a different school by late January 1993. Once again, he improved within a few days after the change.

In March 1993, when he returned to his previous school for 15 minutes, he developed tingling in his upper lip and began to gag. He thought he would vomit. His eyes swelled, and he was forced to leave the school.

At that same time, his father remained in the school for about eight hours. He developed asthma, itchy eyes, and shortness of breath from that exposure. The father's muscles ached so severely during the next few days that he felt as if he had competed in a bicycle marathon race. After staying in the school for four hours, *AB*'s mother also had problems breathing, an ache from her shoulder to her wrist, and a sore throat. That night she could not sleep.

The boy's problems, unfortunately, did not subside completely even though he was no longer exposed to the original school. By then he had developed the so-called "spreading phenomenon." Many new chemical odors, as well as some previously well-tolerated emissions, now began to cause symptoms. For example, in April 1993, this child entered a newly painted department store where carpets had been recently laid, and within 15 minutes he had right leg and thigh cramps and was forced to leave the building. This history indicates that he has multiple chemical sensitivities which had their onset in the original school building. Unfortunately, the problem not only persists, but it also has become more extreme because he experiences symptoms in many buildings where the quality of the air is poor.

When he was tested with an allergy extract prepared from the problem school's air, he developed droopy eyes, extreme fatigue, and the same type of abdominal pain he manifested in that school. A placebo allergy injection did not cause symptoms.

His blood showed a slight decrease in the protective white blood cells called "T" cells. His elevated level of immunoglobulin E was typical of that of other allergic children. He had formed antibodies against the fat (myelin) coverings of his own nerves.

He also had some mild problems with the transmission of the nerve impulses to and from his brain. His brain imaging (SPECT) test showed mild changes compatible with and typical of the sort of damage caused by a neurotoxic exposure. The brain's blood flow and function were not normal.

How was he 20 months later? He continued to be bothered by a wide variety of chemical odors. A whiff of perfume could cause him to develop abdominal pain, nausea, stiffness in his neck and joints, and a severe headache. He said that he felt as if it would "blow off the top of his head." His eyes still burned and watered. He continued to need naps and was too tired even to play soccer. He was discouraged. His new school was better for his health, but he missed his many friends and teachers at the other school.

The prime question at the present time, of course, is related to his future. Will his nerves, brain, muscles, digestion, and immune blood function return to normal after comprehensive environmental medical care? If he can be detoxed more effectively, more chemicals in his body can be eliminated. Who will pay the travel and living expenses for several weeks of treatment? How long will it take before he can go into public places, i.e., stores, churches, restaurants or movie theaters without developing symptoms? Even if he appears well, at some future time will a sudden, large, accidental, unavoidable exposure to a chemical make him prone to a more serious form of environmental illness? Unfortunately, we don't have the answers at this time. We only know that *AB* is far from alone in his struggle with this illness and that he appears to be improving.

Case Study #2: Teacher CD

CD had a history of asthma, eczema, mold allergy, and hay fever. The following complaints, however, began a few weeks after she returned to school in September, 1992:

- headaches, stuffiness, frequent throat-clearing, sore throat
- nightmares, feelings of panic, mood swings, depression
- dry burning eyes, blurred vision
- fatigue, sleepiness, confusion, irritability
- burning airway
- flushed ears
- excessive gas, diarrhea, bloating
- tingling in her tongue, hands, fingers, and toes
- numbness in her cheeks and fingers
- excessive perspiration, problems urinating

Most of her symptoms would begin on weekdays during the morning. She would feel "intoxicated" by afternoon and then would develop numbness of the arms, slurred speech, and an inability to concentrate, write, spell, or even use a calculator. There were times when she could not even drive her car home from school because of her weakness, fatigue, dizziness, and poor coordination.

By late November, 1992, she was forced to leave the school because her symptoms were worse. In addition, she now had sinus problems, a bad taste in her mouth, fullness in her ears, which were often red, ringing in her ears, a painful tight chest, nausea, hives, spots before her eyes, and problems reading. All of these symptoms routinely improved when she was away from the school and were worse when she was in school. In addition, however, she now developed the dreaded "spreading phenomenon." She began to experience symptoms from minute exposures to a wide range of chemicals.

She became ill after a single-blinded challenge test with a drop of an allergy extract made from a piece of carpet from the school. This test provoked a metallic taste in her mouth, cold hands, a sore itchy throat, fatigue, a stiff neck, headache, numb cheeks, pain in her upper right thigh and right foot, shortness of breath, droopy eyes, and irritability. She also developed slight cramps in her right hand and her right wrist hurt. She was much better after she received the correct neutralizing or treatment dilution of the school carpet allergy extract.

Special neuromuscular tests indicated mild mood and behavior abnormalities, and a neuropsychologic evaluation showed changes that were causally related to toxic exposure. Her blood contained some volatile organic compounds. A brain imaging (SPECT) test revealed small defects scattered throughout the cortex of the brain and one localized larger focus of the type seen in association with neurotoxic damage. (See *Figure 1-7*.)

A year after comprehensive environmental allergy care, *CD* was about 75% improved. She could not return to work, however, because she could not tolerate minute chemical exposures. For example, she could only shop for

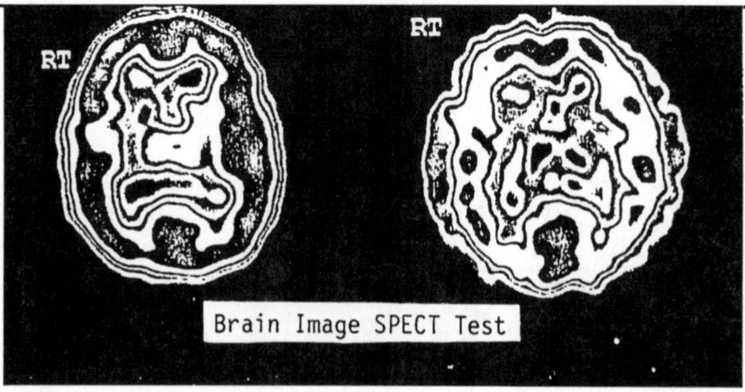

Figure 1-7.
Brain changes due to neurotoxic chemicals.

a very limited period of time in a mall. She would become dizzy and spaced out. Her bladder and visual problems persisted. She now had an intention tremor of her right hand.

She is taking nutrients, sauna treatment, massage, and exercise, and is receiving allergy extract therapy. Her home is as environmentally safe as she can make it. She tries to eat organic food, to drink glass-bottled water, and to take oral nutrients, but she can scarcely afford this extra expense. She would probably improve faster and more completely if she had intravenous nutrient therapy, which she cannot afford. Like most of the teachers at her school, she has been turned down for social security and has reapplied. She must attend Workers' Compensation hearings every 10 weeks, but many medical bills remain unpaid. Her debts continually rise. Her worries include the "spreading phenomenon," and she wonders if she will ever be able to practice her profession again or if she will have to find other employment. How can she pay her bills? When will her endless array of illnesses subside?

 The school officials have informed her that she must return to the school that caused the original problems if she is to use the legislation provided by the Americans With Disabilities Act to help her in her plight. This is an unrealistic requirement, because any exposure to the very chemicals that caused her illness would certainly further impair her already tenuous state of health and would jeopardize her professional activities.

Case Study #3: Teacher EF----A Success Story

Middle-aged teacher *EF* had a long history of typical allergies. She had been in the same classroom for four years. During that time she noted she was always ill from October to May with bronchitis, pharyngitis, sinusitis, laryngitis, congestion, and colds. She started each day with nose clearing and coughing. Her chest was heavy, and she always had too much mucus. These problems subsided whenever she was not in school. The teacher previously assigned to the same classroom had had such severe headaches that she sometimes had to lie on the floor behind her desk during school hours because the pain was so extreme.

EF was embarrassed to admit that she never felt really well and always had a long list of medical complaints. Her illness became extremely severe in May and June 1992. At that time her voice became so hoarse she could barely whisper, and she could not speak aloud for a full month. At that time, the combination of only two open ventilation ducts in the whole school, an extremely old carpet, lavatory disinfectants that smelled of strong chemicals, and pollinating grass was simply too much.

She improved during the summer and felt well, just as she did whenever there was a school vacation. By October, however, after returning to the same room her usual infections began again. Her ears felt full, and she heard ringing sounds. Her muscles ached, and her feet were numb. She had burning, tearing eyes, and visual problems, but the worst symptoms were the excruciatingly painful migraines. She felt that her head would explode because of the throbbing, stabbing pains. She admitted she was a bit hyperactive, and was irritable at times. She had excessive abdominal gas. She had so many health problems that her school principal commented to others about her "complaint of the week." Others were skeptical about her endless array of "psychosomatic" symptoms.

Because she felt ill at school and better at home, she finally realized that something in her school building was making her ill. She learned that one of the students also had symptoms. After a time, a new school superintendent fortunately—if reluctantly at first—not only listened, but also took appropriate action. This change in official attitude appeared not to be related to the teacher's complaints so much as to the symptoms of the student who became very ill, particularly in *EF*'s room. The student's atypical fatigue was extreme and his behavior grew most unusual and inappropriate.

 The superintendent wisely decided to investigate some of the factors that both the teacher and student claimed made them ill. By the time an HVAC (heating/ventilation/air-conditioning) firm evaluated the school, *EF* was so ill that she would develop a flushed face and severe breathing problems within minutes after entering her classroom. In May 1993, the majority of the ventilation ducts, which had been closed for years, were opened and clean new filters were installed. As many odorous chemicals as possible were removed from every classroom and environmentally safer cleaning agents and disinfectants were used. An air purifier was placed in both the teacher's and the student's room. When it was time to purchase new carpeting, they used the "canary in the coal mine" principle. The affected student checked pieces of carpet to see which one was well tolerated. Then the school carpeted one room and because the boy did not become ill in that room, the more expensive carpet was purchased for the entire school in hopes that this would resolve the problem.

The teacher also improved by securing the help of an environmental medical specialist, Kalpana Patel, M.D., in Buffalo, New York. She made changes in her own home similar to those suggested to the school. She drank pure, glass-bottled spring water and tried to eat organic foods that were less chemically contaminated. She took nutrients to strengthen her immune system and to help her body detoxify chemicals. She became more knowledgeable about when and why she was ill and usually could pinpoint the probable cause of a sudden flare-up. She is now well except at those times when she is accidentally exposed to some chemical, which happens much less frequently now, because her classroom, school, and home are more environmentally safe.

When she had challenge allergy testing with an extract made from her school air and the original school carpet, she reacted with a hoarse voice and breathing difficulty of the type noted in her classroom. This was relieved in a few minutes by the correct dilution of the allergy extract. She was also tested and treated for some typical allergenic substances.

By the half-way mark of the present school year, *EF* has not developed the typical repetitive illnesses that began each previous year in October. Not only is she better, but others who happen to be in her classroom or the classroom in which the student became ill are in much better health than they were before the changes were made. *EF* is not a prisoner in her own home wishing she were well enough to return to work and trying to exist on Workers' Compensation or social security. There is no pending legal action.

In this case, the school administration's approach was practical, sensible, and far-sighted. *EF* is working and does not have to be replaced. The student feels better and can remain in school, not needing home teaching. The solution to the situation has helped other children and teachers who had symptoms and illness related to their daily school exposures. There is no pending litigation. The school administration and school board chose very wisely, and the results show how a few sensible changes and precautions can defuse a potentially serious medical and legal powder keg. The school administrator is to be commended and emulated. He has helped everyone in the school, because of his decisive and proper action.

Although the rewards were immense for the school and the faculty generally, let us consider the teacher for a moment. She was not compensated for the lost time, the weeks and months of illness, or many of the previous or present doctors' bills and expense for medications. She is able to work, but she also remains labile and uneasy. Her illness can be triggered too easily and too quickly by minute exposures such as a student's stuffed animal that smells of tobacco smoke, a girl's hair spray, or a whiff of a deodorizer spray. When her throat is in spasm and her breathing is difficult, she wonders if she will be all right in a few minutes. How will she feel five or ten years from now? We don't know the answers, but we are grateful that she realized that her students' health, as well as her own, was in jeopardy and tried to prevent their developing the illness that she had.

The response of this school illustrates that it is both cost- and health-effective to find and eliminate the causes of environmentally-related school health problems. Recognition of their existence and rapid sensible correction of the major sources of the complaints can prevent an immense amount of stress, heartache, and illness. Denial and cover-up will only backfire and delay what will eventually have to be done anyway, and meanwhile, both students and teachers can be significantly and needlessly harmed.

Videos of a number of allergic students' and teachers' reactions to allergy testing with extracts from school air, school carpets, and a variety of other environmental allergic factors are available. (See MISCELLANEOUS RESOURCES section of this chapter, below: PARF.) One video also will demonstrate what happens to some mice when they are forced to breathe air blown over a toxic school carpet.

REFERENCES

Ashford, N.A., and C. Miller, 1991, *Chemical Exposures: Low Levels And High Stakes*, New York: Van Nostrand Reinhold.

Bower, John, 1993, *Healthy House Building: A Design and Construction Guide*, Unionville, IN: The Healthy House Institute.

Colborn, T., and C. Clement (Eds.), 1992, *Chemically Induced Alterations in Sexual and Functional Development: Wildlife Human Connection*, Princeton, NJ: Princeton Scientific Publishers.

Council on Scientific Affairs Report, 1985, "Effects of Toxic Chemicals on the Reproductive System," *Journal of the American Medical Association*, Vol. 253, #23, pp. 3431-3437.

Forbes, W., *Integrated Pest Management for Public and Private Schools*, Albany: NY Coalition for Alternatives to Pesticides (NYCAP). (Draft).

Forbes, W., 1991, "From Spray Tanks to Caulk Guns: Successful School IPM in Montgomery County, Maryland," *Journal of Pesticide Reform*, Winter 1990-1991, pp. 9-21.

Green, N. W., 1991, *Poisoning Our Children: Surviving in a Toxic World*, Chicago: The Noble Press.

Krohn, J., M.D., F. A. Taylor, and W. M. Larson, 1991, *The Whole Way to Allergy Relief and Prevention*, Pt. Roberts, WA: Hartley and Marks.

Levin, A., and M. Zellerback, 1985, *Type 1—Type 2 Allergy Relief Program*, New York: The Berkley Publishing Group.

Rapp, Doris J., M.D., 1989, "Double-blind Case Report of Chronic Headache Due to Foods and Air Pollution," Abstract 13, *Annals of Allergy,* 40, p. 289.

Rapp, Doris J., M.D., 1991, *Is This Your Child? Discovering and Treating Unrecognized Allergies*, Buffalo: Practical Allergy Research Foundation.

Rapp, Doris J., M.D., 1995, *Is Your School Safe for Students and Teachers?* Buffalo: Practical Allergy Research Foundation.

Rapp, Doris J., M.D., 1989, *The Impossible Child: In School, At Home*, Buffalo: Practical Allergy Research Foundation.

Rea, W. J., M.D., 1991, *Chemical Sensitivity*, Vol. I, Chelsea, MI: Lewis Publishers, Inc.

Rea, W. J., M.D., 1994, *Chemical Sensitivity*, Vol. II, Chelsea, MI: Lewis Publishers, Inc.

Rea, W. J., M.D., 1977, "Environmentally Triggered Small Vessel Vasculitis," *Annals of Allergy*, 39, pp. 245-251.

Rea, W. J., M.D., *et al.*, 1984, "Pesticides and Brain-Function Changes in a Controlled Environment," *Clinical Ecology*, 1:3, pp. 145-150.

Rea, W. J., M.D., *et al.*, 1987, "Toxic Volatile Organic Hydrocarbons in Chemically Sensitive Patients," *Clinical Ecology,* 5:1.

Rea, W. J., M.D., and M. J. Mitchell, 1982, "Chemical Sensitivity and the Environment," *Immunological Allergy Practice,* September/October 1982, pp. 245-251.

Rea, W. J., M.D., and G. H. Ross, M.D., 1989, "Food and Chemicals as Environmental Incitants, *Nurse Practitioner*, Vol. 14, #9, pp. 17-40.

Rea, W. J., M.D., and C. W. Suits, 1980, "Cardiovascular Disease Triggered by Foods and Chemicals," in *Food Allergy: New Perspectives*, Springfield, IL: Charles Thomas Publishing.

Rousseau, D., W. J. Rea, M.D., and J. Enwright, 1989, *Your Home, Your Health, and Well-Being*, Vancouver, BC: Hartley and Marks.

Small, B. M., 1985, *Recommendations for Action on Pollution and Education in Toronto*, Goodwood, Ontario: Small & Associates.

Small, B. M., 1982, *The Susceptibility Report: Chemical Susceptibility and Urea Formaldehyde Foam Insulation*, Goodwood, Ontario: Small & Associates

LABORATORY RESOURCES

AccuChem Laboratories, Richardson, Texas, Enviro-Health Systems, Inc. Phone: 214-234-5412. Blood and urine evaluations of chemicals.

Advanced Metabolic Imaging/North Dallas, Inc., Theodore R. Simon, MD, 12200 Preston Road, Dallas, Texas 75230, Phone: 214-490-0536. Brain imaging to evaluate blood flow and function.

Anderson Laboratories Inc., 30 River Street, Dedham, MA 02026-2948, Phone: 617-364-7357; Fax: 617-364-6709. Health effects of indoor air and product offgassing; diagnostic support provided for physicians.

Antibody Assay Laboratory, 1715 E. Wilshire, Suite 715, Santa Anna, CA 92705, Phone: 800-522-2611. Specializes in immunology; works with attending physicians.

MISCELLANEOUS RESOURCES

American Environmental Health Foundation, William Rea, MD, 8345 Walnut Hill Lane, Suite 225, Dallas, Texas 75231-4262, Phone: 800-225-2343; 214-261-9515; Fax: 214-691-8432.

E. L. Foust Co., Box 105, Elmhurst, IL 60126, Phone: 800-225-9549; Fax: 708-834-5341. Vapor barrier. Free catalog.

Environmental Education and Health Services, Inc., Mary Oetzel, 3202 W. Anderson Lane, No. 208-248, Austin TX 78757, Phone: 512-288-2369. Safe building/design consultant.

Environmental Health Services, 3202 West Anderson Lane, #208-249, Austin, TX 78757.

HealthComm, Inc., Jeffrey Bland, Ph.D., 5800 Soundview Drive, Gig Harbor, WA 98335. ULTRACLEAR.

National Center for Environmental Health Strategies, *The Delicate Balance*, Mary Lamielle, Director, 1100 Rural Avenue, Voorhees, NJ 08043, Phone: 609-429-5358.

New York Coalition for Alternatives to Pesticides (NYCAP), P.O. Box 6005, Albany, NY 12206-0005, Phone: 518-426-8246; 518-426-9331.

PACE Chemical Industries, Inc. 710 Woodlawn Drive, Thousand Oaks, CA 91360, Phone: 805-499-2911. Crystal Aire sealant.

Practical Allergy Research Foundation (PARF), P.O. Box 60, Buffalo, NY 14223-0060, Phone: 800-843-3440. General information, books, pamphlets, and videos.

2

WHY CHILDREN ARE MORE SUSCEPTIBLE TO ENVIRONMENTAL HAZARDS

by William J. Rea, M.D., F.A.C.S., F.A.A.E.M.

In this chapter, Dr. Rea, Director of the Environmental Health Center in Dallas, explores the many facets of children's susceptibility to environmental hazards, from pre-natal pollution exposure to contaminated air at home and in school. In Dr. Rea's analysis of each of these causes, you will find answers to many questions, including:

☐ *Why do teachers often say the hour after lunch is "the worst" period of the school day?*

☐ *Why do some children behave inappropriately or have trouble learning during the early hours of the school day?*

☐ *How can some chemicals found in school buildings impair both adults' and children's memory?*

☐ *Why should a child's complaint be recognized as an early warning of environmental contamination?*

☐ *What can schools do to avoid activities that irritate children's nervous and immune systems?*

There are many reasons for children's susceptibility to environmental hazards, including: genetic abnormalities; the state of nutrition and total body pollutant load in the mother's uterus; the state of nutrition and total body pollutant load at the time of exposure; the immature immune system; an inability to deal with addictive exposures; the imperception of parents and teachers relative to the child's exposure; a difficulty in hearing the child's complaints; inadvertently contaminated living quarters; schools contaminated, both intentionally and unintentionally, with pollutants over which the child has no control; clothing forcibly contaminated by law or inadvertently contaminated by processing and materials; a poor diet, additive- and sugar-rich, and deficient in many vitamins, minerals, and amino acids; social customs that ignore environmental factors (i.e., psychological explanations for physical phenomena), immunization shots; the frequent use of antibiotics, cortisone, and other symptom-suppressing medications *often* administered in lieu of finding and eliminating the causes of symptoms; and finally, children's immature nervous systems. Each of these causes will be discussed separately.

GENETIC ABNORMALITIES

Over 2,000 metabolic genetic defects have now been identified, in addition to long-known anatomic ones. It is reasonable to assume that most children have one or more of these defects, which are "time bombs" waiting for the right combination of environmental triggers to manifest their pathology. One example of a metabolic genetic deficiency is the condition known as phenylketonuria. If the environmental trigger of phenylalanine is avoided in the diet, children with this deficiency will grow to adulthood unharmed. If the condition is triggered by meat or Nutrasweet® or other foods containing phenylalanine, susceptible children will develop brain damage. Other examples of individuals with metabolic genetic deficiencies are the slow oxidizers and the slow acetylators. When the genetic defect is present, these last two groups may be unable to detoxify toxic chemicals entering the body and thus may suffer an increase in total body pollutant load which may result in learning disability and hyperactivity.

STATE OF NUTRITION AND TOTAL BODY LOAD IN THE MOTHER'S UTERUS

It has now been shown that due to the child's poor liver detoxification systems, poor kidney function, or poorly developed detoxification systems in other areas of the developing fetus, toxins may have accumulated in the child's body before birth. The activity of the mother during pregnancy may result in a bioconcentration of the toxics in the fetal tissue (i.e., if the mother drinks her coffee from a styrofoam cup, she may retain one part per billion of the styrofoam while her fetus may retain two or three parts per billion). Such a bioconcentration can occur for many chemicals, thus increasing the fetus's toxic load and causing more vulnerability to any new environmental exposure. It is well known today that alcoholic or drug-addicted mothers produce babies already carrying a toxic overload and prone to disease. These babies are, in fact, addicted.

Excess toxic load depletes nutrients such as vitamins, minerals, and amino acids, thus allowing vulnerability to disease, learning disability, and poor brain function.

IMMATURE IMMUNE SYSTEM

At birth a child has his or her mother's immunity which has been passively transferred through the placenta and continues to be fed to the child in the mother's milk. It takes a period of time to stimulate the immune parameters until the child is more resistant to disease. If the mother is unable to breast-feed the child, then the child will be more prone to environmentally induced diseases caused by infection and chemical exposures. The child may become sensitive to foods and ambient environmentals that wouldn't normally bother him or her, and may also be prone to recurrent ear infections, hyperactivity, and learning disabilities.

INABILITY TO DEAL WITH ADDICTIVE EXPOSURES

Although children are not usually taught how to recognize addictive behavior in themselves and how to deal with and eliminate it, they should be trained to recognize and control it. All humans are prone to some type of addiction, whether it be to drugs, alcohol, food, or exercise. The child is not generally taught that throughout life he or she will experience exposures that may be temporarily pleasing, giving him or her an immediate boost that will be followed later by a letdown. We frequently see chocolate addicts, soft-drink addicts, and other sugar-addicts whose addiction affects their learning capacity strongly and adversely. They develop mood swings and attention deficits that grossly impair their ability to learn. Often these children have stuffed-up noses, attacks of sneezing, and sinus pain, causing a need for symptom-suppressing antihistamines, cortisone compounds, and antibiotics. All children should be taught that there is a need for variety in their diet and other environmental exposures. They should be schooled in the fact that if a substance makes them high when ingested or inhaled, they may develop adverse withdrawal effects later. They also should learn that they will pay the price of nutrition deprivation with the inability to function well. In every school there are many glue, gasoline, and lighter fluid sniffers, and their behaviors, if allowed to go on long enough, may cause brain damage and inappropriate behavior of various kinds.

DIFFICULTY IN ADULTS HEARING THE CHILD'S COMPLAINTS

It has been our experience that children often know which environmental factors bother them. Frequently they are sensitive to substances such as the odor of perfume, cigarette smoke, gas from stoves, cleaning solutions, pesticides, dust, newsprint, copy paper, and fumes from the swimming pool. No one asks these children about their sensitivities, however, and often adults pay no attention when they complain. On one occasion, the author observed that when a pesticide was sprayed in the classroom, although 50% of the children complained, the teacher disregarded their complaints because she misinterpreted them as mass hysteria. She even ignored her own symptoms that occurred after the spraying. Children have wonderful environmental sensors that should be utilized by teachers and parents to keep the classroom and home free of pollutants.

CONTAMINATED LIVING QUARTERS

Often a child's room at home may be contaminated and the boy or girl may suffer the after-effects when he or she gets to school, being unable to function well until late morning or early afternoon because it takes children's physiology a long period of time to clear their systems of the the home's pollutants. Children may sleep with dogs or cats or stuffed animals to which they have become sensitive, and they will have hangovers in the morning similar to those an alcoholic experiences. They also may be exposed to other harmful emanations such as the fumes from pesticides, natural gas or oil heat, carpets, or formaldehyde from press board, plywoods, and synthetic materials. A child may sleep on a foam mattress that outgasses the fumes of formaldehyde. Also spot removers, detergents, and other depressors may upset the child's physiology and disturb his or her capacity to learn easily. All of these exposures may keep a child depressed or irritated and therefore may impair his or her learning capacity.

SCHOOL CONTAMINATION

The classroom is often contaminated either inadvertently or intentionally. Certainly the type of heat and the conduits that deliver it to classrooms are problems in some schools. Gas and oil heat are the worst offenders. If the system utilizes forced air, the ducts may never have been cleaned and are full of dust, dirt, grime, bacteria, viruses, and mold. Furnaces may leak and the conduits may pick up fumes from the cafeteria and/or chemistry labs. If the ducts are made of or lined with fiberglass, they will fume when heated and the result will be an environment that is not conducive to children's learning. Furnaces should be checked for leaks at least once per year. The ducts should be cleaned at the beginning of the school year during each season when the children are not in school. Maintenance staffs should be sure that air intakes are not located in areas where mold, dust, or fumes can enter easily.

Windows in each classroom should be openable so that outside air can be brought in on days of low pollution and low pollen counts. Floors should be hard, because carpet collects dirt, and the fumes coming from carpets or the glues that secure them and the pads beneath them are often toxic. Since floor-cleaning materials often fume and cause learning difficulties for some children, all such materials should be non-toxic. If markers for the chalkboards are made of synthetics, they should be water-soluble and should not contain toxic substances such as xylene or toluene.

The author did a study with a group of dentists in which they were instructed to write down a simple ditty on a piece of paper. This ditty was well within the memory capabilities of an adult, and the individuals in the test group could write it down from memory without errors. They were then asked to take a sniff of a chalkboard marker which contained the solvent toluene. After one sniff of the marker, 50% of these well-educated professional people could not write down the ditty accurately. They had short-term memory loss, shaky handwriting, problems with hand-eye coordination, and problems with perception. One can easily see that children exposed to these fumes all day could have learning and behavioral problems.

Storage of toxic materials in classrooms may also be a problem. For example, formaldehyde used for embalmed animal storage and alcohols used for other preservative functions can cause some children to have problems with learning. Some of them actually become intoxicated from the fumes of these solutions.

Although hardwood or plastic chairs do not emit fumes, chair seats made of foam rubber *do* emit them. We have seen some students who couldn't remember or think while sitting on chairs with foam rubber cushions.

Copy paper, new books, and other reading materials may also put out fumes. We have observed a patient who simply could not take tests in the classroom using a particular kind of copy paper. Yet when she was placed in the hall with a glass barrier between her and the test, this patient consistently scored in the top third percentile of the United States. *Figure 2-1* shows a reading box that can be used by children who are newsprint-sensitive. In addition, glass desks can be used to screen the student from fumes from books and papers. (See *Figure 2-2*.)

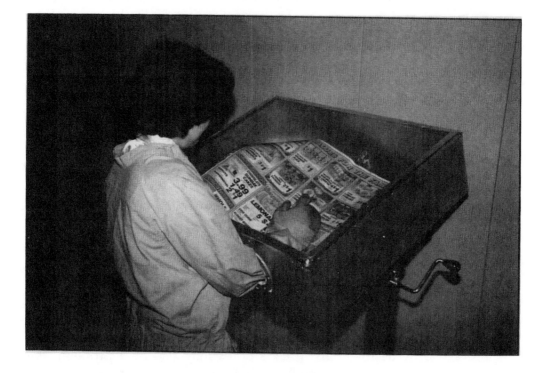

Figure 2-1.
Student using reading box for newsprint-sensitive individuals.

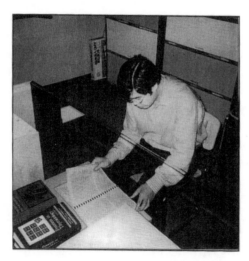

Figure 2-2.
Student working on glass desk for screening fumes from books and papers.

Since the fumes from paper and binding materials will cause learning problems for some students, books, journals, and papers should be kept in cupboards with doors that can be closed. (See *Figure 2-3.*)

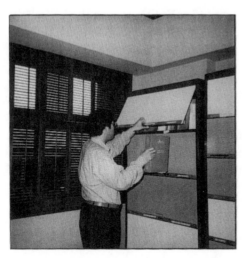

Figure 2-3.
Closed cupboards for screening the chemical fumes from books and journals.

The playground should be kept clean and no artificial fertilizers, pesticides, or herbicides should ever be used there. Care should be taken especially on fields where contact sports are played, since many children and young people have been made ill by exposure to toxic substances emanating from the ground. The author observed one young football player who lost his appetite and rapidly lost weight until he grew so weak he found it difficult to attend school. He also became sensitive to the odors of perfumes, cleaning solutions, markers, photocopied papers, and molds to the extent that when he was exposed to them, he couldn't remember who or where he was. Once it was found that pesticides and artificial fertilizers were causing the problem, the boy was removed from the areas where the solutions were used, and he rapidly regained weight and became a keen learner again. Though he became a track star and a Regency scholar, however, he couldn't walk into the school again without becoming ill. His situation would have been totally preventable had safe maintenance practices been used on the school playing field.

Since they go directly up the olfactory nerve into the brain, perfumes can retard learning seriously. We have observed that children in classes where perfumes or perfumed cosmetics are used by other students or faculty members often have more problems with learning and behavior than those in fragrance-free areas.

FORCIBLE CONTAMINATION OF CLOTHES

Fire-proofing laws often cause contamination of children's clothing. Many clothes are rated for flammability, and to meet rating standards, the fabrics from which they are made are treated with toxic chemicals to make them fire-resistant. Though they are fire-proof, the clothes will outgas constantly, forcing the child who wears them to absorb and breathe potentially harmful fumes. Intake of these fumes may cause learning problems, hyperactivity, or sluggishness. Washing clothes in fabric softeners and detergents also often creates fumes that are not conducive to learning.

CUSTOMS INADVERTENTLY DESIGNED TO IGNORE ENVIRONMENTAL SENSITIVITY

Some families and larger social groups hold the philosophy that perceptions of environmental phenomena are psychological in origin. We have often seen situations in which children's reports of physical phenomena were documented by their teachers as "psychological problems". Though I'm sure the unprovable and unproven "psychological problem" exists, such a diagnosis is clearly often substituted for investigation of a problem. We have seen many children damaged by environmental outgasses because their complaints have been discounted as psychological.

IMMUNIZATION SHOTS

Though in general I advocate immunization shots, caution should be taken in administering them, because some children react adversely to these injections. I have seen at least a half-dozen children who had permanent brain damage because their reactions to their first injections were ignored, and they were forced by a school to take the second round. Some children are sensitive to the egg vaccine is grown on and others are super-sensitive to the actual vaccine. All children, therefore, should be observed carefully when they receive vaccinations of any kind.

POOR DIET

Often, both at home and at school, children are fed a poor diet high in sugar, milk, wheat, corn, and additives. Teachers frequently complain that the hour just after lunch is the worst during the school day, because many children are sluggish, dull, or hyperactive. School staffs should monitor foods served in the school cafeteria and should request that the menu be altered if either sluggishness or hyperactivity is evident in students after lunch.

FREQUENT USE OF MEDICATIONS

Because of modern medicine's dependence on drug treatment for most maladies, many children and teachers are frequently on medications. Chronic use of any medication such as an antihistamine, Ritalin, phenobarbital, Tegretol, tranquilizers, cortisone, anti-wheeze medicines, and many others tend to either dull the brain or cause hyperactivity. Most medication tends to retard learning and will certainly stifle creativity. In the late 20th century enough knowledge is available to define the agents that trigger learning problems and to eliminate them, so that individual students and teachers will be well naturally, not in a state of false, medicated wellness.

IMMATURE NERVOUS SYSTEM

Since the child's nervous system is immature, it is more prone to injury by environmental pollutants than the adult's nervous system is. A classic example of nervous-system injury is that of the child exposed to lead. Because his or her blood-brain barrier is not well developed, he or she will sustain brain damage while the adult exposed to the same amount of lead may have only peripheral nerve damage. It has been shown that children exposed to constant environmental pollution have generally lower IQs and are less creative than those who do not suffer lead exposure.

The routine use of pesticides in the school should be condemned, because most of them are neurotoxins that may well damage the child's nervous system. Pesticides and solvents also tend to damage the child's immune system easily. If pesticides are ever indicated, they should be used the day school is out in the spring so that three months will have elapsed before the children and teachers are exposed to them. The author saw one boy who became extremely paranoid after an exposure to pesticide in the school. He couldn't concentrate, was hyperactive, saw monsters, and thought everybody was against him. He was failing in school and was about to be sent to a mental institution. He was placed in the environmental care unit designed by the scientists and physicians at the Environmental Health Center in Dallas to be as pollution-free as possible. After 48 hours in the pesticide-free air, where pollution was kept to a minimum, the boy wanted to do his school work. In fact, under pollution-free conditions, he spent eight hours per day with excellent concentration on his school work, and he lost all of his other symptoms. When he was given an inhaled challenge test of the pesticide used in his school, after only two whiffs of the "safe ambient dose," all his symptoms, including the paranoia and learning difficulties, returned and lasted for 48 hours. No wonder this child could not learn! A tragedy was averted for him only because the cause of his problem was found early enough.

Many other substances such as those used in dental work, braces, and artificial prostheses can cause nervous system dysfunction. *Figure 2-4a* shows the brain of a 12-year-old who had braces placed on his teeth. The child developed short-term memory loss and inability to concentrate, and he became paralyzed from the waist down. His brain scan shows a typical neurotoxic pattern with holes in the function phase. The boy's problem was traced to the glue used to fix his braces. Once this substance was removed and the child's total environmental load was reduced, he lost his paralysis and regained his brain function. *Figure 2-4b* shows his brain scan after treatment. Now two years post paralysis, he is an A student and is active in sports.

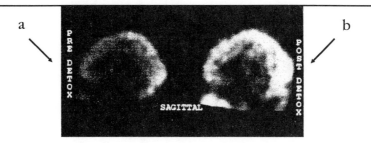

Figure 2-4.

a: Brain scan of 12-year-old with braces before treatment.

b: Brain scan of 12-year-old after treatment. Light areas denote improved brain functions.

SUMMARY

There are numerous reasons why children are more susceptible to environmental pollutants than adults. Most of the pollutants, if recognized, can be dealt with, and reducing them effectively will help create an ideal learning situation for both the child and the teacher.

3

IT'S NOT ALL IN THEIR HEADS:
Managing The Psycho-Social Aspects of Sick School Building Syndrome

by Shirley W. Kaplan, M.A., L.C.S.W.

In this chapter, Ms. Kaplan, who has endured environmental illness (EI) for several years, focuses on the unique psycho-social problems associated with EI and the ways a better understanding of them can help school personnel deal with environmentally sensitive students and colleagues. The author first shares some of her personal experiences as an EI patient and suggests strategies for dealing with the difficulties caused by EI She then goes on to describe specific reactions some children have to environmental toxins that may have a long-term effect on a child's emotional development. In exploring EI and the reasons for both individual and institutional resistance to acknowledging its impact, Ms. Kaplan provides answers to these questions:

☐ *Why do chemical sensitivities have such a devastating effect on school children?*

☐ *What can the parent of an EI child do to help their child in the school setting?*

☐ *How can family members, friends, and professional associates help the teacher who suffers from EI?*

☐ *Why does the general public often feel threatened by those with EI?*

☐ *What can teachers do to raise their student's consciousness about their peers who have EI?*

I have been a psychotherapist for 30 years. My practice includes working collaboratively with schools to treat children who have learning disabilities or behavior problems or both, as well as counseling individuals and families. Eight years ago I was diagnosed with Environmental Illness (EI), a cluster of severe allergies and multiple chemical sensitivities. I can tell you that both my personal and professional life, and my whole approach

51

in dealing with clients' problems, have not been the same since. My experience is not unusual. Every individual, family member, and health or education professional confronting EI is affected in fundamental ways.

My focus in this chapter is on the unique psycho-social problems associated with EI, and the ways in which a better understanding of them can help school personnel deal with the environmentally sensitive student. In short, it is my intention to help the school become part of the solution instead of contributing to the problem. The persistent nonacceptance of EI, the lack of services to treat it, and the unusual nature of the illness—all of these—affect every interaction of the patient with other individuals, and addressing these psycho-social issues is a crucial component of treatment and management. My material is based on my own evolution as a patient, on what I have learned from other EI patients and their families, on my work as a psychotherapist with individual clients, and on my work with schools.

THE PATIENT'S EXPERIENCE

For many years I had headaches that were more or less untreatable. But nine years ago I developed acute cerebral and other symptoms, which were termed "psychiatric," that I knew intuitively could not be emotionally based. I was fortunate. In contrast to most patients I know who have been told for years that "it's all in your head," I got to a clinical ecologist very quickly. I felt a brief relief when I heard the EI diagnosis, because at the same time I learned that there was treatment not only for my acute symptoms, but also for the chronic headaches, fatigue, "brain fog," and other problems I had.

Those not familiar with EI need to know that, especially if an individual is chemically sensitive, his or her whole world is up for grabs. Everything the EI patient eats, breathes, and otherwise comes into contact with has to be evaluated as a possible source of symptoms. For me, finding alternative foods and nontoxic manufactured products was a minor difficulty compared to contemplating major modifications in my home. Most difficult was the way in which the illness became a significant challenge to be reckoned with in every relationship and activity. Suddenly not only my own, but everyone else's perfume, detergent, home, and office became a potential problem for me.

COMING TO TERMS WITH PSYCHO-SOCIAL PROBLEMS

Patients, including myself at the time of my illness, justifiably become "paranoid" about everything in their environment. At the same time, the patient's family and other associates understandably feel that they are hostages to every one of the patient's whims. Families and friends are often confused about what is real and what is imagined. The family atmosphere can become volatile at times, and in spite of the very supportive attitudes of my husband and children, my own family experienced such volatility during my illness. At some point I decided that if we were to survive this experience, I would first have to prioritize changes at a pace my family could adjust to. Second, I needed to understand that they were having emotions and reactions similar to mine, and that their learning was ongoing, just as mine was. Third, we would have to communicate with and educate each other a lot more than we had been doing.

These strategies are necessary for any arena in which the EI patient is functioning—whether with family or friends, at school, or at work. Coping with EI is a lifelong learning process, with mutual adjustments for everyone involved. Eventually our situation *did* stabilize, and at some point I discovered and became actively involved in a Chicago-area EI support group, which currently has about 300 members. Being active in this group and related organizations has been both therapeutic and empowering for me.

Patients, families, and others dealing with EI go through a number of stages, which may be experienced simultaneously or in different sequences. The most common sequence, however, is initial denial, followed by anger and depression, sadness, and, eventually, some degree of acceptance. Typically, when patients and others are at different stages—emotionally out of sync with each other—problems flare up most intensely. For example, when a mother makes great efforts to prepare special meals for a child who is in denial about his or her food allergies, there is a potential scenario for conflict. As each situation arises, patients and their families should recognize that these phases are normal reactions to the illness.

THE CHILD WITH EI

Initially, the diagnosis of EI in a child may provide some relief for the parents, since they now know that the problems are real and treatable—

that it's not all psychological, though certainly emotional problems may be part of the picture. Parents feel validated when they discover it's not all their fault, especially in our society where so much fault is attributed to parents. (We've become accustomed to the attitude that suggests: "When in doubt, blame the parents, especially the mother.")

But the next stage—that of implementing major dietary and environmental changes, and the accompanying emotional roller coaster both within and outside the family—presents the most acute problems and makes everyone involved feel most vulnerable. It is at this time that the family needs to inform and educate other people in the child's world—extended family, friends, school personnel, and professionals. This is a stage in which families need *massive* amounts of emotional support and understanding. Support groups, networks, and professional advocates can be very helpful. For example, an EI child can use a support group to ventilate feelings of anger and frustration safely, or to figure out how best to explain to other kids why hair spray makes her ill or why a chemical odor gives him a headache. In individuals or families where maladaptive psychological patterns have become entrenched, psychotherapy with an EI-knowledgeable or open-minded counselor may be helpful. Unfortunately, because it is not currently recognized as a legitimate illness by some segments of the medical community, EI brings with it terrible feelings of alienation and isolation. We can only hope that, as society and institutions such as schools respond more appropriately, fewer and fewer people will have to suffer these reactions.

WHAT THE CHEMICALLY SENSITIVE CHILD EXPERIENCES

For the chemically-sensitive patient, the psycho-social aspects of the problem are truly formidable, in a class by themselves. Just why do these sensitivities have such a devastating effect? One of our basic emotional needs is to feel grounded, i.e., to feel we have a solid base, with a reasonable degree of control over our thoughts, feelings, and bodies. Also, we need a reasonably predictable environment, one that affirms us as individuals. For children to develop normally, they especially need this grounding and trust.

Even as an adult, however, when I currently react to chemicals or some foods, both my inner and outer worlds become temporarily unreliable. Let me explain. With an unexpected whiff of perfume, or, worse, with an undetectable toxic substance, my brain fogs up. I can't think clearly or articulate words, and I may suddenly become hyper and irritable. Even though I understand intellectually what is happening, I can't count on my own mental resources or trust what is going on in the world around me. In a word, I'm emotionally adrift.

We can very easily understand how these kinds of experiences would affect a child. If these unpredictable fluctuations in a child's emotions and functioning continue without intervention, that child will experience an inner sense of confusion and chaos. Combine that with the understandably negative reactions of others, whether frustrated parents and teachers or angry playmates, and soon enough the child may internalize the view that he or she is different and *bad*. Negative self-image and poor self-esteem may follow. Maladaptive or aggressive behavior may develop to compensate for confused and inadequate feelings. The child is also angry that his or her world is so unreliable. The result may be personality and behavior problems which are secondary to the illness, even in an emotionally healthy family.

Now let's look at the problem from the non-patient's point of view. When members of the general public are confronted with the chemically-sensitive patient, they are apt to feel threatened. And it's important to understand some of the reasons why. One reason is the fear that the same thing might happen to them. After all, we all more or less breathe the same air and are exposed to the same chemicals in the environment. A second, more complicated reason goes something like this: in the process of growing up, as part of our development, we all learn to respect people's boundaries, who they are physically and emotionally. As children we're taught that it is rude to comment on or criticize someone's personal attributes, their appearance, their clothes, and certainly their smell.

Smell is our most primitive sense. At first a person may become defensive, or even belligerent, when an EI patient complains about his or her smell because he or she—like most of us—perceives smell as such a definitive personal attribute. So when we, as patients, need to ask someone to give up a particular hair spray, or change a detergent, that request is experienced as—and in fact is—an intrusion into what other people consider their personal space. Such a request may be experienced as something beyond normal civility. Let me emphasize, however, what is *really* abnormal is our civilized society's current ability to produce such an array of harmful substances that people can and do literally become toxic to one another.

What I refer to as the three D's——defensiveness, denial, and discrediting of the patient——are typical initial reactions of non-patients. Those interacting with the patient——whether they be family, friends, classmates, or teachers—need time and opportunities to change their reactions, by going through an ongoing learning process, just as EI patients themselves do.

I hear EI patients complain, "They just don't get it!" Well of course they don't, at least not right away. But if they persist in not getting it, in spite of our best efforts, then it's unlikely they ever will. In that case, patients and their families need to change strategies. Often pragmatic negotiation without the expectation of any understanding is the only answer. As the problems of EI patients are increasingly recognized in our society, it is my hope that the attitudes of non-patients will change.

THE SICK BUILDING IN THE COMMUNITY

Institutions, too, are threatened by EI, in more complicated ways. Factors such as power and economic interests play a major part in the institutional response to EI, as do bureaucratic rigidity and belief systems. A typical example of the complexity of response to an environmental issue involves a recently built, newly occupied $53 million county courthouse. The county board denied that problems existed in the building and for many months stonewalled on making necessary corrections, in spite of ongoing complaints—from minor to very serious—by a majority of workers, ranging from janitors to judges. Only after a number of emergency evacuations and cases of workers being rushed to hospitals, not to mention lawsuits, did the county finally acknowledge that the courthouse was a sick building. One and a half million dollars was voted to correct the problem, and the correction is now in progress. Numerous lawsuits have been brought by workers because of alleged disabilities, and by the county against the architects and general contractor. Clearly, the initial resistance to acknowledging and correcting the problems has a great deal to do with the economic issues involved.

A very instructive psychological aspect of the sick-building problem also reared its ugly head in this case. Early on, when several supervisors threatened a walkout, they were characterized by the county board chairman as "irrational." Such an uninformed defensive posture is among the most serious difficulties associated with sick buildings. The attempt to discredit people and invalidate problems by implying that environmental hazards are created by irrational minds—"it's all in their heads"—generally increases the time and money required to cure the building.

We can assume that the county board dealing with the sick courthouse was forced finally to take the problem seriously because of lawsuits and negative publicity. As these indoor environmental hazards are increasingly acknowledged and thereby avoided, we hope legal measures will not be so necessary to bring about change.

It is also important to recognize how individuals functioning within institutions are threatened, especially those professionals whose belief systems are challenged. Even the best-intentioned professionals may be brought to an understandable disequilibrium, and therefore an initial resistance, when the working assumptions and theories they may have held lifelong are questioned. One's professional belief system often not only relates to the way one works, but also becomes an integral part of one's identity.

In the mental health field there is a long-standing history of an incredible range of syndromes that were considered to be psychological in origin. These include autism, schizophrenia, and "psychosomatic" illnesses such as asthma, ulcer, eating disorders, and learning and behavior problems, to name but a few. The implied psychological bases have been blamed either directly or indirectly on bad parenting, and the fault has been attributed particularly to the mother. In recent years, the focus has shifted to include neurological and genetic factors. However, nutritional and environmental factors that may contribute to some of the problems in a major way are typically not accepted or even considered in the mental health field. Pharmaceutical solutions seem to have the current monopoly, however, and we see an alarmingly high—and increasing—proportion of the adult and child population taking psychotropic drugs that are being prescribed not only by psychiatrists but also in rapidly growing numbers by pediatricians, internists, gynecologists, and other specialists.

Clearly, there is a major lag in recognizing and treating those learning, behavior, mood, and other health disorders caused by allergic, nutritional, and environmental factors. To provide a truly healthy, supportive school environment, all educational professionals, including social workers, psychologists, consultants, and other specialists, urgently need to be educated about EI and its causes.

THE PARENT'S ROLE

Typically, the parent of an EI child initiates the request that the school provide for the special needs of the child. In mild to moderate cases, such requests can be handled at the classroom level, with the help of understanding and accommodating teachers. Once beyond the classroom, however, when special services and cost-conscious administrators become involved, the task for the parent and child may become much more difficult. Considering the kind of resistance the EI condition may evoke, a parent dealing with a school administration on behalf of a child must be credible, knowledgeable, and confident, and must have whatever supporting documentation is necessary to inform and educate the school's personnel. The situation requires that parents *not* present themselves as hostile, but remain goal-oriented and purposeful, while being prepared to deal with an array of negative responses. This is a pretty formidable task for most parents, especially if they are in the midst of coping with all the other demands at home that we've discussed. Support groups and networking can be very helpful to parents, as is an accessible team of professional advocates such as that discussed in *Chapter 16* of this book.

TEACHING AND LEARNING ABOUT EI

School provides an environment not only for formal education, but also for developing and maintaining peer relationships, managing a broad spectrum of authoritarian relationships, and learning how people and problems are treated within an institution. It is important that the child with special needs be responded to appropriately in order that his or her learning and development be nurtured to the maximum degree possible. It is also important, however, that all children develop compassion for the disabled and, in the process, learn to empathize with the limitations and vulnerabilities of all people.

It seems that children respond easily when the adults in their environment, by example and by direct teaching, set the tone of acceptance. Some time ago I read a moving newspaper story about how a school had mobilized itself on behalf of a new student with severe facial disfigurement, with an incredibly positive response from the whole school, especially the children. This example seems to me to illustrate how it is possible for school personnel to take on a leadership role, and thereby stimulate an atmosphere of acceptance of the student or teacher with EI.

Teachers should feel free to set up appropriate hands-on projects in which children can learn to understand EI at their own developmental levels, and can work out cooperative strategies to help classmates with EI. In this way, not only will the EI child's symptoms be ameliorated, but also—and most importantly—secondary psychological damage will be minimized for the child. In the process, all children benefit, as psychological and moral values are strengthened in the cooperative milieu. Since environmentally induced problems are clearly on the rise, we can only hope that the positive scenario I have outlined will prevail.

Part Two

Causes and Treatment of Sick School Building Syndrome

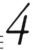

TOP TEN CONCERNS FOR A HEALTHFUL SCHOOL ENVIRONMENT

by Norma Miller, Ed.D.

A recent research project at Texas Women's University identified ten areas of most serious concern to environmental specialists studying the ecology of contemporary school buildings. In this chapter, Dr. Miller discusses these ten concerns, draws the reader's attention to other important studies, and recommends ways to introduce and maintain in school buildings the conditions most conducive to the good health of students, teachers, and other school staff. Dr. Miller answers in detail a number of questions vital to today's educators, parents, and community leaders, including:

□ *Why are certain building and remodeling processes and the products utilized in them dangerously toxic?*

□ *When should school remodeling projects be undertaken?*

□ *How can school maintenance workers help preserve the good health of all those who occupy a school building?*

□ *How does the heating, ventilating, and air conditioning (HVAC) system affect the health of students, teachers, and others in schools?*

□ *Why are some products better suited than others for maintaining a nontoxic atmosphere in schools?*

□ *What do you look for on the labels of art supplies to be sure you are using nontoxic products?*

Would you give a 50-pound child the same dose of medicine you'd give a 200-pound adult? Probably not. Yet many children are exposed at school to toxic substances that may not harm an adult, but which can be harmful to a developing child. The environmental quality of school facilities may affect the learning ability of some students, and the students who are most at risk—those with asthma, learning disabilities, hyperactivity, or multiple chemical sensitivities—need optimum ecological conditions at school.

Recently, research was done at Texas Woman's University to establish some ecological guidelines for a healthful school building. In this study the Delphi technique—a research method that elicits the opinions of experts to project information on a specific subject—was used to design a series of three questionnaires. Sixty environmental specialists from 26 states and two other countries participated in the study, giving their opinions on the construction and maintenance of healthful school buildings. They agreed on ten areas of major concern listed below in the order of their importance:

1. heating, cooling, and ventilation
2. pest controls
3. cleaning products
4. chemicals
5. fragrances
6. site selection
7. lighting
8. remodeling the school building
9. floors
10. art supplies

CONCERN ONE: HEATING, COOLING, AND VENTILATION

In 1989, the Maryland State Department of Health published the *Indoor Air Quality Management Program* in which heating, ventilating, and air-conditioning systems (HVAC) are described as the lungs of the school building that control the quality of the indoor air, thus affecting the health, learning ability, and productivity of the students. In school rooms equipped with individual thermostats and windows that can be opened, many ventilation problems can be alleviated. Of course, when both teachers and students are prevented from controlling the ventilation in classrooms, frustration often ensues.

Those planning the HVAC system in a new school should consider placing the HVAC unit in a separate building a few feet removed from the classrooms. This forethought applied to the design of the facility can prevent students' exposure to the fumes of downdrafts or unburned combustion gases and can also diminish their contact with the electro-magnetic field created by the central HVAC unit.

The HVAC ductwork should always be carefully maintained—cleaned, disinfected, or encapsulated if hazardous materials cannot be removed. Some ductwork has been found to contain—alone or in combination—mold, mildew, asbestos, pollen, viruses, bacteria, lead, insect parts, carbon, or fiberglass particles. Fiberglass-lined ductwork is difficult to vacuum since fiberglass particles may become dislodged and circulate in the school when the HVAC fan is operating. However, sheet metal ductwork can be cleaned thoroughly.

"The number one problem with HVAC systems in schools is that the fresh air supply has been completely closed off," according to Thad Godish, Director of the Indoor Air Quality Research Laboratory at Ball State University. The second problem is that the HVAC unit is not clean. The condensation drip pan needs to be cleaned regularly. When the drip pan is not kept clean, slime will collect and microorganisms can grow in it. (Godish 1994)

Good filters are a necessity for HVAC systems, and a medium-efficiency filter should be used in schools. Each filter should be cleaned or changed every two months, because filters that are not cleaned regularly may have molds growing within them. While mold levels in the school room itself may be low, the molds growing within the filters may release allergens into the classroom. (Godish 1994) According to another authority, A. S. Levin, " 'antigen' is a broader term that includes viruses and bacteria as well as inhalants; an allergen is a specific antigen (pollen, dust, formal-dehyde, and so forth) that causes allergies." (Levin 1983)

Dirt on cooling and heating coils decreases their effectiveness. Surface contamination of heating and cooling coils has been found to reduce their efficiency in transferring thermal energy by as much as 30%. (Wheeler 1992)

Heating-cooling units used for individual rooms are often full of filth. Unit ventilators should be cleaned thoroughly every two months, and they can be upgraded with better filters. Classroom unit ventilators usually are supplied with one-inch-thick coarse fiber filters that have a low efficiency and limited dirt-holding capacity. Filtration can be improved by installing a replaceable one-inch pleated extended-media filter. An excellent guide useful for keeping the school HVAC system clean is the Maryland State Department of Education's technical bulletin entitled *Air Cleaning Devices for HVAC Systems in Schools* (1992).

Upgrading air filtration may require extra work and may incur added cost. The result, however, will be improved indoor air quality (IAQ) in schools. As the 1992 Maryland Technical Bulletin states, improved IAQ may result "in a more effective teaching environment, less absenteeism and fewer complaints." (Wheeler 1992)

For further information on HVAC systems and indoor air quality, see *Chapter 5*.

CONCERN TWO: PEST CONTROLS

Many people believe that if a pesticide has been registered by the Environmental Protection Agency (EPA), it can be considered harmless to humans. The EPA, however, generally does not have chronic toxicity or chronic exposure data for nonagricultural pesticides. The long-term exposure risks to pesticides are unknown because most of the chemicals they contain have not been reassessed in accordance with current scientific standards. A U.S. General Accounting Office publication (1986) states that the EPA believes that no pesticide can be considered "safe." According to legislation enacted in 1972 by Congress to ensure that pesticide risks are adequately studied, any pesticide must be re-registered after testing has shown that it will not cause adverse effects on the environment. The reassessment process has been slow, and since 50,000 pesticides must be reassessed, it will continue into the 21st century. Meanwhile, pesticides remain on the market as testing for chronic toxicity continues. In a survey of the schools in New York state, it was found that 87% of the schools used pesticides, all of which "contained substances which may cause immediate or long-term health problems." (Volberg, Surgan, Jaffe, and Hamer 1993)

How can schools eliminate pests and protect the health of students and faculty? A few states have passed laws that mandate the use of nontoxic pest controls. In Texas, Integrated Pest Management (IPM) will be the preferred method of treatment for all schools by September 1995, and the Dallas Independent School District is implementing IPM in schools in 1994.

IPM, though not a new technique, is a systems approach that seeks to reduce pest damage to tolerable levels but does not necessarily eradicate a pest species. It first uses the least toxic methods of pest control. Only after all nontoxic methods have proved to be ineffective is a chemical pesticide introduced. Jeff Mitchell uses IPM in his science classes at Eddyville School in Lincoln County, Oregon. He has written, "IPM is a creative and challenging example of the scientific thinking and application that all universities encourage science educators to impart." His idea of the "systems approach" is that a scientist looks at the total picture, not just the organism or economic justification in isolation. (Mitchell 1988)

Educators may sometimes discourage the use of nontoxic pest control methods. An interviewer at a convention for pest control operators found that many of the exterminators were willing to use less toxic pest control methods. They expressed the opinion, however, that at most schools a small minority of very vocal staff members would panic at the sight of one insect and would demand an overkill treatment with a pesticide. School staff members who are afraid of insects may need to be retrained to understand IPM methods in order to provide an environment that is nontoxic to both students and faculty.

The nonprofit Bio-Integral Resource Center (BIRC) in Berkeley, California has been developing guidelines for using IPM in schools. This project will identify the least toxic methods for managing pests found in school buildings and other urban environments. One outcome of the project will be a practical how-to manual for implementing IPM programs in schools. The manual is expected to be available from BIRC shortly.

For further information on managing pests in schools, see *Chapter 12.*

CONCERN THREE: CLEANING PRODUCTS

Products used to clean schools should not leave toxic fumes in the indoor air. Most scouring powders are corrosive and contain toxic irritants such as ammonia, ethanol, or chlorine bleach. Disinfectants may contain naphtha, cresol, lye, and formaldehyde. Cresol "attacks the liver, kidneys, spleen, pancreas, and central nervous system; it may be absorbed through inhalation or through skin." (Turiel 1985) If toxic chemicals are used (that is, when school is not in session), windows should be opened and central air circulation should be turned off to prevent the spread of fumes throughout the building.

The dust mite is a well-known allergen. According to Thad Godish, current studies in Europe are showing that *dust* itself is also a significant allergen. Therefore, school furnishings should be wet-wiped rather than dusted. (Godish 1994) The vacuum cleaner is another source of dust. "There is a temporary increase in potential exposure to allergens associated with the vacuuming process." (Pope, Patterson, and Burge 1993) Typical vacuum cleaners only recirculate dust, which comes out of the vacuum bag in smaller particles only to be recirculated and inhaled more deeply into the lungs where it can do great damage. An industrial-quality vacuum cleaner with a high efficiency particulate absolute (HEPA) filter is a necessity for a school that has wall-to-wall carpeting.

Waxes and floor strippers contain toxic chemicals that can linger for days inside a schoolroom. Floor waxing should be done in the summer or during a long vacation period, and the school should be adequately aired out before the students return.

A good quality floor wax that has been maintained properly should not have to be stripped. Because a low grade wax leaves a soft residue, it needs to be stripped every six weeks. It saves time and money not to strip floors, however, and because of the cost and the toxic chemicals used in stripping, the decision to strip a floor should always be made jointly by the maintenance staff and the administrative office. (Hill 1994) Schools can take a lesson from the excellent maintenance practices of the LBJ Library in Austin, Texas, which did not have its floors stripped for three years.

What procedures can schools use to reduce the frequency of floor-wax stripping? Lee Hill suggests the following routine:

- Use only high quality liquid wax.
- Let the waxed floor dry from three to seven days, and keep all traffic off the floor during that time.
- When the floor is thoroughly dry, burnish it with a high-speed buffer. Use a liquid made specifically for high-speed burnishing. Since burnishing heats the wax and makes it harder, *do not use liquid wax at this stage.*
- To maintain it well, continue to buff the floor with a high-speed buffer, *but never add liquid wax.*

■ When the floor is dirty, use a soft buffer pad and mild soap to scrub the surface at a low speed. Then rinse-mop the floor three to four times. Any soap that is left on the floor will prevent the next layer of wax from adhering to the surface. Use a pH-neutral liquid in the rinse water to tell when to change water. (The water will change color when it is time for replacement.)

■ After the floor is rinsed and allowed to dry, a coat of high-quality liquid wax can be applied. When the wax is dry, it should be burnished.

A floor maintained in this manner may need to have the wax stripped only once in a five-year period. (Hill 1994)

For further information on using the least toxic cleaning products, see *Chapter 7.*

CONCERN FOUR: CHEMICALS

The copy machine emits ozone. Chemicals are used in the science lab. Radon seeps through the cracks in the basement. And volatile organic compounds (VOCs) may be found in every classroom.

School buildings need to be tested for radon and lead, and the levels of each need to be measured. In addition, management and maintenance personnel should implement plans to keep the school environment free from carbon monoxide, carbon dioxide, and volatile organic compounds (VOCs).

The Maryland State Department of Education has published several guides for managing chemicals in schools. One of them entitled, *Guidelines for Controlling Indoor Air Quality Problems Associated with Kilns, Copiers, and Welding in Schools,* proposes the use of appropriate hoods to remove contaminants at the point of origin. (Turner and Lippy 1991)

When kilns are fired at high heat, emissions may include carbon monoxide, sulfur dioxide, ozone, or nitrogen dioxide. A canopy hood for local exhaust ventilation should be used above the kiln, and, if possible, the kiln should be fired when children are not at school. (Turner and Lippy 1991)

The Maryland State Guidelines also identify each of several duplicating processes as "a source of indoor air contaminants which pose potential health hazards for equipment operators and building occupants."

(Turner and Lippy 1991) Photocopiers, spirit duplicating machines, mimeograph machines, diazo dyeline (blueprint) machines, and electronic stencil markers are listed among the culprits. A by-product of photocopying is ozone which can cause headaches, irritation to mucus membranes, or impaired vision. Spirit duplicating machines release methyl alcohol vapors into the ambient air, and overexposure to them has caused burning of the eyes, drowsiness, vomiting, and dizziness. Blueprint machines use ammonia which, when released into the air, is an irritant of the mucus membranes and the eyes. Ventilation rates and appropriate exhaust hoods for each duplicating process are recommended in the Maryland State Department of Education Indoor Air Quality Management Program.

Aerosol cans are another source of chemical hazard. The National Institute of Drug Abuse estimates that 450,000 teenagers 12 to 18 years of age are inhaling fumes from aerosol cans. Kathy MacIntyre, Executive Director of the International Institute for Inhalant Abuse, reports the death in 1992 of a six-year-old child, caused by inhaling vapors from an aerosol can. It should be noted, too, that chemical inhalants are sometimes hidden by abusers in pop cans or asthma inhalators.

The school staff is advised to remove all solvents from the school building, since some students having easy access to these substances may abuse them by inhaling them. Correction fluid or felt markers should also be stored securely, because students may also sniff them to get a high.

For further information on radon and asbestos, see *Chapter 8*; for more on lead, mold, and formaldehyde in schools, see *Chapters 13* through *15*.

CONCERN FIVE: FRAGRANCES

According to the U.S. Food and Drug Administration (FDA), fragrances cause 30% of all allergic reactions. When exposed to perfume, more than 70% of asthmatics develop respiratory symptoms.

Is the learning ability of children affected by perfume? William J. Rea, M.D., Director of the Environmental Health Center in Dallas, has discovered in challenge testing of children at his clinic that perfume often shuts down learning capacity, and he advises teachers not to use perfume or chemical fragrance products at school. (Rea 1992) Since many types of chemicals can affect a child's immune system, other experts also advise teachers to avoid scented soaps and hair sprays, after-shave lotions, perfumes, and colognes. (Crook and Stevens 1987)

Experts have long recommended that in order to correct the environment for allergic students, no air fresheners should be used in a healthful school. (Mandell & Scanlon 1979) Air fresheners often contain irritant chemicals that coat the mucus membranes and actually pollute the air. One authority says, "A few air fresheners contain chemicals that diminish the ability to smell." (Turiel 1985)

The Single Photon Emission Computed Tomography Machine (SPECT) is used to map flow of blood in the brain. Dr. T. Simon states that if a child has inhaled a noxious chemical like chlorine, a SPECT image will show whether the child might experience trouble in the upcoming hours. Dr. Simon also uses the SPECT scan to study the effects of perfume on the brain. A baseline of blood flow in a patient's brain is first established by a SPECT scan. Then, at a later date, the patient is given perfume to sniff, and a second SPECT scan is done to measure blood flow. In this study many patients have shown abnormal blood flow in the brain after exposure to perfume. (Simon 1992)

Numerous cases of students who have an allergic reaction to fragrances have been documented by physicians. School attendance can improve, and academic achievement may also increase if an effort is made to remove all perfumed products from the classroom setting.

For tips on how to create an allergy-free classroom, see *Chapter 18.*

CONCERN SIX: SITE SELECTION

Schools should not be built near major highways, railroads, airports, television or radio stations, microwave towers, high power electrical lines, toxic dumps, or garbage incinerators.

While no urban site is completely safe, careful site selection can lessen school pollution significantly. Dr. E. J. Fenyves, a physicist at the University of Texas at Dallas, has said that a school building located 1,000 feet from a highway will have approximately 10% of the pollution of a building situated 300 feet from the same highway (Fenyves 1991). Vehicles on highways produce exhaust fumes, noise, and sometimes, toxic spills.

Toxic spills also occur on railroad tracks. The Department of Transportation listed 482 hazardous cargo rail accidents in 1992 (Calvin 1994), and in about 8% of the accidents, hazardous materials were released from derailed cars.

Because of the possibility of a toxic spill, one southwestern city moved a school from a location across the street from a railroad track to a safer site. The entire student body, which was composed of teenage mothers who brought their babies to school with them, was moved to another building in a safer location.

Noise, too, can hinder learning. According to a recent report, a few years ago trains roared by 80 times a day outside Public School 98 in Manhattan. The reading scores of sixth graders on the side of the school nearest the train tracks were a year behind those of the class on the farther, and quieter, side of the building. "Once sound-deadening pads were put on the train tracks and acoustical ceiling tiles were installed in the classrooms, the discrepancy in reading scores disappeared." (Lang 1991)

Airports are also a source of noise that distracts students from their lessons at the same time that it exposes them to microwave radiation. Radar may extend a few miles from an airport, and the microwave radiation associated with it has been shown to be biologically harmful. (Zaret 1988)

It may be possible to incinerate hazardous waste without releasing health-threatening products into the atmosphere. This is possible, according to D. W. Moeller, "if the operating temperature of the incinerator is sufficiently high, and if there are adequate distribution and mixing of the combustion air, production of these compounds can be avoided or reduced to very low levels." (Moeller 1992) The same authority also cites an alarming 1990 EPA survey in which data available on 725 hazardous waste disposal sites showed that nearly 50% of more than 4 million people living within one mile of these sites were young children, women of childbearing age, and elderly citizens. Some of these people reported such adverse health effects as respiratory problems, eye irritation, neurological complaints, and dermatologic problems. The ground water at approximately three-fourths of these sites was contaminated. More research is needed to study the possible health effects on populations living near hazardous waste incinerators.

A healthful site should always be selected for an optimum school environment. For further information on considerations for designing and building new schools, see *Chapter 20*.

CONCERN SEVEN: LIGHTING

Natural light is the most healthful. Yet today many school rooms have no windows and must be lighted by artificial light. Daylight, which consists of all the subtle changes of sunlight from dawn to nightfall, would be more healthful and would promote learning in classrooms. Until the second half of the twentieth century when cheap electricity and fluorescent lighting became available, architects used daylight as the primary source of illumination in all buildings. (Lechner 1991) In the 1950s, daylighting became a minor issue because electricity was inexpensive and because of the perceived superiority of electric lighting. "At first only the energy implications were emphasized, but now daylighting is also valued for its aesthetic possibilities and its ability to satisfy biological needs." (Lechner 1991)

Michael Terman, Director of the Light Therapy Unit in Columbia-Presbyterian Medical Center, and President of the Society for Light Treatment and Biological Rhythms, said recently, "No question, much school lighting is deficient from my vantage point. Inadequate daytime light exposure can foster problems such as lethargy which works against educational objectives." His research has been used to develop a new futuristic system "with gradually modulated dawn, daylight, and dusk simulation (with advanced microprocessor controls). A key underlying concept is that the on-line modulation of light level—above and beyond enhanced absolute intensity—may serve to enhance alertness and performance." Dr. Terman believes that optimum design of whole-room lighting in schools requires expert consultation and supervised installation; this is "more than standard lighting companies and architectural firms are currently able to offer," he says. (Terman 1994)

Whole-room light installations are not the only option, Dr. Terman continues. "Since individuals differ in their responsivity to various lighting levels," he is interested in the development of local-area lighting such as "work station" models. The level of light at each work station could be adjusted to the individual's needs. Hughes Lighting Technologies has patented a portable illuminator product that can provide selectable light intensities with minimum glare. The portability of this light allows it to be positioned at tables, desks, or computer consoles. Terman believes that the "work station" model approach to light would be more economical than whole-room systems. (Terman 1994)

For further information on lighting in schools, see *Chapter 10*.

CONCERN EIGHT: REMODELING

Remodeling often includes the installation of new floors, painting, or roof repairs. New synthetic floor tiles and carpeting will outgas volatile organic compounds (VOCs) for some time. When new floors are to be installed, schools should specify that only low-level VOC-emitting adhesives be used. According to the Maryland Department of Education's 1993 technical bulletin *Carpet and Indoor Air Quality in Schools* (pp. 5-6):

> The State of Washington employs a 90-day flush-out program. After carpet installation the HVAC system in the unoccupied building is operated at maximum outside air, 24 hours a day for 30 days. Washington's mild climate permits the use of maximum outdoor air ventilation with very little energy penalty. After 30 days, the furniture is installed and the building HVAC system is operated for an additional 60 days at maximum outside air.

The ingredients of paint include benzene, toluene, fungicides, xylene, naptha, kerosene, and coal tar. Although none of these products should end up inside the lungs of school children, gas engineer Francis Silver has written that if a paint product that evaporates "is sprayed into the air or spread over a large surface inside a building, a substantial portion of that product will end up inside the occupants of that building." (Silver 1980)

Roofing repairs may expose students to adhesives known to contain central nervous system toxins or to roofing tars containing carcinogens. These materials may be particularly toxic to young children.

In an article in a 1992 issue of *American School & University*, James Giachino listed safety, noise, odors, dust, and moving walls and windows as important concerns when remodeling is done at school. For safety there should be a clear separation between the construction activities and the occupants of the building. Remodeling of the school building can expose the occupants to many toxic products, so it should be done at those times in the school year when school is not in session or during the summer months.

If school is in session, no work should be done over or under occupied classrooms. Remodeling work in these areas and the use of concrete jackhammers and tamping machines should be scheduled for after-school hours if at all possible. Since construction causes many airborne particles, more money should be allowed for periodic cleanup of construction areas in an occupied school than would otherwise be necessary if school were not in session.

Giachino believes that in the learning environment, even mild odors can be disruptive. While an odor-free environment may not be possible, noxious chemicals should be used only when a school building is unoccupied.

When walls and windows are to be moved, Giachino's rule is to remove and remodel only as much as can be completed in the summer.

For further information on environmental concerns for school remodeling activities, see *Chapter 20*.

CONCERN NINE: FLOORS

Floors in school buildings should be durable and easy to clean, and they should not expose students and faculty to toxic substances. For those areas where traffic is heavy, ceramic tile, terrazzo, or brick are good choices. In other areas, synthetic tiles, wood, and carpet are often used.

Although carpet has many aesthetic and acoustic properties, some adverse health reactions from wall-to-wall carpeting have been reported. In particular, carpeting is a reservoir of indoor allergens, and dust mites thrive in it.

In 1993, the Institute of Medicine published *Indoor Allergens*, a report of the allergy problems many citizens of the United States face. The executive summary states, "a first-ever risk assessment in this field shows a positive relationship between cumulative exposure to mite allergen and the risk of sensitization." (Pope, Patterson, and Burge 1993) Allergy symptoms can be reduced by avoiding the allergen. One recommendation for avoiding the dust mite is the use of polished wood floors. The University of Virginia Allergy Clinic's *Instructions for Reducing Exposure to House Dust Mites* recommends that all floors have a primary polished surface such as wood or vinyl. If there is carpet, it should be movable. (Pope, Patterson & Burge 1993)

Dust-mite exposure is significant in the development of asthma. The Institute of Medicine report estimated that asthma-related illness in the United States costs $6.2 billion annually, and asthma is the cause of much student absenteeism. Children included, about one third of the people in the United States show evidence of allergy to dust mites.

Thad Godish thinks that carpet should not be installed in schools, because it is ideal for dirt deposit and hence is a major source of pollutants. If carpet is used in schools, Godish recommends steam-cleaning two to three times a year using an unscented detergent. (Godish 1994)

Good ventilation is needed after carpet is shampooed. In one school in which the wall-to-wall carpeting was shampooed in the summer and the building closed up until fall, the carpet had to be removed before school started in the fall because of an overgrowth of mold. A hard-surface floor with an area rug that can be taken out to be cleaned is more healthful.

For further information on school floor coverings, see *Chapter 9*.

CONCERN TEN: ART SUPPLIES

Children should not use professional-grade art materials, and elementary schools should have only art supplies specifically designed for children. On nontoxic art products the label should read: "conforms to ASTM-D4236." The "Labeling of Hazardous Art Materials Act," which became effective in 1990, requires that toxic art products be labeled with a warning of the hazard. Teachers are not prevented by this law from having such hazardous materials as rubber cement and spray fixatives if they are used only when the children are not in the classroom, and if these materials are locked away from the children. When toxic substances are used by a teacher, the room should be aired out before the children return.

Toxic art materials enter the body through inhalation, ingestion, or skin contact. The art room should be well ventilated with appropriate exhaust hoods, and students should not eat food there. All students should wash their hands thoroughly at the end of art projects.

The Arts and Crafts Materials Institute has designed two labels for nontoxic products. "AP" means an *approved product*, and the presence of those letters on a label means that the art product is nontoxic when absorbed through the skin, inhaled, or ingested by mouth. "CP" means *certified product* and when it appears on a product label it designates quality and non-toxicity. "HL" (*health label*) indicates the presence of toxic substances and is a warning in accordance with the guidelines of the American Society of Testing Materials/Arts and Crafts Materials Institute.

The following measures can help art educators to select less toxic art materials for children:

■ Always select products that are specially designed for children.

■ Use water-based rather than solvent-based glues and drawing supplies.

■ Avoid paints or inks that contain cadmium, lead, or chromium. (McCann 1985)

■ Do not use aerosol sprays with carbolic acids or any products containing the following: benzene, benzidine dyes, cadmium/silver solder, carbon tetrachloride, chloroform, cyanide solutions, lead chromate, perchloroethylene, phenols, trichloroethylene, uranium oxide, or zinc chromate (Shields 1989). Airbrush and aerosol art products cause a significant exposure to paints and solvents and should not be used around children.

■ Food-scented art supplies should be avoided, since children may be tempted to eat these items. (Jacobson 1984)

■ Dry clay contains silica which may damage the lungs. A good substitute for young children is modeling beeswax or homemade "play dough," which is free of preservatives and perfume. (Dadd 1987)

SUMMARY

This handbook provides a wealth of information on how to identify, minimize, and eliminate the environmental hazards in and around schools. *Figure 4-1* lists the "top ten concerns" along with cross-references to other chapters in this volume where you can find an extended discussion of that topic. All of the stakeholders—whether they plan and maintain school building or attend, teach, administer, or send their children to schools—will need to work together to provide the ultimate "healthy" school environment.

REFERENCES

Calvin, T., 1994, "Poisoned Cargo," *Family Circle* 107, no. 2: 100-103.

1	Heating, cooling, and ventilation	See Chapter 5.
2	Pest controls	See Chapter 12.
3	Cleaning products	See Chapter 7.
4	Chemicals	See Chapter 8, 13, 14, and 15.
5	Fragrances	See Chapter 18.
6	Site selection	See Chapter 20.
7	Lighting	See Chapter 10
8	Remodeling the school building	See Chapter 20.
9	Floors	see Chapter 9.
10	Art supplies	Although several of the other chapters discuss art supplies, this chapter probably offers the most detail on this concern.

Figure 4-1.
Top ten concerns for a healthful school environment and where to find addition information in this handbook.

Crook, W. G. and L. J. Stevens, 1987, *Solving the Puzzle of Your Hard-to-Raise Child*, Jackson, TN: Professional Books.

Dadd, D. L., 1987, "Art Hazards in the Home," *Everything Natural*, May/June: 8-12.

Fenyves, E. J., Personal communication, May 30, 1991.

Giachino, J., 1992, "Men at Work: Kids in Class," *AS&U* 64, no. 12:24-25.

Godish, T., Personal communication, January 4, 1994.

Hill, L., Personal communication, January 8, 1994.

Jacobson, L., 1984, *Children's Art Hazards*, New York: Natural Resources Defense Council.

Lang, S.S., 1991, "Hidden Hazards of Chronic Noise," *Family Circle* 104, no. 15: 51-52, 57.

Lechner, N., 1991, *Heating, Cooling, Lighting*, New York: John Wiley & Sons.

Levin, A. S., 1983, *The Type 1/Type 2 Allergy Relief Program*, Los Angeles: Jeremy P. Tarcher, Inc.

Mandell, M., and L. W. Scanlon, 1979, *Dr. Mandell's 5 Day Allergy Relief System*, New York: Thomas Y. Crowell, Publishers.

Maryland State Department of Education, 1993, *Carpet and Indoor Air Quality in Schools*, Baltimore: The Department.

McCann, M., 1985, *Health Hazards Manual for Artists*, New York: Nick Lyons Books.

Miller, N. L., 1991, *Ecological Perspectives on a Healthful School Environment: A Delphi Study,* University Microfilms No. 92-19640

Mitchell, J., 1988, "Science, Students, and Living Lightly: IPM in Eddyville Public School," *Journal of Pesticide Reform* 8: no. 1: 2-6.

Moeller, D. W., 1992, *Environmental Health*, Cambridge: Harvard University Press.

Pope, A. M., R. Patterson, and H. Burge, Eds., 1993, *Indoor Allergens*, Washington, D.C.: National Academy Press.

Rea, W.J., Personal communication, 1992.

Shields, G.M., 1989, "Looking Great Without Poisoning Yourself," *Health Med Notebook* 1, No. 5.

Silver, F., 1980, "Ecology of Household Supplies," *The Household Environment and Chronic Illness*, edited by G. O. Pfeiffer & C. M. Nikel. Springfield, IL: Charles C. Thomas Publisher.

Simon, T., Personal communication, October 24, 1992.

Terman, M., Personal communication, January 7, 1994.

Turiel, I., 1985, *Indoor Air Quality and Human Health*, Stanford: Stanford University Press.

Turner, R.W. and B. E. Lippy, 1991, *Guidelines for Controlling Indoor Air Quality Problems Associated with Kilns, Copiers, and Welding in Schools*, Baltimore: Maryland State Dept. of Education.

University of Virginia Allergy Clinic, *Instructions for Reducing Exposure to House Dust Mites*, Charlottesville, VA: The University.

Volberg, D.I., M. H. Surgan, S. Jaffe, and D. Hamer, 1993. *Pesticides in Schools: Reducing the Risks*, New York: State of New York.

Wheeler, A. E., 1992, *Air Cleaning Devices for HVAC Systems in Schools*, Baltimore: Maryland State Dept. of Education.

Zaret, M. M., 1988, "Electromagnetic Energy and Cataracts," *Modern Bioelectricity*, edited by A. A. Marino, New York: Marcel Dekker.

5

HEATING, VENTILATING, AIR CONDITIONING, AND AIR QUALITY PROBLEMS

by Joseph Lstiburek

Indoor air quality (IAQ) is an important component of the indoor air environment of a school, and the heating, ventilating, and air conditioning (HVAC) system is a vital factor in maintaining acceptable indoor air quality. In this chapter, Mr. Lstiburek discusses the aspects of building construction, occupancy, and maintenance that result in harmful concentrations of pollutants in schools. He also shows how effective HVAC systems combine source control and removal of pollutants to improve indoor air quality. As he presents information about moisture and humidity, cross-contamination of fresh air, air pressure control, air flow balance, and many related problems and procedures, he answers questions that building maintenance personnel and administrators face every working day:

□ *How can the HVAC system function most efficiently and cost-effectively to maintain the health and comfort of school-building occupants?*

□ *How can maintenance personnel work most effectively to maintain the HVAC system and control pollution at its sources in the school building?*

□ *What is the relationship between of indoor air quality and the comfort of students, teachers, and others in the school?*

□ *How do people in the building contribute to contaminated air?*

Heating, ventilating, and air conditioning (HVAC) systems, as the name clearly indicates, involve both thermal comfort (heating and air conditioning) and the dilution of interior pollutants (ventilating). The HVAC system includes all heating, cooling, and ventilation equipment serving a building, including their associated distribution systems (furnaces, boilers, chillers, cooling towers, air handling units, exhaust fans, duct-work, filters, etc.).

The five principle functions of a building's HVAC system are:

■ To maintain thermal comfort under operating conditions.

■ To provide fresh air to the *head space* of building occupants in sufficient quantity and quality to dilute pollutants generated by occupants, furnishings, and the structure itself. This involves the outdoor air supply and determines the effectiveness of the ventilation system.

■ To facilitate source control of pollutants by providing adequate interzonal and interstitial pressure control. This involves system operation, maintenance, and commissioning/balancing.

■ To facilitate source control of pollutants by providing both *capture at source* exhaust ventilation at locations where pollutants are gen-erated and by preventing reintrainment of this local exhaust.

■ To facilitate source control of pollutants by providing air cleaning. This involves the filtration of particles and gases, as well as the dehumidification of airborne moisture.

COMFORT AND AIR QUALITY

The ultimate objectives of a successful environmental system are to provide for the comfort and welfare of the occupants of a building and to prevent an accumulation of unpleasant and/or harmful pollutants.

Indoor air quality (IAQ) is only one of the components that define the indoor environment of a school or any other building. Indoor environment also involves the interrelationship of comfort factors such as temperature and relative humidity; physical stressors such as noise and lighting; and psycho-social factors (personal relationships, peer pres-sures, work stress, etc.), as well as chemical, particulate, and biological concentrations. In addition, comfort factors and physical stressors affect perceptions of indoor air quality at the same time that they help define the indoor environment. A further complication is often the difference between real indoor air quality and that perceived by building occupants. The complexity of these interrelationships is illustrated in *Figure 5-1*.

Thermal comfort must be maintained within a building for an acceptable indoor environment to exist. Occupants who are uncomfortable will complain. If an interior is too hot or too cold, or if it is too dry or too

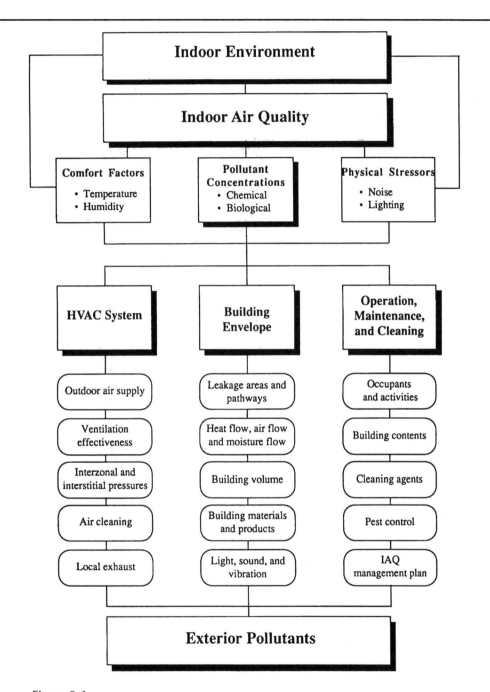

Figure 5-1.
The interrelationships between indoor environment, indoor air quality, and comfort factors.

damp, comments from occupants may not be significantly different from those of people exposed to elevated levels of pollutants. In other words, many indoor air quality complaints may in fact be misdiagnosed comfort complaints.

Many variables interact to determine whether occupants are comfortable. In its Standard 55-1992: *Thermal Environmental Conditions for Human Occupancy*, the American Society of Heating, Refrigerating, and Air-Conditioning Engineers (ASHRAE) describes the temperature and humidity ranges comfortable for most people involved in various activities. Some of the variables discussed in Standard 55-1992 are:

■ uniformity of temperature (temperature stratification, convection)

■ radiant heat transfer (cold or warm surfaces such as windows)

■ relative humidity

■ activity level, age, and physiology of occupants

■ clothing levels

There is considerable debate among researchers, building scientists, engineers, and health professionals concerning recommended levels of relative humidity. Interior relative humidities that are too low are uncomfortable, and interior relative humidities that are too high are unhealthy. A consensus is emerging that the critical relative humidity for biological activity to occur at a building's envelope surface is 70%. Where relative humidities above 70% occur at surfaces, mold growth, dust mite growth, decay, or corrosion can result. Therefore, conditions should be maintained within a building in such a way that the critical 70% (or higher) relative humidities at building envelope surfaces do not occur. Due to climate differences, interior conditions that must be maintained to avoid the critical surface relative humidities vary from region to region and from one time of year to another. They also vary with the thermal resistance of the building envelope.

In general, relative humidities should be kept as low as comfort levels and HVAC equipment will allow. Although people are rather insensitive to variations between 25% and 60%, relative humidity variations within this range *do* affect perception of temperature. In other words, interior relative humidities should be maintained as low as possible and interior temperatures adjusted within the parameters specified in Standard 55-1992 to provide thermal comfort. Relative humidities below 20% are uncomfortable to most people and should be avoided. During cool spells interior relative humidities should range from 25% to 35%. During warm periods interior relative humidities should range from 50% to 60% if equipment allows. In hot, humid climates it may not be economical or practical to maintain relative humidities below 60% during those periods when air conditioning must be used.

DILUTION, OUTDOOR AIR SUPPLY, AND VENTILATION EFFECTIVENESS

For a healthy indoor environment, the principal focus should be placed on concentrations of pollutants. In simple terms, the greater the pollution concentration, the greater the risk. Pollutant concentrations are determined by two factors----*source strength*; and *rate of removal*----and HVAC systems impact both.

Source strength is determined by the rate of pollutant entry into a conditioned space from the exterior, the rate of pollutant generation within the conditioned space, and the rate of pollutant offgassing from the materials used in construction and furnishing of the building. (See *Figure 5-2*.)

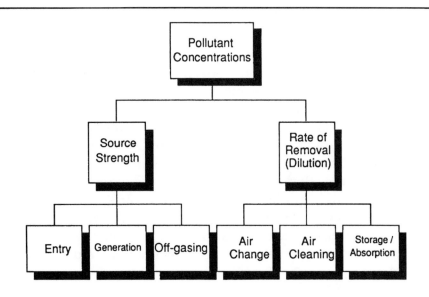

Figure 5-2.
Pollution concentration.

Removal or Dilution of Pollutants

Removal or dilution is typically determined by air change, air cleaning, and storage of pollutants. Air change can be considered a combination of natural ventilation (infiltration/exfiltration) and mechanical (controlled) ventilation. Air cleaning usually occurs through the filtration of particulates and some gases, and by the removal of moisture (dehumidification). Storage of pollutants involves the furnishings and surface coverings such as carpets that absorb pollutants and/or become receptors for particulates.

In general, if the rate of entry, generation, and offgassing of pollutants exceeds the rate of removal, concentrations will rise; and if the rate of removal exceeds the rate of entry, generation, and offgassing, concentrations will fall. The key is to maintain pollutant concentrations at levels sufficiently low to avoid problems.

One simplistic approach is to provide mechanical ventilation to control pollutant concentrations. The greater the source strength, the greater the mechanical ventilation required. The problem with this approach is that the ventilation air, which must come from the exterior, must be heated or cooled, and humidified or dehumidified depending on the climate. In some locations the air must also be cleaned (filtered) prior to use within a conditioned space.

The conditioning of air consumes energy and increases operating cost. The greater the rate of dilution by mechanical ventilation and infiltration/exfiltration, the greater the operating cost and the capital outlay for equipment to provide the dilution and conditioning. Furthermore, dilution by itself is very inefficient as a solution to indoor air pollution. Any powerful pollutant source will overpower even very high ventilation rates. In hot, humid climates, dilution itself can become the problem. The greater the rate of dilution in these climates, the greater the entry rate of moisture. Because moisture allows mold and other biological agents to multiply quickly and get out of control, it is a major indoor pollutant. In cooler climates that require seasonal heating, high dilution rates during the seasons when heating is on can lead to excessive loss of interior moisture, and in order to compensate, humidification may be necessary.

Source Control of Pollutant Concentrations

Another simplistic approach is to provide source control to diminish pollutant concentrations. If pollutants are prevented from entering conditioned spaces, are not generated within conditioned spaces, and are not offgassed from building materials and furnishings, then dilution by mechanical ventilation and infiltration/exfiltration is not required. Source control is not entirely effective, however, because the major pollutant source in a building enclosure happens to be people.

People can be considered as evaporatively cooled, unvented combustion appliances. They burn a hydrocarbon fuel (food) and generate three principal by-products of combustion: carbon dioxide, moisture, and odors, depending on diet and activity. When deodorants, perfumes, clothes, and hair sprays are added, people become thermal cracking towers, and analogies can be made to petroleum distillation. It has been said that if people were not allowed into buildings, we wouldn't have pollution problems. It is also obvious that source control for people is not practical.

Combining Source Control and Removal

Combining source control and removal is the preferred approach and ultimately is the most cost-effective and energy-efficient. Source control and air cleaning can be provided for all the pollutant sources except people. Ventilation can then be provided for the people, which might be rephrased, "You ventilate for people not for buildings." The higher the ventilation rate, the higher the operating and energy costs will be. Therefore, schools have a great incentive to reduce ventilation rates to save operating costs and energy. Ventilation rates, however, should not be lowered beyond those required to control the pollutants generated by the people themselves (carbon dioxide, moisture, and odors).

All other pollutant sources can be managed by source control and air cleaning. There is also a great economic incentive to provide source control and air cleaning for all non-human sources, since ventilation (the only other alternative) increases operating costs and the capital outlays for installation and maintenance.

RANDOMLY LEAKY BUILDINGS CANNOT PROVIDE AN ACCEPTABLE INDOOR ENVIRONMENT

First, let's quash the notion that random leakage openings and the effects of wind and stack to provide air change through infiltration/exfiltration will ensure dilution that is either constant or available when required. It will not. For health reasons, all buildings need controlled mechanical ventilation, regardless of their tightness.

Times Have Changed

Maintaining an acceptable indoor environment by natural means such as wind, is unacceptable by today's standards. In the past, energy was inexpensive, and natural means, such as wind, were relied upon to bring fresh air into buildings. Building envelopes were leaky, so that in cooler climates—those that required indoor heating—indoor moisture and other indoor pollutants could move outdoors through the leakage openings around windows and doors without causing serious problems. In warmer climates, air conditioning was not common, and extensive natural ventilation was needed for minimal comfort. The introduction of air conditioning in these warmer climates resulted in a significant reduction in natural ventilation.

Building enclosures have become significantly tighter over the past several decades, and mechanical cooling and heating are common in all climate zones. At the same time, hundreds of thousands of new chemical compounds, materials, and products have been introduced to satisfy the growing consumer demand for goods and furnishings. Interior pollutant sources have increased while the dilution of these pollutants through air change by natural ventilation has decreased.

Natural Ventilation

Natural ventilation—infiltration/exfiltration—driven by the stack effect and wind through random openings or through deliberate, discrete openings such as openable windows, doors, ductwork or holes, is not adequate to remove pollutants and odors from an enclosure on a continuous basis. The lack of consistency of the stack and wind-driving forces that causes this discontinuity adds significantly to the annual energy consumption for heating and cooling. Natural ventilation reduces the ability of occupants to control ventilation rates while at the same time seldom providing ventilation effectively to the critical *breathing zone* or head space.

Natural ventilation that may be adequate at a certain moment, may not be adequate at another time when there is no wind, when there is a change in wind direction, or when an insufficient interior to exterior temperature differential exists. In typical building envelopes, the normally random distribution of leakage openings influences the exfiltration/infiltration process that is responsible for the rate of natural ventilation. This random or accidental distribution of leakage openings resulting in accidental leakage does not provide assurance that adequate air change can take place.

The random distribution of leakage openings in a typical building causes the instantaneous infiltration/exfiltration rates in the building to vary substantially. Because wind pressures, stack pressures, and pressures induced by air-consuming devices influence natural ventilation rates, a building or areas of a building can have adequate natural air change at one time and inadequate air change at another. The variation can be so substantial that the infiltration/exfiltration rate may be on the order of several hundred cubic feet per minute (cfm) during a wind gust, and just moments later, zero cfm if the wind suddenly dies down and the majority of the randomly distributed leakage openings accidentally and temporarily fall along the neutral-pressure plane. Furthermore, there is seldom provision under natural ventilation for air change to be effective enough to improve the air quality in the breathing zone.

CONTROLLED VENTILATION

"Controlled ventilation" is the provision of a controlled driving force to remove pollutants and supply ventilation air through deliberate, discrete openings. This driving force can be provided on a continuous basis or, as necessary, depending on the level of pollutants and odors within an enclosure.

The principle behind acceptable indoor air quality and providing controlled ventilation to achieve it is very basic: *ventilate for occupants and provide source control and air cleaning for everything else.* This is the single most energy-efficient and cost-effective approach.

How much air must be supplied to accomplish this? ASHRAE Standard 62-1989: *Ventilation for Acceptable Indoor Air Quality* recommends 20 cfm per person.

Once a ventilation rate is determined by occupancy the basic requirements for ventilation should be applied, including provisions for

- air exhaust
- air supply
- continuous operation during occupancy
- distribution

One of the key requirements is the quantity of exterior air supplied to the *head space* of a room. Head space refers to the zone in each room where occupants' heads are likely to be located. For example, while seated at a desk, the head space location is between three and five feet above floor level. Head space zones are the locations where occupants obtain their "fresh" air for respiration. Test and balance information typically determines the flow rate of air (including fresh air) into rooms, spaces, and common areas, but does not determine flow rate of exterior supply air to the head space region. The amount of fresh air delivered to the head space compared to the amount of fresh air delivered to the room as a whole is referred to as the *ventilation efficiency*.

AIR PRESSURE CONTROL

Four factors are required for an air-pollution problem to exist:

- a pollutant
- a receptor or occupant
- a pathway connecting the pollutant to the occupant
- a pressure difference to push the pollutant down the pathway to the occupant

HVAC systems are often implicated in three of these factors. First, the HVAC system itself may be contaminated with pollutants such as mold growing in duct linings or bacteria growing on coils and in filters. Second, the HVAC duct distribution system is often the most common pathway for pollutants within a building. It is sometimes referred to as the "pollutant interstate." Finally, the HVAC system is often instrumental in creating air-pressure relationships between zones and building cavities that facilitate the movement of pollutants.

Air Pressure Differentials

Air pressure differentials are of major significance in the transfer of pollutants from special-use areas such as cafeterias, as well as those resulting from spillage and backdrafting from combustion appliances. They may also permit radon ingress. Managing air-pressure relationships determines the effectiveness of the HVAC system in containing pollutants in the vicinity of their origin and exhausting them from the building without letting them impact on other areas.

If more air is supplied to a room than is exhausted from it, the excess air leaks out of the space and the room is said to be under a positive air pressure. If less air is supplied than is exhausted, air is pulled into the space, and the room is said to be under a negative air pressure. Different rooms in a building can have different air pressures. Entire buildings can be under a negative or positive pressure. Finally, spaces such as floor cavities, exterior wall cavities, and interior enclosures formed by partitions can also be under a negative or positive air pressure.

The tighter a building envelope or enclosure, the less air required to pressurize or depressurize the conditioned space. Leaky buildings require a great deal of air from the outdoors in order to achieve pressurization. In the humid south, pressurization of conditioned spaces is desirable in order to exclude exterior humid air that can lead to mold growth. Air that is brought in from outdoors in order to achieve pressurization must be dehumidified and cooled, however, and the more air that is brought in, the greater the cooling load and the greater the operating cost. It is therefore desirable to construct tight building envelopes in order to minimize the amount of air required to provide pressurization.

Many building enclosures have exhaust systems and air consuming devices such as dryers and cook tops that extract air from a building. This air must be replaced with *make-up air*. If it is not, depressurization of the conditioned space occurs, resulting in infiltration. See *Figure 5-3*. More air should be mechanically supplied to a building, than is extracted under all operating conditions.

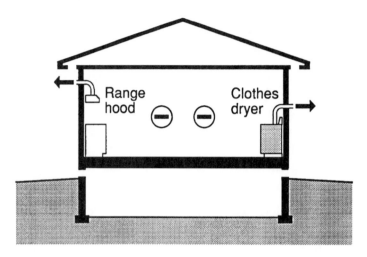

Figure 5-3.
Some appliances extract air from a building.

Make-up Air

In some facilities, attempts are made to supply make-up air passively through packaged terminal air conditioners (PTACs) or packaged terminal heat pumps (PTHPs). These are the typical units common in schools. Often located in walls under windows, they extract air from the building via a central exhaust system. For air to be drawn into the room through the PTAC or PTHP, a negative pressure created by the central exhaust system must exist in the room. Unfortunately, air is also drawn into the room through random leakage openings in the building envelope, as well as through the PTAC or PTHP.

Some PTAC and PTHP units supply make-up air by means of a fan in order to deal with the negative pressure problem of passive make-up air openings. Usually this air is supplied only when the unit is operating. The duty cycle—or "on" time—of these units is typically 20% to 30%, though the central exhaust from such a special-use area as a bathroom is usually on continuously. In other words 70% to 80% of the time make-up air is not being supplied and the conditioned space is under a negative pressure relative to the exterior. It is necessary to coordinate the exhaust fan operation with the duty cycle of the PTAC and PTHP units in order for this strategy to work, and since such a coordination is almost impossible, negative air pressures often result.

Make-up air should be conditioned. In other words, incoming air in cool climates should be heated in cool periods, and it should be cooled and dehumidified in hot climates during hot seasons. In the humid south, the moisture should be removed from incoming air----conditioned to dew point 55----prior to its use in the building.

Passive inlets or window units in humid climates typically provide unconditioned air containing substantial moisture. Recent experiences of serious mold and biologically-related indoor air problems in the humid south have underscored the need to supply make-up air mechanically and condition it prior to use. In addition, more air should be supplied than is extracted. Providing a passive supply of unconditioned air may be just asking for trouble. Recent experiences have shown that if you don't supply the make-up air deliberately, the building will supply it for you. When the building supplies it, it does so accidentally through random leakage areas that may be in the worst possible locations from an IAQ perspective.

AIR HANDLERS, DUCT LEAKAGE, AND UNBALANCED FLOWS

Air handlers create air pressure differences in buildings in two ways, through *duct leakage*, and *unbalanced flows*.

Most forced air duct systems leak substantial quantities of air. Field investigations have shown that 10% to 15% leakage of duct flow is typical. Leakage of 25% to 35% of duct flow is not uncommon. The effect of duct leakage on building enclosure pressures and air quality can be significant. For example, in a simple single zone system, if leaky supply ductwork is installed in the attic or crawl space of a building, or on the rooftop, air is extracted out of the building, depressurizing the conditioned space. This leads to the infiltration of hot, humid air and very likely to mold and other biologically-related problems, particularly in the south, as well as to the infiltration of radon and soil gas in all climates. (See *Figures 5-4* and *5-5*.) Furthermore, negative air pressures can lead to the spillage and backdrafting from combustion appliances.

If leaky return ductwork is installed in an attic (or on the rooftop), air is supplied to the building from the attic, pressurizing the conditioned

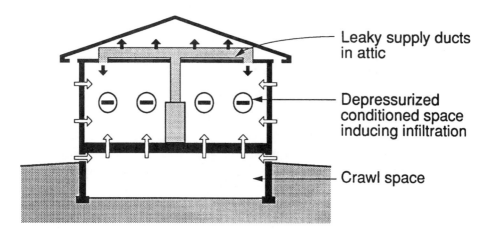

Figure 5-4.
Depressurized conditioned space with leaky supply ducts in the attic.

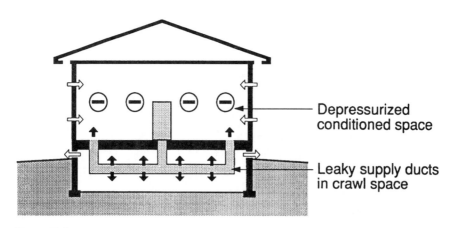

Figure 5-5.
Depressurized conditioned space with leaky supply ducts in the crawl space.

space. Infiltration of hot, humid air in hot climates, or of radon and soil gas in all climates does not occur, but the pressurization is accomplished with hot, humid air which significantly increases interior moisture levels. If the cooling system is unable to remove this moisture, mold and other biological growth will also result.

Unbalanced flows often occur when the supply and return of air to individual rooms are not equal. This typically occurs when supply air registers are located in each room and the return is located in a hallway. When the room doors are closed, air is not able to access the return, so the rooms become pressurized and the hallway becomes depressurized. (See *Figure 5-6.*)

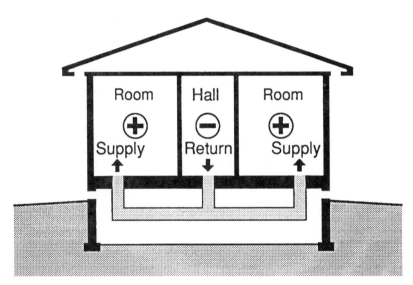

Figure 5-6.
Unbalanced air flows occur when supply and return units are located in different areas.

In large facilities the pressure relationships can become very complicated. One zone of a building may become pressurized, while another zone becomes depressurized. Furthermore, leakage of ductwork enclosed within building cavities can lead to the depressurization or pressurization of the cavities themselves. This is very common in facilities where individual room air handlers with leaky housings are built into exterior corners or into dropped ceiling locations where demising wall cavities are connected directly to exterior walls. It is not unusual to have a room at a positive air pressure relative to the exterior, while the wall cavities are at a negative air pressure relative to the exterior. (See *Figure 5-7.*)

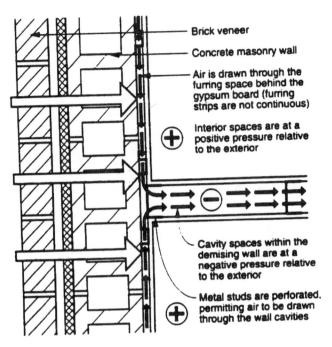

Figure 5-7.
Moist outside air can be drawn into the cavities within buildings even though the interior space is positively pressurized. This is caused by negative pressures within wall cavities created by an air-handling system with leaky return ducts.

Negative air-pressure fields in enclosed spaces such as building cavities can extend great distances away from air-handling equipment because of the perforated nature of most framing systems coupled with service chases----the conduits containing electrical, plumbing, and mechanical apparatus.

When the amounts of supply and return air are the same in a room or a facility, no air pressure differential occurs. Many facilities are *commissioned* by balancing contractors who measure air flows in and out of spaces. Since traditional air balancing is limited to the measurement of air flows into and out of supply and return registers, it is not effective in identifying duct leakage and air pressure relationships in conditioned building spaces and cavities. Zonal air pressure differentials are rarely measured. Furthermore, subtracting the sum of the return flows from the sum of the supply flows will not determine quantities of outside air or pressure relationships because duct leakage of the conditioning unit and the exhaust ducts is not considered.

Air pressure relationships should be determined with smoke pencils and digital micromanometers. Relationships between rooms and the exterior as well as between building cavities and the exterior should be determined with air handling equipment on and off, as well as with exhaust systems on and off.

Although mechanical systems can pressurize building enclosures near the exterior with conditioned air, duct leakage from return systems and air handlers enclosed in building cavities and service chases can depressurize demising walls and other cavities. If these cavities are connected to the exterior they become pathways for the infiltration of pollutant-laden air.

It is important to recognize that the more tightly a building enclosure is constructed, the less air flow is required to establish an air-pressure differential. Building enclosures should be built tight, not just to eliminate openings and pathways, but to make it easy to control air pressures with minimum air flows. An ideal level of tightness would be that at which the ventilation air-flow requirements resulting from human occupancy are sufficient to provide air pressure control. This is typically not possible unless building envelopes are constructed to high levels of tightness.

REINTRAINMENT OF EXHAUST VENTILATION/FRESH AIR SUPPLY

The level of *reintrainment*—or cross-contamination—occurring between building exhausts, air intakes, and air leakage sites in the building envelope is also important. The concern with reintrainment of exhaust air back into the building is that with this additional component of recirculation, there may not be adequate amounts of uncontaminated outdoor air entering the outdoor-air intakes to achieve acceptable ventilation rates.

One of the most common IAQ problems related to the HVAC system is the placement of fresh-air intakes at locations where pollutant sources—such as cooling towers, dumpsters, or loading docks where trucks and busses are idling—are also present. (See *Appendix* to this chapter.)

CONTROL OF POLLUTANTS

To facilitate control of a pollutant, you need to identify its sources. The major pollutants in conditioned spaces——exclusive of the moisture, carbon dioxide, and odors generated by occupant respiration——in order of impact are:

■ combustion products

■ biological agents (mainly moisture-related)

■ radon

■ formaldehyde and other volatile organic compounds (VOCs)

■ particulates

■ heavy metals (mercury, lead)

Each of these pollutant categories responds to one or more strategies involving source control and removal or dilution.

Source control of pollutants (see *Figure 5-8*) involves the following strategies:

■ Exclusion (control of air pressures; materials and furnishings selection; encapsulation; housekeeping; maintenance; and operation)

■ Capture at source (fume hoods; local ventilation; and negative-pressure containment rooms such as bathrooms, spas, etc.)

Removal or dilution of pollutants (see *Figure 5-9*) involves the following strategies :

■ Air change (controlled mechanical exhaust and supply)

■ Air cleaning (dehumidification and filtration of particles or gases)

Applying the principle of *ventilation for occupants, not buildings* leads to the use of source control and air cleaning for the identified pollutants, exclusive of those generated by respiration. Controlled ventilation is then provided for the moisture, carbon dioxide, and odors generated by the respiration of occupants.

Combustion Products

Exclusion and capture at source are the most effective methods of dealing with combustion products. Negative pressures created within conditioned spaces as a result of duct leakage, closing of interior doors, and

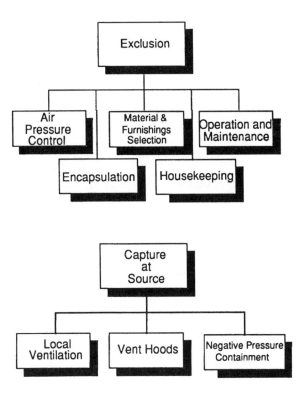

Figure 5-8.
Source control of pollutants.

competition for air from air-consuming devices such as exhaust fans, range hoods, and clothes dryers can lead to the spillage and backdrafting of traditional chimneys when they are used with gas- and oil-fired furnaces and water heaters. These types of chimneys and the combustion appliances that use them should not be installed in conditioned spaces. In other words, they should be excluded.

Sealed combustion and power-vented gas, oil and wood appliances eliminate concerns about spillage and backdrafting of combustion appliances. Hence, they demonstrate capture at source. No unvented combustion appliances of any kind (for example, kerosene heaters) should be installed within conditioned spaces; they should be excluded. Capture at source is an effective method of dealing with kitchen/cafeteria

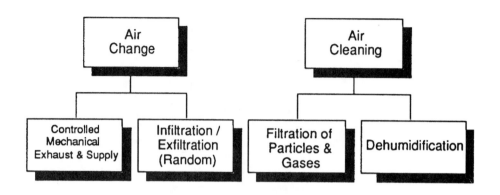

Figure 5-9.
Removal of pollutants.

appliances. Exhaust range hoods should be installed with all gas cook tops.

Environmental tobacco smoke (ETS), classed as a known human carcinogen, constitutes such a strong pollutant source that often the only practical management strategy is source control. Dilution of ETS is not economically feasible in most commercial and institutional facilities. Source control typically manifests itself in two ways: smoke-free buildings (exclusion) or smoking rooms maintained under a negative air pressure relative to surrounding spaces and ventilated and conditioned independently of the rest of the facility (capture at source).

Biological Agents (Moisture-related)

Controlling indoor moisture levels, surface temperatures, and moisture movement will provide source control of biological agents such as mold, bacteria, and dust mites. In cool climates the major moisture sources in buildings, exclusive of the occupants, are foundations. A correctly designed and constructed foundation excludes pollutants and hence has a major impact on indoor air quality issues linked to moisture-related biological agents. In hot climates, the infiltration of hot, humid air is the single largest moisture source, greater even than occupants and foundations. Infiltration of moisture-laden air below grade in all climates; infiltration of hot, humid air above grade in hot climates (or during hot periods); and exfiltration of, warm, moisture-laden interior air in cool climates (or during cool periods) are major concerns. Accordingly, it is desirable to control air pressures within buildings in order to control air-transported moisture (exclusion), and the most desirable air pressure relationships—depending on the climate and/or the heating/cooling process—are:

- pressurization of all below-grade spaces
- pressurization of building enclosures during air-conditioning seasons

Furthermore, all moisture-producing appliances such as clothes dryers should be vented directly to the exterior in all climates (capture at source). Unvented space heaters and other unvented combustion appliances generate significant amounts of moisture as well as other pollutants and should never be installed within conditioned spaces (exclusion). Bathrooms, washrooms, and any other moisture-generating rooms should be mechanically vented directly to the exterior in all climates (capture at source). Firewood should never be stored indoors (exclusion).

In cool climates or during cool periods, dilution by controlled ventilation (air change) can be utilized to remove moisture from building enclosures. In hot climates or during hot periods, dilution by controlled ventilation (air change) cannot be utilized to remove moisture from building enclosures. Dilution by dehumidification through air conditioning (air cleaning) should be used during hot periods or where exterior vapor pressures are high (for example, in the Pacific Northwest during those periods when heating is required).

Radon

In order for radon to enter a space three factors must be present:

- Radon in the soil surrounding the building
- An opening or pathway
- A driving force (an air pressure difference or a concentration gradient)

It is appropriate to assume that radon will almost always be present in the surrounding soil. It is also reasonable to assume that openings and pathways will be present in all building enclosures, notwithstanding the best attempts of builders, designers, and contractors to control them. Accordingly, control of the air pressure driving force constitutes the best approach for managing radon entry. Below-grade spaces should be pressurized with respect to the surrounding soil (exclusion). At the very least, air-handling systems, combustion appliances, and exhaust systems should be prevented from depressurizing below-grade spaces through duct leakage, make-up air and combustion, and draft control. Sub-slab depressurization is also recommended in all climate zones. Passive radon vents should be installed with the option of continuous mechanical exhaust. This air pressure control strategy for radon source-control is fully consistent with the air pressure control strategy recommended for air-transported moisture in all climate zones.

Formaldehyde and Other Volatile Organic Compounds (VOCs)

Formaldehyde is one of the most common industrial adhesives in current use. It is a VOC typically occurring in two forms:

- urea formaldehyde
- phenol formaldehyde

Phenol formaldehyde is much more stable than urea formaldehyde and is not water-soluble. Accordingly, phenol formaldehyde is typically used as an adhesive in exterior-rated building materials such as plywood, waferboards, and oriented stran boards (OSBs) that are exposed to rain. Urea formaldehyde is water-soluble and offgases readily at room temperatures. Increases in interior relative humidity and temperature significantly increase urea formaldehyde offgassing. Urea formaldehyde is used in the manufacture of particleboard, which is typically found as floor underlayer material, in cabinetry, and in furniture. It is also a key component in many surface finishes and is commonly used as a preservative. It is a potent human irritant linked to multiple chemical sensitivities. It is also an animal carcinogen, as well as a suspected human carcinogen.

Products containing urea formaldehyde should not be used within building enclosures (exclusion), or if used, the urea formaldehyde should be sealed or encapsulated to reduce emission source strength. For example, paint can be applied as a sealer on the exposed surfaces of cabinetry and furniture made of particleboard.

Gradual replacement of formaldehyde-containing products with those of lower pollutant capacity should be undertaken whenever possible. For example, urea formaldehyde-based products should be replaced with phenol formaldehyde-based products and those, in turn, should be replaced with urethane-based products and so on.

Carpeting rarely contains formaldehyde. Some carpeting, however, contains numerous other VOCs that may pose risks to susceptible individuals. Most of these VOCs have a rapid decay rate and pose little risk several months after installation. Unfortunately, problems can occur within the first few months or if defective products (carpets with high VOC loading) are installed. Of considerably more concern are the adhesives used to secure carpets and floor coverings to heavily-traveled floor surfaces. More often than not, the carpet or floor covering is blamed for a pollutant source problem created by a highly toxic adhesive used in conjunction with a relatively clean or uncontaminated floor covering.

One of the most serious concerns arising from VOCs comes not from the building products or furnishings themselves, but from maintenance and cleaning methods and materials. It has been said that in North America we clean for appearance, not for health. In other words, the surfaces may look clean, but in the act of cleaning, we may have poisoned them. Many cleaning agents are extremely toxic, and these substances are almost always stored in kitchen or bathroom cabinets. Offgassing from cleansers has been linked to corrosion of stainless steel heat exchange surfaces in high-efficiency combustion appliances and it has caused severe reactions in human beings. In many cases occupants choose to use more powerful substances than are necessary to accomplish the cleaning task effectively. For example, ammonia is used to clean window glass when vinegar diluted with water would be adequate. Source control in these cases involves user education that will enable the person doing the cleaning to match the strength of a cleaning agent to the size of the task and will encourage storage of cleaning and maintenance agents outside of conditioned spaces, perhaps in a garage or shed.

Many air fresheners are VOCs that perfume the air or coat the linings of the respiratory/olfactory system to mask an offending odor. Deadening of the senses is a typical outcome of the use of air fresheners, which in any case are not an acceptable solution to indoor pollution problems.

Synthetic, Natural And Benign Materials

It has been said that there are no bad materials, only bad uses. The use of a material has to be put into the context of a system. *The appropriateness of use* then takes on a critical meaning. There are really no truly benign materials, only degrees of impact. There may be no alternative to a particularly toxic material in a specific system, but the use of that material in that system may pose little risk and it may even provide a significant benefit to that system. For example, the use of bituminous damp-proofing on the exterior of a concrete foundation wall enclosing a pressurized basement is a beneficial one with little risk involved.

Society has benefited immeasurably from the use of tens of thousands of materials, compounds, chemicals, agents, and products many of which have been developed in the last half century. It is impractical to avoid including manufactured and synthetic agents in construction. Concerns have been raised, however, about the use of these products with respect to their impact on indoor environments (offgassing, etc.), and it is felt by many that synthetic materials should be avoided, and that *natural* or *green* materials should be used. Although natural materials are somehow felt to be safer, many of them contain VOCs and are potent irritants that pose hazards to human health. Allergic reactions to the odors emanating from cedar closets and chests are common.

In fact, what does *natural* or *green* mean? Radium and radon are natural materials. We doubt that any rational human being would suggest that these two substances be used in construction, even though radon gas, in place of argon gas, would prove an excellent insulator in sealed glazing systems and radium could be used on thermostat dials to make them easy to read at night.

The guiding principle to employ in selecting a product containing a particular synthetic or natural agent is that as long as that agent remains in the building product during its useful service life it does not enter or affect the human system through respiration or physical contact. Products that do not offgas are preferable to those that do. Products which offgas a little are preferable to those that offgas a great deal. Less toxic alternatives should be used in place of more toxic materials, and all of these choices need to be placed in the context of the system or assembly that contains the material.

When considering volatiles, the offgassing decay rate also needs to be considered. For example, most interior latex paints contain significant quantities of VOCs. They are usually the vehicle for the pigment and the resin in the paint. They offgas or evaporate very rapidly as they dry and leave behind a relatively benign surface finish that offgases very little after several weeks. These VOCs dissipate very quickly and typically pose very little real risk to most occupants over the useful service life of the paint finish. They may, however, pose a real risk to the painters as an occupational hazard. Accordingly, if a product containing a VOC that offgasses is used, it is preferable that the offgassing occur in a short time frame and that occupational risks be considered as well as risks from short-term early occupancy in a building in which the product is used.

The principle of product substitution should be employed wherever possible. Products containing compounds and chemicals that are volatile should be replaced by products containing less volatile agents. VOCs should be replaced by semi-volatile organic compounds, and semi-volatile organic compounds should be replaced by non-volatile organic compounds. If a compound or product does not contain any volatile agents, it is likely that the constituent materials will not be emitted from the product and enter the human respiratory system or be absorbed through the skin. Finally, if volatile agents are used, it is preferable that they have very rapid decay rates and that their "dwell" time in a particular product be limited.

Particulates

Particulates can be controlled by air cleaning (filtration) and by exclusion (encapsulation or product substitution). Of particular concern are respirable particles, or materials that can enter the lower reaches of the human respiratory system.

Particles that can be inhaled are usually smaller than 20 microns. Particles between 10 and 20 microns are typically deposited in the upper respiratory system (nasopharyngeal region). Those that can reach the lower respiratory tract (tracheobronchial and pulmonary regions) are in the less than 10 micron size range and are classed as respirable.

Respirable particles can pose a health risk when they interfere with the lungs' ability to exchange gases and when they cannot be easily removed or broken down by body defenses.

Asbestos fibers meet this criteria and as such are believed by some to pose a serious health risk. Fiberglass fibers used in cavity and attic insulation and as a lining on mechanical system ductwork do not. Part of the concern with asbestos fibers is their aspect ratio. They resemble tiny spears one to two microns in diameter and four to six microns in length. Once these tiny spears become embedded in the mucus lining of the lower respiratory system, they are very difficult to clear and cannot be broken down by the body. Thus they contrast with fiberglass "twigs" or "rocks" that are typically 15 microns in size or larger and as such cannot access the lower respiratory system. Fiberglass particles can also be cleared more readily by the body and can be broken down or dissolved.

Fiberglass fibers are easily aerosolized and may be a significant irritant for sensitive individuals. Fiberglass cavity insulation encapsulated by gypsum board or located above gypsum board ceilings typically poses little risk unless the fibers find their way into a mechanical system or into a conditioned space. Although fiberglass fibers in ductboard and acoustical lining do not readily become aerosolized, the materials constituted from them can become hosts for dust and biological agents, especially should wetting or condensation occur. Careful cleaning protocols must be employed with such products, and should they become contaminated or wet and biological growth occur, removal and replacement may be the only option.

Carpeting is typically the major source for particulates in indoor environments. Vacuuming and traffic aerosolize particles collected by carpeting as well as the carpet fibers themselves. If dust mite infestation is also present, both the dust mites and their feces will also become aerosolized. Installation of central vacuum systems with extraction fans located in garages are an effective method of source control as is the use of a high efficiency particle arrestance (HEPA) vacuum system that captures respirable particles. Finally, the use of flooring materials such as wood and tiles is also an effective source control.

Carpets should be maintained with periodic steam extraction in accordance with professional standards. Owner-conducted carpet shampooing can create more problems than it solves, including perfuming the carpet and providing moisture that facilitates dust-mite growth. Dust mites can be killed and removed if steam accesses deep into carpet piles and particulates are removed under high suction. Dry extraction and other dry cleaning methods should also be considered. To prevent reinfestation and growth of dust mites, carpet micro-climates should be maintained at below 70% relative humidities.

Filters in most air-handling systems are installed to protect equipment, not people. Typical filters are "bolder catchers" that capture 50 to 100 micron and larger particulates that can clog and contaminate fans and heat-exchange surfaces. Dust mites are in the 30 to 40 micron size range and dust-mite feces are in the 15 to 30 micron size range.

Electronic or electrostatic filters tend to be very efficient. They can contribute to ozone production at very low air flows, however, and they require regular cleaning to remain effective. Their principle attraction, aside from their effectiveness, is that they do not restrict air flows as much as HEPA filters. The new generation of HEPA filters, about to be introduced for use in residential and commercial systems, promises to address this flow-restriction issue.

Air flow through a filtered system can be as important a consideration as filter efficiency. Air with a given volume circulated in a room more frequently through a low-efficiency filter can be as free of pollutants as the air in a comparable room circulated less frequently through a more efficient filter. In some cases air-flow rates can be used to compensate for less efficient filtration. A high circulation rate helps improve the capture of large particles. Higher efficiency filters, however, will capture particles that are so small they may never be arrested by lower efficiency filters.

Heavy Metals

Mercury, lead, and cadmium are commonly referred to as heavy metals and are recognized as extremely toxic substances. Cadmium is not typically found on construction sites. Mercury, however, has a long history of use as an effective mildewcide or biocide in paints, gypsum board, joint compound, and many other products. Lead, once considered a pigment, was used in paints and was a key constituent of solder used in plumbing systems for many years. The use of mercury and lead as mildewcides and biocides is strictly regulated, and it is not likely that these two agents will turn up in new products and materials. Their prior widespread use, however, makes them a concern when rehabilitation of existing structures takes place and when recycled materials are used in new construction.

CASE STUDY ONE: A SINGLE STORY MASONRY SCHOOL BUILDING OVER CRAWL-SPACE FOUNDATION

Description of Facility and History of Problems

The facility in question is a single story masonry school building constructed over a crawl space foundation. It consists of several wings constructed at different periods over the past 60 years. Each wing has a separate foundation system, although communication is possible between the various crawl space foundations. The crawl space in the affected area consists of a perimeter cast concrete foundation wall on concrete strip footings. The floor deck consists of cast concrete supported on precast concrete beams which, in turn, are supported on the perimeter foundation walls and interior cast concrete bearing walls. The crawl-space floor surfaces are uncovered earth. Crawl-space ventilation consists of numerous 8" x 12" vents, distributed in an approximate ratio of 1/1500 between vent area and floor area.

A teacher in one of the classrooms of the affected area of the facility complained of mold odors, headaches, fatigue, and flu-like symptoms. Discussions with the teacher indicated that similar complaints were also common among the students.

Investigation and Testing

In the classroom occupied by the affected teacher and students, deterioration of plaster and baseboard surfaces were visible along interior and exterior walls. The deterioration was most intense at the baseboard level, and decreased in intensity with height. Paint had peeled from the plaster at many locations. Water markings were observed on the plaster surfaces. The plaster was soft to the touch and disintegrated when probed. When the plastic covering over the wood baseboard trim was removed, noticeable musty odors were encountered. The wood was soft and "punky." Significant decay of the wood was observed. When the wood baseboard was pulled away from the wall, the intensity of the musty odors increased significantly.

Visual observations revealed a joint between the concrete floor slab and the masonry perimeter wall. Other joints were observed in the concrete floor slab at the interior concrete foundation walls. Smoke pencil testing indicated substantial air flow between the crawl space and the classroom through these exposed joints. Readings taken with a digital micromanometer indicated that the crawl space was operating at a 4 Pascal positive air pressure with respect to the classroom. (See *Figure 5-10*.)

Removal of deteriorated plaster verified wall construction. Specifically, interior plaster was installed over wood furring strips creating an air space (or channels) between the plaster and the masonry wall. Removal of ceiling tiles indicated that the plaster finish extended just above the dropped ceiling level and that the air space (or channels) between the plaster and the masonry wall was open at the top and connected to the air space above the dropped ceiling. This wall geometry created "chimneys" which extended from the crawl space to the air space above the dropped ceiling.

Discussion with school district staff and examination of photographs of the affected area indicated that no ground cover was present in the crawl space. According to staff, the top surface of the soil appeared dry. In addition, many of the steam lines in the crawl space were reported to be uninsulated due to ongoing asbestos mitigation work. Crawl space temperatures in excess of 100 degrees Fahrenheit were typical according to staff.

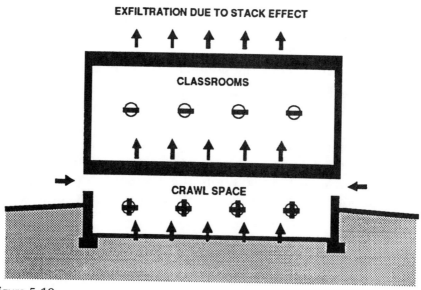

Figure 5-10.
Crawl space operating at a positive air pressure in relation to the classrooms.

Crawl space vents were sealed and an exhaust fan was installed in the crawl space exhausting air to the exterior. The access opening connecting the affected crawl space and the adjacent crawl space was also sealed. Air pressure differentials between the affected classroom and the crawl space were monitored. Extracting approximately 650 cfm of air from the crawl space by means of an exhaust fan depressurized the crawl space 4 Pascals with respect to the classroom area. This was shown to result in a flow reversal of air between the crawl space and the classroom area. Air could be shown to flow from the classroom area into the crawl space when the exhaust fan was operating, rather than from the crawl space into the classroom.

Discussion and Conclusions

The complaints from the teacher and students were due to musty odors resulting from the deterioration wood trim and other building materials. These odors and deterioration were due to excessive moisture migrating from the crawl space under the classrooms into the interstitial spaces of interior and exterior walls as a result of the air pressure relationship between these spaces and the crawl space.

According to the rationale followed to determine the pollution source, for an odor or IAQ problem to occur, four factors are necessary:

- a pollutant
- a receptor (occupant)
- a pathway (connecting the pollutant to the occupants)
- a pressure difference (to push the pollutant down the pathway to the occupant)

It is obvious that occupants must be present in order for a problem to exist or for it to be detected. It is clear that although removing occupants is an effective short-term solution, this strategy is not an appropriate long-term solution. The receptors in this case were the teacher and students.

The primary pollutant was moisture, and this moisture led to the creation of the secondary pollutants which were mold and other biological agents. Removing the pollutant would be a very effective source-control approach to indoor air quality problems.

If pollutants and receptors are isolated from each other by "perfect" barriers, then problems can also be eliminated. In this case the pathway connecting the moisture pollutant and the receptor were the openings connecting the crawl space and the channels between the plaster surfaces and the masonry walls.

Finally, the driving force was an air-pressure difference between the crawl space and the classrooms. This air-pressure difference was created by a combination of the stack effect (heated air rising) and the exhaust operation of the classroom ventilators.

Moisture, the primary pollutant, in the soil of the crawl space was evaporated in the elevated temperatures of the crawl space. Warm moisture-saturated air migrated through openings in the floor slab into the air space created by the plaster and wood furring (the pathway). The air was pulled into the space between the plaster and wood furring as a result of its temperature and the building's stack effect, combined with the operation of the classroom ventilators (the driving force). The moisture-saturated air cooled once it was in the furring space, which led to condensation and saturation of the building materials at this location (see *Figure 5-11*). The saturation of the building materials resulted in their deterioration and the creation of odors and other biological agents (the secondary pollutants). These secondary pollutants entered the classroom and reached the teacher and students (the receptors).

The crawl space soil surface was dry because of the rapid rate of evaporation of moisture (vapor diffusion) from the upper soil surface into the crawl space enclosure resulting from the heat from the uninsulated steam lines. Where it was possible to probe several inches beneath the crawl space floor surface, the ground material was damp to the touch, supporting this hypothesis.

Crawl space vents removed moisture and the ambient (exterior) vapor pressure was lower than the vapor pressures in the crawl-space enclosure. The rate of moisture removal by ventilation, however, was judged to be extremely low due to the small number of vents, their location, and the small cross sectional areas.

Moisture levels within enclosures are determined by a combination of moisture source strength (rate of moisture generation or entry) and air change or ventilation (rate of moisture removal). If the rate of moisture generation or entry is higher than the rate of moisture removal then high enclosure moisture levels can occur. The levels of airborne moisture in

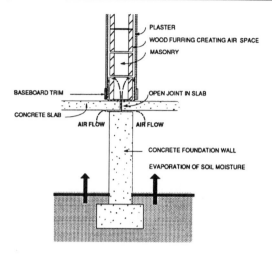

1. MOISTURE IN SOIL EVAPORATES DUE TO ELEVATED TEMPERATURE OF CRAWL SPACE

2. MOISTURE SATURATED AIR MIGRATES THROUGH OPENINGS IN SLAB INTO MASONRY WALL AND FURRING SPACE DUE TO AIR PRESSURE DIFFERENCE BETWEEN CRAWL SPACE AND CLASSROOMS

3. MOISTURE SATURATED AIR COOLS ONCE I N FURRING SPACE, DEPOSITING MOISTURE AND LEADING TO DETERIORATING PLASTER AND BASEBOARD TRIM.

Figure 5-11.
The migration of moisture from soil to plaster and trim, causing deterioration.

the crawl space were high because the rate of moisture generation or entry in the crawl spaces was higher than the rate of moisture removal by ventilation. This was consistent with the observations of low moisture removal (poor ventilation) and the lack of an effective ground cover.

Recommendations for Rehabilitation Measures

It was recommended that all four factors active in air quality and odor problems (receptor, pollutant, pathway and pressure) be controlled in this case:

- For the short term, removal of the receptors was advised. Students and teachers should not be allowed access to the affected classroom until the rehabilitation measures have been implemented.

- Source control for the primary and secondary pollutants should be undertaken. The secondary pollutants should be removed by stripping the damaged portions of the interior plaster surfaces and removing all wood baseboard trim. The carpets should be lifted and examined for deterioration and cleaned with a HEPA vacuum.

■ The primary pollutant, airborne moisture from the crawl space, should be controlled at the source. Crawl space enclosure moisture levels could be reduced in only two ways: by limiting moisture source strength (moisture entry) or by dilution (moisture removal by ventilation or dehumidification). A desired result would be a rate of moisture entry lower than the rate of moisture removal, or a level of moisture accumulation in building materials that does not lead to deterioration. In order to achieve this desired result, it is our belief that it is practical to control the source strength (moisture entry by evaporation from the ground) and not rely on dilution (moisture removal by ventilation).

A temporary polyethylene ground cover should be installed immediately. A permanent stabilized, reinforced polyethylene ground cover should be installed after mechanical system work was completed in the crawl space. (See *Figure 5-12.*) As part of this work, all steam lines should be insulated.

■ The pathway for the primary pollutant (moisture) should be sealed by installation of foam sealants after damaged and deteriorated materials had been removed at baseboard locations.

■ Finally, the driving force for pollutant transfer—specifically, the air pressure relationship between the crawl space and the classrooms—should be altered by the installation and operation of an exhaust fan which should run continuously. (See *Figure 5-13.*) In order to facilitate air pressure control the crawl space vent openings should be closed.

CASE STUDY TWO: MULTISTORY SCHOOL BUILDING ON SLAB FOUNDATION

Description of Facility and History of Problems

The facility in question is a multistory school building constructed over a slab foundation in the early 1970's. The facility consists of three levels, with the first level built into sloping terrain forming a walk-out. The upper two levels overhang the lower level approximately 25 feet on three sides.

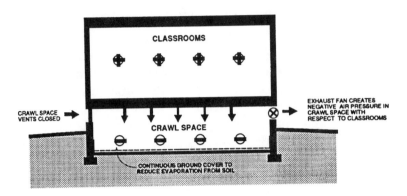

1. AIR PRESSURE RELATIONSHIP BETWEEN CRAWLSPACE AND CLASSROOMS CHANGED BY EXHAUST FAN

2. GROUND COVER REDUCES SURFACE EVAPORATION OF MOISTURE

Figure 5-12.
Exhaust fan and continuous ground cover reduce surface evaporation of moisture in crawl space.

Staff members and students have been complaining of odors, headaches, fatigue, and nausea.

Investigation and Testing

Observations revealed that both the fresh air intake grills and stale air exhaust registers of the air-handling systems were located in close proximity to each other under the overhang portions of the second and third levels which sheltered the loading dock area. Cars and trucks were parked in this location while making deliveries. The dumpster for the facility was also located under this overhang. Staff members took their smoking breaks under the overhang. A pungent odor was noticed at this location and traced to a sewer manhole immediately adjacent to the overhang. In addition, a central vacuum system exhaust was located under the overhang and was operating during the observation period.

Inspection of the rooftop air-handling systems indicated plumbing vents, washroom fan exhausts and the terminus of the boiler vent stack all located in close proximity to the fresh air intakes of the rooftop air handling systems. In addition, standing water and condensate were pooling adjacent to the fresh air intakes creating an odorous warm

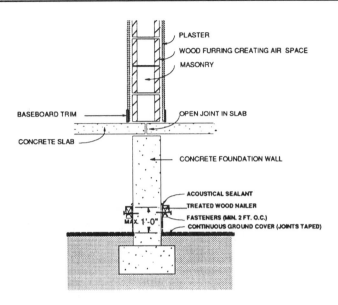

Figure 5-13.
The continuous operation of an exhaust far will act as a driving force for pollutant transfer.

slime-like broth. The roof top air handling systems were sheltered from winds by screens forming enclosures. The plumbing vents and washroom fan exhausts were located within these enclosures.

Discussion with building staff indicated that most of the environmental complaints came from the common areas on the second and third levels and that truck exhaust odors were frequently smelled in the common areas above the overhangs during cold weather, and sewer/decay odors were detected intermittently throughout the year.

Air pressure testing with a digital micromanometer indicated that the facility was operating under a positive air pressure relative to the exterior (1.5 to 3 Pascal).

Air pressure testing was also conducted in the boiler room area relative to the exterior. When one of the three boilers fired, the air pressure in the boiler room dropped 3 Pascals relative to the exterior. The combustion air grill was observed to be 50% covered with a loose fitting piece of plywood. The filter in the grill was caked with contaminants and was black from this material.

Tracer gas testing was conducted using sulfur-hexafluoride (SF6) as the tracer gas and a gas chromatograph (Miran 101) as the detector. SF6 was released outside the facility under the overhang area near the dumpster and sewer manhole. Within three minutes, SF6 was detected in both the office and the common area on the third level. Concentrations were highest in the office area.

Discussion and Conclusions

The complaints from the staff and students were due to odors resulting from the reintrainment of boiler flue gases, exhaust ventilation, washroom exhaust, plumbing vent stack exhaust, and central vacuum system exhaust, combined with the intake of sewer gas, dumpster odors, automobile and truck exhaust, tobacco smoke, and bioaerosols from standing water/slime. The fresh air intakes located under the overhang as well as those located in the screened-in regions on the roof draw pollutants from the exterior into the facility.

The rationale for these conclusions, like that in Case Study One, depends on the existence of four factors:

■ a pollutant

■ a receptor (occupant)

■ a pathway (connecting the pollutant to the occupants

■ a pressure difference (to push the pollutant down the pathway to the occupant)

Again, the receptor was the collective occupants of the building.

In this case, the primary pollutants are believed to be:

■ sewer gas

■ dumpster odors

■ reintrained combustion products from the boilers

■ automobile and truck exhaust

■ tobacco smoke

■ central vacuum system exhaust

■ plumbing vent stack odors

- reintrained washroom exhaust
- bioaerosols from standing water/slime
- reintrained exhaust ventilation

Removing the pollutant sources was deemed to be a very effective approach to controlling indoor air quality problems.

In this case, the pathway connecting the pollutants and the receptors was the facility's existing mechanical ventilation system. Tracer-gas testing showed that gases released at the overhang area are quickly drawn into the facility through the building's ventilation system.

The driving force was an air pressure difference in the mechanical ventilation system induced by the system's fans. Air that was contaminated was drawn from the exterior into the facility, pressurizing it. As the ventilation rate increased, the quantity of contaminants entering the facility also increased.

Recommendations for Rehabilitation Measures

It was recommended that source control for the pollutants be undertaken as follows:

- The mechanical ventilation should be redesigned and modified so that fresh air could be introduced into the facility from above the upper roof areas rather than from under the overhang.
- The rooftop screens sheltering the rooftop air-handling systems should be removed or replaced with air-permeable screens.
- Drainage of condensate from roof top units should be facilitated.
- An extension should be added to the existing boiler flue-pipe system.
- Loading, unloading, parking and/or deliveries should be forbidden under and immediately adjacent to overhang areas.
- The dumpster should be relocated farther away from the facility.
- The blockage of the combustion air opening in the boiler room should be removed.
- The filter in the combustion air opening in the boiler room should be replaced.

APPENDIX

Case Study: Solving Vehicle Exhaust Problems

The Minnetonka School District, in suburban Minneapolis, has posted new signs (see *Figure 5-14*) in the bus loading areas and in the delivery zones of all nine schools in the district. These signs notify the drivers of school buses and delivery trucks that their vehicles will no longer be allowed to idle near the school causing exhaust fumes to fill the outside air and contaminate the school buildings.

This action was prompted by the principal of one elementary school after receiving a parent's letter. The parent was concerned because during a visit to the school she noticed a strong smell of exhaust fumes in the corridors and classrooms that was caused by a milk truck idling near the building. In her letter to the principal, she made a number of suggestions to minimize exhaust fumes in and around the school building including posting "NO IDLING IN THIS AREA" signs at delivery points.

The principal responded by distributing the letter throughout the district. Supervisors from the health, safety, and maintenance department developed an action plan. They were aware of the exhaust fume problem and recognized that it needed to be addressed in the Minnetonka schools. Soon after, members of the maintenance staff were seen in delivery areas telling drivers to turn their vehicles off. In addition to the signs, letters are being sent to the bus companies and vendors informing them that they must comply.

The signs were in place by November 1994, slightly more than two months after the suggestion was made to the school principal. Children and staff in the Minnetonka schools will breathe cleaner air because a conscientious school staff responded to one constructive letter sent by a parent.

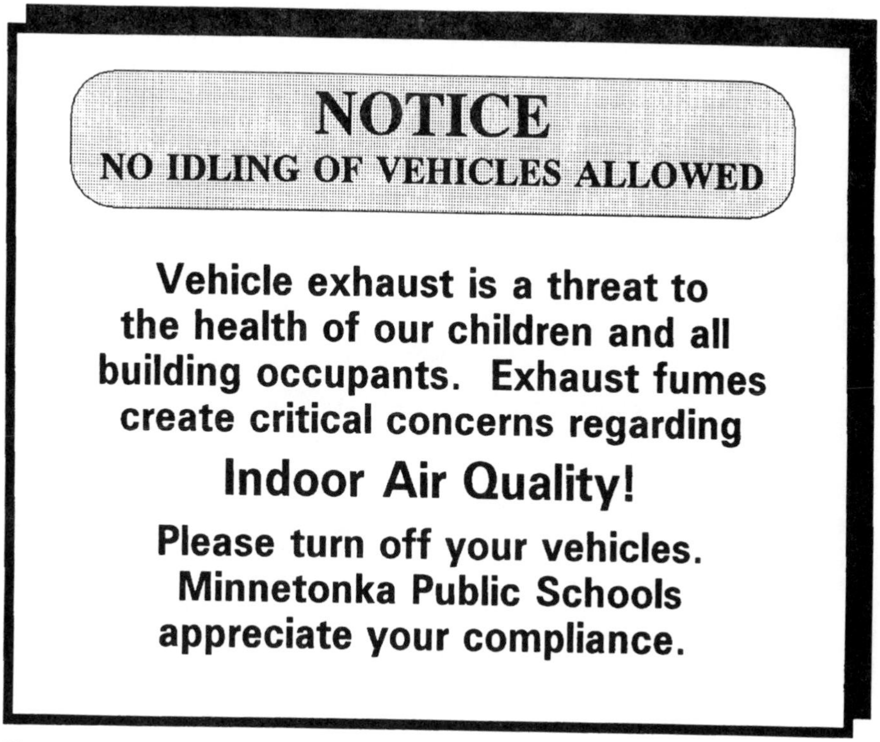

NOTICE
NO IDLING OF VEHICLES ALLOWED

Vehicle exhaust is a threat to the health of our children and all building occupants. Exhaust fumes create critical concerns regarding

Indoor Air Quality!

Please turn off your vehicles. Minnetonka Public Schools appreciate your compliance.

Sign Dimensions are 30" Wide x 24" High

Figure 5-14.

"No idling of vehicles allowed" signs are now posted at Minnetonka schools because a conscientious school staff responded to a letter sent by a parent.

6

HOW INDOOR AIR QUALITY AFFECTS PRE-EXISTING HEALTH PROBLEMS

by Mary Ann Block, D.O.

In this chapter, Dr. Block discusses how health problems can be further exacerbated by poor-quality indoor air in classrooms and other school areas. In a striking analogy, she equates health to a mountain slope and shows that many people unknowingly spend much of their lives far down that slope on the brink of illness. She shows that poor air quality often plays a significant role in pushing brink-sitters over the edge into full-fledged disease. In addressing the effects of poor air quality on pre-existing health problems, she answers a number of questions for the reader, including:

☐ *How does an accumulation of exposures to environmental pollutants affect pre-existing disease such as asthma, enuresis, and attention deficit hyperactivity disorder?*

☐ *Why do the symptoms triggered by poor air quality differ so widely?*

☐ *Why is it difficult to pinpoint the specific environmental trigger of a school-child's recurring symptoms?*

☐ *How can teachers and parents together take steps to diminish a child's environmentally-triggered symptoms?*

There are differences between the indoor air problems existing in old and in new schools. Some obvious problems found in older schools are dust, dust mites, bacteria, fungus, pollens, and even tobacco. The gerbil or pet mouse often found in primary classrooms can leave behind fur and dander. The heating, ventilating, and air conditioning system (HVAC) harbors these particles and provides a wonderful medium for the growth of bacteria and viruses. Cleaning products and other volatile organic compounds (VOCs)—particularly pesticides, which may have been used over the years—accumulate and spread throughout a school building through the HVAC system. Maintenance, repairs, and remodeling create problems similar to those usually associated with newer schools.

While newer school buildings can contain the same pollutants as the older ones, they also may have their own set of problems associated with the use of building construction products containing formaldehyde and other VOCs used in carpeting, paint, fabrics, and cabinets. Whether the school is old or new, one of the keys to preventing it from becoming a sick school building is to have an adequate ventilation system and the proper amount of fresh air circulating throughout the building.

PRE-EXISTING HEALTH PROBLEMS

> The U.S. Clean Air Act specifically recognizes that some individuals in the population are sensitive to air pollutants and indicates that such individuals need to be protected. . . . Frequently, those with preexisting illnesses are part of the sensitive population because they may often respond, sometimes hyperrespond, to a pollutant exposure that may not affect most people. (Lebowitz 1991)

It is well recognized that different people placed in the same environment will have different reactions to that environment. For example, if a group of people is exposed to formaldehyde, those who already have a chronic illness, such as asthma, will respond with more symptoms than those who have no history of chronic illness. A very wide range of possible reactions can occur if there is a pre-existing illness, even if that preexisting illness is in remission. Because of the differences in individual reactions to indoor air, students and teachers themselves are the best ones to determine if the air quality in the school is a problem.

Pre-existing health problems can range from asthma to ear infections; from stomach problems to behavioral problems. Since pre-existing health problems are extremely varied, the illnesses that poor indoor air quality can trigger are also extremely varied. They all have one thing in common, however: they can be triggered from occurrences in the environment. Let's take a look at why this might happen.

Figure 6-1 illustrates the Mountain of Health/Brink of Disease concept and shows why health problems stemming from pre-existing illnesses can be easily triggered. Everyone has the capability of good health. But it is known that what a person is exposed to or not exposed to, even before conception, can affect her/him for the rest of her/his life. For example, the importance of a vitamin called folic acid has only recently

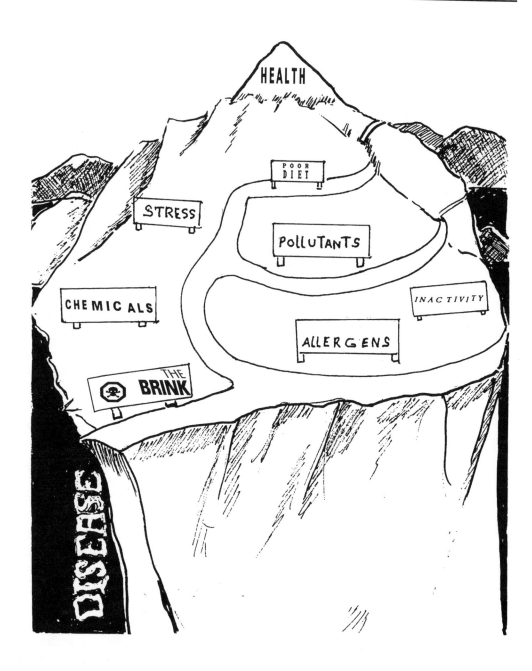

Figure 6-1.
The Mountain of Health.

been understood. If a mother is deficient in folic acid prior to becoming pregnant, the probability of her child having a neural tube defect that affects the child's spinal cord is increased by 60%. (Rush 1992) It is only now beginning to be understood what nutrients in our diet and chemicals in our environment can do. It is also known that if a mother smokes cigarettes, her child will be more likely to have a decreased birth weight and an increase in associated problems. If the mother does not breast feed, the child is more likely to have upper respiratory problems. (Minchin 1987) There are many other examples of the effects that diet and environment can have on an unborn and newborn child.

All the "external" situations illustrated on the Mountain of Health (poor diet, pollutants, stress, chemicals, allergens, and inactivity) affect the internal workings of the child, and help determine how well adjusted she or he will be to the world just before or after birth. Each challenge can start the child on a downhill road toward disease. While many people may recognize that they have traveled quite a distance down that road by the time they reach middle age, it is usually thought that children are very healthy. Unless there is an obvious illness, even a person in the older population is thought to be basically healthy. But nothing could be further from the truth. Health is not merely the absence of disease, and there is a very long road that must be traveled between good health and disease. Many sit there on the Brink of Disease, thinking they are perfectly healthy when they are actually subject to an illness just waiting to happen. They sit on that brink because most health problems come about slowly. The human body has a remarkable ability to compensate, so an individual only gets sick when his or her body is so overloaded that it can no longer compensate. All of those hazards represented on the Mountain of Health are avoidable. Because people often do not feel an instantaneous decline in health when they are exposed to hazards, without the immediate negative feedback they continue the exposure. But the exposures affect everyone and eventually accumulate to such an extent that they push an individual further down the slope of the Mountain of Health until he or she reaches the Brink Of Disease. Many people live most of their lives on the brink. It doesn't take much to throw them over the edge into full-blown disease. Sometimes the disease is fairly minor, such as a cold or sore throat, but at other times it is deadly serious, perhaps cancer or a heart attack. Often one can take a medication to make the symptoms go away and then can climb back up to the brink, remaining there until another exposure occurs. But at other times, the situation is much more serious and there is no return. Death or a permanent disablement occurs. A pattern of falling off and returning to the brink will continue throughout life until there is no return to the brink. Those who are able to see the fall-off as a warning sign and decide to change their lifestyles permanently can not only remain on the brink longer, but also have the chance to climb back up the Mountain of Health.

The variability in response of different individuals to the same environmental insults may well be due to the Mountain of Health/Brink of Disease phenomenon. Since different people are at different places on the mountain, each person's reaction will be very different from that of other people. One who is on the brink will show symptoms in response to an environmental trigger much sooner and will be pushed over into the Cavern of Disease much more quickly than the person who is higher up the mountain who may slide down the mountainside one level, perhaps not even noticing a change at all.

As mentioned above, a child having no specific and obvious illness is generally thought of as healthy. Nutritional biochemist Jeff Bland, Ph.D., has stated that "from a biochemical perspective, 80% of an organ's reserves is lost before a diagnosed disease is evident." (Bland 1993) We spend an entire lifetime slipping down this mountainside, away from health and toward disease. The slide down starts even before conception.

If the mother has eaten improperly during pregnancy, has smoked or been exposed to side-stream smoke, has drunk alcohol, or has had poor prenatal care, the child will have begun a slide away from health even before birth. Then if the child is not breast fed, or is breast fed while the mother continues to eat or drink improperly, he or she will experience further problems. Ninety percent of all children will have at least one ear infection, while 75% will have three or more. (Jung 1991) Ear infections would not be so prevalent if children's bodies were working better. But the 90% who have ear infections have slid all the way down the road into disease. Although they can be pulled back up to the brink and will usually outgrow the problem as they get older, they remain on the brink, continuing to be susceptible to other health problems unless actual lifestyle changes are made.

With all of these children teetering on the brink, it should come as no surprise that many different physical insults will cause them to become ill. A child who has had many of the exposures illustrated on the Mountain of Health, has a high probability of falling off the brink repeatedly. Additional environmental problems in the school and class-room are the last straw for some children.

ASTHMA

It is now accepted that asthma is an illness exacerbated by the environment. The most common triggers appear to be allergens, viruses, exercise, cold, and stress. While each of these seems to be totally unrelated to the others, if you consider the Mountain again, you can see why any of these triggers might bring on an asthma attack. If a child is prone to asthma and has had continuous bouts with hyperactive airway problems, then she or he is showing signs of being right on the brink and can be pushed off the Mountain by almost anything. Since these triggers are common in our society, the child who is susceptible can easily react to one of them. In the past few decades there has been a substantial increase in asthma morbidity and mortality, particularly in the school-age child. One study indicates that between 1964 and 1983, there was a doubling or tripling of the number of cases of asthma in school-age children, though not in infants or adults. "This increased incidence in asthma may be a result of some unidentified environmental factor. This is the age group in which airborne allergens are the predominant cause of asthma." (Yunginger 1992) If a school-age child is sitting on the brink with a history of asthma, it may take only a small amount of an airborne allergen to push her or him over into an asthma attack.

Anyone with a history of asthma is a strong candidate for exacerbation of the illness from exposure to poor quality indoor air. It is not uncommon for children with asthma to react negatively to the introduction of new carpet or construction activities in the school. Even low levels of irritants can cause someone with a history of asthma to move quickly into a full-blown asthma attack. Since asthma is defined as a reversible airway obstruction, it is easy to see how one can move back up from disease to the brink by the use of asthma medications. If the underlying cause of the reaction is not eliminated, however, another exposure will push the child right back into the critical area.

Case #1: Asthma

Jason is a nine-year-old boy who came to see me because he was experiencing frequent breathing problems. His parents often had to take him to the hospital emergency room for breathing treatments, and he missed a great deal of school because of this. With Jason's history of asthma, his parents suspected that allergies were the most significant trigger for his attacks. After I explained to Jason and his parents the importance of clean air to his well-being, they cleared their home of the most common allergens. The boy responded very quickly, having fewer asthma episodes. His parents observed that since they had cleaned up their home Jason's attacks appeared to be triggered only at school. When they talked to Jason's teacher and principal about the situation, there was no attempt to remedy it, because the school administration felt it would be impossible to accommodate Jason's needs for the elimination of dust and molds and the cleaning chemicals currently in use. Jason did so much better on the weekends and on vacations when he was at home where his environment could be controlled that his parents decided to teach him at home. During the past year in which he has been schooled at home, his asthma attacks have occurred less and less frequently. When he does have an attack it is much less significant than were those in the past, and his hospital visits have become very infrequent.

Case #2: Asthma

Fourteen-year-old Kay is similar to Jason in that she, too, has asthma. She has had allergy problems all her life, and she has obviously been standing on the brink for a very long time. Allergies and exercise trigger her asthma. Construction work in the gym of Kay's school has resulted in poor air quality in the area where she must exercise. Since the construction started, she has had to increase her daily breathing treatments considerably. Perhaps if Kay had been exposed to only one trigger at a time, her breathing problems would not have been so excessive, but having to exercise in an area where air quality was poor due to construction work, guaranteed that she would be thrown from the brink into a full-fledged disease, asthma. Her situation was easier to remedy than Jason's: we simply excused her from her physical education classes until the construction was completed.

ATTENTION DEFICIT HYPERACTIVITY DISORDER

The influence of the nervous system on the immune system is one that has been recognized for centuries. Today there is evidence that the opposite effect, that of the immune system on the nervous system, also occurs. Our immune cells produce chemicals which communicate with our nervous system. (Dunn 1989) A challenge to our immune system, such as an allergic reaction in which histamine is released, can result in the release of neurochemicals that influence the way we feel and act.

The relationship between our immune system and our nervous system brings up another health problem that appears to be on the rise in our children, Attention Deficit Hyperactivity Disorder (ADHD). The most common treatment by pediatricians for ADHD is medication with a drug such as Ritalin. Confirmation that there has been a rise in the diagnosis and treatment of ADHD in recent years came with the announcement in November, 1993, that the company that produces Ritalin expected to run out of the drug before the end of the year.

The relationship between ADHD and allergies or chemical sensitivities has been debated for years. In 1989, Paul Marshall of the University of Minnesota wrote of the relationship between ADHD and allergy from a biochemical perspective. He hypothesized that allergic reactions result in an autonomic and central nervous system imbalance similar to the changes seen in a child with ADHD. This imbalance, he postulated, leads to a poorly regulated arousal system, and attention problems are the result. It appears that the child who is attention-deficient has a hyper-stimulated cholinergic system. Too much cholinergic stimulation has been associated with depression, nightmares, lethargy, sleepiness, for-getfulness, difficulty in—or slowed—thinking, visual problems, fatigue, loss of interest in work, difficulty remaining alert, and even psychomotor retardation. These are often the symptoms of a child who has been diagnosed with ADHD. (Marshall 1989)

Case #3: ADHD

Robert was lucky to have an astute mother. Although he had completed kindergarten without any problems and with no complaints from his teacher, when he started first grade, things were quite different. His parents were constantly receiving notes from the teacher about his inappropriate behavior. He was very disruptive, refusing to stay in his seat, and talking when he shouldn't, and his teacher had even moved his desk right next to hers with no effect on his disruptive activities. In fact his behavior seemed even worse after the move. After several weeks, Robert's parents went in to see his teacher about this strange behavior, which seemed particularly odd to them because they had never had any such problems with their son at home. His kindergarten teacher and preschool teachers had never complained either. The parents were quite upset. When they sat down across from the teacher, the strong cologne she was wearing became extremely obvious to both of them. Fortunately for Robert, his mother had just read Doris Rapp's book *Is This Your Child?* and had learned from reading it that anything a child eats, touches, or smells can affect the way she or he acts. As courteously as possible, Robert's mother told the teacher about what she had learned from Dr. Rapp's book and went on to express her concerns about the teacher's cologne. She suggested that the teacher not wear any fragrances for a few weeks and see what happened. The teacher agreed and in a short time Robert's behavior problems had ceased. His parents took this as a warning to clean up more of their home environment so that Robert could move away from the edge of the brink. Then, if he were exposed to a fragrance beyond the range of his control, the accumulation of chemical irritants being reduced, he might not react in the same extreme manner as he had to the teacher's cologne.

Case #4: ADHD

David, much like Robert, was also sensitive to fragrances, a fact which his parents had discovered before he entered school. While they were able to keep the home environment fairly fragrance-free, David was too often exposed outside the home to odors that would trigger a dramatic behavior change. By modifying David's diet, his parents were able to move him further back from the brink. Though they, too, had read one of Dr. Rapp's books and stayed alert to what their son ate, touched, or smelled, they were mystified by David's latest outbursts at school. The teacher and principal having been eye-witnesses to some of his earlier outbursts caused by indoor air pollutant exposures, were very cooperative with David and his parents. They could not figure out, however, what might be causing a recurrence of his inappropriate behavior, and they conferred with his mother about the problem. When she visited the school, she observed that while David's classroom had always had a computer, a new computer table had recently been purchased. This was the culprit. It was made from particle board which contains a significant amount of outgassing formaldehyde, the smell of which was very obvious when she entered the classroom. After she had brought the problem to the attention of David's teacher, the computer table was removed and David's outbursts disappeared.

ENURESIS

Case #5: ADHD and Enuresis

John is a seven-year-old boy who originally came to see me at the age of five because of severe behavior problems. His behavior was so extreme that his parents were afraid he was going to harm himself. On one occasion he had opened the car door and attempted to get out while his mother was driving on the freeway at 55 miles per hour. Although he was extremely bright, it seemed he did not understand the consequences of his behavior. Modifying John's diet and treating his inhalant allergies had made a big difference. He soon began making straight A's in school and behaving very well, but when some remodeling began in his school, he reverted to his unpleasant behavior. The dust and construction seemed to move him back to the brink, and new carpet pushed him all the way over. John not only had a change of behavior, but he suffered from upper respiratory problems as well. At that point, he came to see me much more frequently for coughs, colds, and watery and itchy eyes. Another problem that the carpet brought about was enuresis, or bedwetting. He had not had a bedwetting episode since his first visit to see me and now the problem was back, and he and his parents were noticeably distressed. His teacher was sick from the new carpet also, his mother reported, but they could not get school officials to do anything about it. The school administration simply did not understand the significance of the new carpet and its impact on John. He was missing school because of illness, and his self esteem was greatly affected by the return of the bedwetting. The next time John came to see me, he hardly looked like the same child I had been treating. He had lost weight, had large dark circles under his eyes, and appeared depressed. Something needed to be done, but even a letter from me did not change the school's position. Fortunately, school will be out soon for the summer, and as of this writing, we can only hope that over the vacation the carpet will outgas enough to make the classroom tolerable for John and his teacher next year. If not, his parents tell me they will put John in another school.

GASTROINTESTINAL PROBLEMS

In Texas, school starts in late August or early September just as the ragweed season reaches its peak. Many school children have an allergy to ragweed that manifests itself in ways other than hay fever symptoms.

Case #6: Gastrointestinal Problems

Katie was a child with ragweed allergy. Everyone thought that she had a school phobia, because each fall when school started she would develop severe stomach cramps, nausea, and vomiting. Her mother was told by school administrators that Katie did not like school and was just using the stomach pains as an excuse to stay home. School phobia being the diagnosis, the child was referred to a psychologist. Katie's school phobia always improved by November, and then was forgotten until it recurred the next fall. After becoming aware of the effects on Katie of different pollutants in the environment, her mother began cleaning up their home and changing the family diet. Katie was also treated for her allergy to ragweed. As a result, Katie moved back up the Mountain of Health, and the next fall she did not experience stomach problems.

EAR INFECTIONS

Case # 7: ADHD and Ear Infections

Jennifer age 10, had chronic ear infections as a young child. When antibiotics failed she had tubes placed in the ear canal to help drain the fluid. The tubes fell out rather quickly and were replaced twice. By the age of six, she no longer had ear infections. In school, her teachers say she doesn't pay attention, seems to daydream and had trouble following directions. When the teacher is talking, Jennifer often "doodles" or plays with the ribbons in her hair.

Ear infections become less frequent by the time a child reaches school age and are quite rare by the age of nine. This is probably because the eustachian tube becomes more vertical as we grow and fluid can then drain more easily. This lessens the chance of having a fluid medium in which the bacteria can grow. However, children who have had multiple ear infections and/or tubes inserted multiple times in the ears may have an increased likelihood of having scar tissue on the ear drum.

Any of the substances in *Figure 6-2* can cause eustachian tube inflammation and swelling and increase the likelihood of having fluid in the ear. Having fluid in the middle ear for long periods of time can also lead to learning problems. Allergens such as those listed can cause learning problems. Most children I see in my office are still tactile learners. This means they learn best by touching things. But school learning is mostly auditory and visual. A child who had ear problems when young may tend to be less dependent on hearing as a learning sense. When she/he enters school the child will use touching instead of listening to try to learn and will be at a disadvantage in the classroom.

Jennifer "doodled" and played with her hair because she was actually trying to pay attention and learn. Because she had become less dependent on her hearing as a learning sense because of her chronic ear problems, she was unable to process information satisfactory through the ears. The "doodling" and ribbon playing actually helped her pay attention better. It gave her a tactile means of "listening." A child who has had chronic ear infections may need special help in learning to be a auditory learner. If we could use all of the senses, particularly tactile, auditory, and visual to teach our children, I believe we could reach more of them.

Substances causing problems in the classroom	Problems that can occur from any of these substances
Dust Mites	Allergies
Dust	Asthma
Trees	Bronchitis
Weeds	Headaches
Grass	Hyperactivity
Molds	Attention Deficit Disorder
Cleaning Chemicals	Learning Problems
White Board Markers	Skin Rash
New Carpet	Runny Nose
Particle Board Furniture	Watery Eyes
Hamsters/Birds/Rabbits	Agitation
Chalk	Irritability
Fresh Paint	
Air Fresheners	
Perfume/Cologne/Aftershave	
Food	

Figure 6-2.
List of substances that my cause problems in the classroom and examples of the types of problems that can result.

CONCLUSION

The problem is clear and it is real. Indoor air quality does indeed affect pre-existing health conditions, and the question we must ask is, *What will be done about it?* Children are being exposed and affected constantly. A few of the conditions our children can suffer from contaminated air have been illustrated. In some cases, a cooperative and understanding school administration has turned a potentially serious, long-term problem into a short term incident in which no real damage has occurred. It will become increasingly important to educate school administrators and staffs to the potential effects of poor indoor air quality so that warning symptoms will never have to become chronic problems. Frequently, doing something quickly will keep a child's symptoms and inappropriate behavior from escalating into a problem that will have more far-reaching consequences. Rectifying a problem early as Robert's parents and teachers did, will help keep a child like Robert healthy and spare him or her from long-term expensive medical treatment. Cooperation by the administration at Jason's school might have kept him in the public school system. Although his parents might be excellent teachers, Jason liked going to school, and there may be long-term psychological effects for him if he is unable ever to return to his public-school classroom. But if he is physically sick when he attends school, then the effects on him will be psychological as well.

Although home schooling is not an infrequent choice for my patients and their parents, it is rarely a first choice. It is a choice made only when the child is continuously ill from the environment at the school itself. Some parents and their children thrive on home schooling, but it is certainly not for everyone. The interactions between some parents and their children actually make it totally impossible for home schooling to occur, which leaves the parents very few options. Some switch to a private school situation. Although small private schools may sometimes be more accommodating than a large public school system, the reverse can also be true if the private school is too small and does not have the funds to accommodate one child's problems. Usually though, a parent can find a private school that understands or, being motivated to fill up a classroom, will make the appropriate accommodations.

If these options are not workable, there is another one to consider. If a parent cannot determine exactly what in the air is bothering the child, or if the school cannot find an environmental cause of the problem, a child can be tested and treated with an allergy extract made of the school air itself. Just as we test and treat people for other inhalant allergies such as trees, weeds, and grasses, we can test and treat the child for whatever is in the air of her or his school.

Since each child comes into the classroom with a specific position on the Mountain of Health, she or he will react to the school environment in a specific way. Some children will already be on the brink when they arrive, and it is imperative that the classroom itself not be the agent that throws that child into the Cavern of Disease. Children must be able to study and learn without being exposed to potential hazards in the air of their classrooms.

REFERENCES

Bland, Jeffrey, 1993, Maui, Hawaii: Functional Medicine Symposium.

Dunn, A. J., 1989, "Psychoneuroimmunology for the psychoneuroendocrinologist: A Review of Animal Studies of Nervous System-Immune System Interactions," *Psychoneuroendocrinology*, Vol. 14, No. 4, pp. 251-274.

Jung, T., 1991, "Otolaryngologic Approach to the Diagnosis and Management of Otitis Media," *Otolaryngologic Clinics of North America*, Vol. 24, No. 4, pp. 931-945.

Lebowitz, M. D., 1991, "Populations at Risk: Addressing Health Effects Due to Complex Mixtures with a Focus on Respiratory Effects," *Environmental Health Perspectives*, Vol. 95, pp. 35-38.

Marshall, Paul, 1989, "Attention Deficit Disorder and Allergy: A Neurochemical Model of the Relationship Between the Illnesses," *Psychological Bulletin*, Vol. 106, No. 3, pp. 434-446.

Minchin, M., 1987, "Infant Formula: A Mass, Uncontrolled Trial in Perinatal Care," *Birth*, Vol. 14, No. 1, pp. 25-34.

Rush, D., 1992, "Folate Supplements and Neural Tube Defects," *Nutritional Review*, Vol. 50, No. 1, pp. 25-26.

Yunginger, J. W., 1992, "A Community-Based Study of the Epidemiology of Asthma," Department of Pediatrics, Internal Medicine and Health Science Research, Mayo Clinic and Foundation, pp. 888-894.

7

INTEGRATED CLEANING MANAGEMENT

by Annie Berthold-Bond

Cleaning and cleaning supplies that use harsh chemicals can be the cause of environmental illness and discomfort. In this chapter, Ms. Berthold-Bond develops the concept of an Integrated Cleaning Management program. She gives tips about safe cleaning substances, many of them old-fashioned home remedies, and she lists resources that custodial staff can contact for evaluations of chemical products. Directing her discussion and recommendations to school administrators, as well as maintenance workers, she answers questions that arise in all schools about keeping a safe and clean environment for students and staff.

☐ *What are the steps that should be taken in a school to achieve integrated cleaning management?*

☐ *What are the advantages of an in-house cleaning staff over contracting out the cleaning?*

☐ *How can schools work together to maintain cleaner buildings?*

☐ *What regulations concerning cleaning products must be met?*

☐ *How should "green" cleaning products be chosen?*

☐ *How are folk recipes useful for cleaning chores in today's schools?*

In preparation for writing this chapter on cleaning, I decided to visit the Director of Facilities of the public schools in my town, to find out how cleaning is done in buildings in my school district. I also wanted to know if environmental health issues are considered at all in my local schools. I am embarrassed to say that I had a stereotype in my mind and expected to find a contemporary version of the school janitor from my childhood—friendly but conservative, concerned about children's safety, but not pro-active. (I was in high school at the end of the 1960s, when people's ideas seemed clearly distinguishable just by the length and style of their hair.) Much to my astonishment, I met the facilities director of 1990s, in this case Mr. Kirk Williams.

Mr Williams is extremely sophisticated about indoor air pollution issues, pro-active on every issue that concerns the health of the children and staff, and, most surprising of all, he goes out of his way to *think up* ways to reduce the use of chemicals in his schools. And Mr. Williams has no personal agenda about environmental health that has motivated him to be so progressive in his ideas on the subject. Instead, he represents the new breed of facilities manager—in charge of every aspect of indoor air quality in schools, including choosing less toxic products. While forced to work on a limited budget, he is responsible for meeting *and understanding* the many government and state regulations regarding school environments; and, most importantly, for protecting the health of all the occupants of the buildings in his charge. In other words, the modern-day superintendent of buildings and grounds, known in my school district as the Director of Facilities, is a person with enormous responsibilities and, in Mr. Williams' case, with great capabilities. My meeting with him has convinced me that the only way to succeed in developing higher standards for healthy indoor air in schools is to work squarely within the system, to ensure that any person holding the position of Director of Facilities, or its equivalent, understands the responsibilities of the position, and to provide him or her with as many tools as possible for selecting less toxic products for use in cleaning the school.

CERTIFICATION OF FACILITIES MANAGERS

Even while I was thinking about how fortunate my town is to have such a pro-active Director of Facilities, I was aware that many communities are not so lucky. Further, the more I spoke with Mr. Williams about his responsibilities, the more aware I became of how crucial his role is for the health of the entire school system. If the Director of Facilities is not involved in the decision to use or not use each and every chemical being considered for maintaining a school building, is not educated about what these chemicals are, and does not know how to train every employee in the safe use of chemical substances, then control over the quality of indoor air in schools is jeopardized. The person holding this position should be required pass examinations that include concerns of indoor air pollution and be certified by the state as qualified for the job. The New York State Association for Superintendents of School Buildings and

Grounds has a voluntary certification program requiring a Director of Facilities to study and pass exams in 27 different disciplines (including environmental health). All states should develop such a program.

FIVE STEPS TO INTEGRATED CLEANING MANAGEMENT

I was introduced to the concept of good current cleaning management by Mr. Williams in my local public school. His procedure sounded so much like Integrated Pest Management (see Chapter 12) that I thought I would call it Integrated Cleaning Management. The illuminating aspect of this concept is that with a little bit of thought, a lot of hazardous cleaning chemicals can be eliminated or significantly reduced because the problems they are meant to solve are solved instead by common sense, not by the application of powerful chemicals. Another nice aspect of the new attitude towards cleaning is that one can achieve success pragmatically, using a five-step checklist. (See *Figure 7-1.*)

□ **See how to reduce the need for cleaning products**

□ **Determine the cleaning need**

□ **Choose the least toxic approach**

□ **Use as little cleaning products as possible**

□ **Make sure the program is cost effective**

Figure 7-1.
Checklist for Integrated Cleaning Management

For every job that must be done, the person in charge can approach the task with this checklist to come up with a more progressive, less toxic, solution. To help make this method seem real to you, let's see how to approach the task of cleaning tile floors using the check list.

1. See How to Reduce the Need for Cleaning Products

Dirt Defense. The first line of dirt defense is to have little or no dirt. To succeed in this program one needs to determine where the dirt comes from. In the case of the tile floors, the dirt is tracked into the school, onto the floors, from outside. If every student entering a school walks through dirt and mud on the way into the building, he or she will invariably track the dirt onto the floors. By growing grass around the building, correcting areas of erosion, and erecting railings along walkways to keep students on clean pavement, facilities managers will ensure that significantly less dirt is tracked into the school.

Second, if the school invests in a high quality tract mat to collect the dust, and it is placed where all students must walk over it while entering the school, then a significant amount of dust will be removed from the shoes.

Third, the remaining dirt can be swept with a manual push-sweeper and removed entirely, not merely relocated to another part of the floor. If these three steps are taken, there will be very little dirt left to be cleaned up by means of a cleaning agent.

Networking. At this point one can take time out to measure the amount of dirt tracked in from outside and ask if there is any way to reduce it even more, by making changes at its source. This could be a time to use a network of Directors of Facilities developed from certification programs (see below) to determine what successful strategies have been used to reduce the amount of dirt tracked into other schools.

2. Determine the Cleaning Need

What is appropriate for cleaning this floor now? After step one has been completed, although dirt on the floors has been reduced, what there is requires attention. It is crucial now that one determine what needs to be cleaned and only choose appropriate products to do the job. I heard recently of one custodian who cleaned the floors with a disinfectant. What needed to be disinfected? Nothing. The floors had ground dirt on them, not blood, vomit, or any other source of bacteria. In fact, the floors at this stage need nothing more than the mildest of detergents, and in many cases probably just a damp mop. In other words, avoid the overkill approach practiced so often. In the case of the disinfectant used on the floors, the tragedy is that for no reason other than good intentions, the school was infused with a disinfectant that is also labeled as a pesticide because the habit of overkill was instilled in a custodian by a lifetime of advertisements.

Only use what is appropriate for the job of cleaning the floor. More is not necessarily better.

3. Choose the Least Toxic Approach

A damp mop may be enough. By this point in the project—before cleaning the floor with a mild detergent—two chemical products could have been used. One is a spray for the track mats to help attract dirt, and the other is a treatment for the mop to help provide dustless cleaning. Is either of these products necessary? Would buying a higher quality track mat eliminate the need for what must be a toxic tracking spray? (It is hard to imagine a benign chemical able to attract dirt and collect it on the mat!) What chemicals are in the dustless sweeping product? Would slightly dampening the mop with water achieve the same results?

If it is determined that the floors need a small amount of detergent, choosing the most harmless for health and the environment is appropriate. The detergent is only needed to cut the slight amount of oil in dirt.

4. Use As Little Cleaning Products As Possible

When you need more than a damp mop. After all the loose dust is removed, it may seem straightforward to get a bucket, mop, detergent and water. But here is where sharing the equipment with other schools fits beautifully. There are automatic floor scrubbers available now that require little or no detergent at all. The scrubbers clean thoroughly. If a detergent is deemed necessary, as small an amount as is recommended on the label may be used. If your school district can't afford a scrubber, your administration might join those of neighboring districts to buy one.

5. Make Sure the Program is Cost Effective

Every school is under budget constraints these days. By pooling equipment, relying on common sense about where and when to use cleaning products, and choosing to use only the smallest amount possible of chemicals, the five-step approach to cleaning tile floors should be more cost-effective than traditional methods.

WHEN YOU CAN'T CHOOSE LESS TOXIC PRODUCTS

Solvents

According to Monona Rossol, editor of *Acts Facts*, The Monthly Newsletter from Arts, Crafts and Theater Safety (181 Thompson Street, #23, New York, NY 10012-2586, 212/777-0062), there are no safe solvents. "The safest solvent available is alcohol, and that causes birth defects." Of particular concern to Rossol is the switch many are making to citrus solvents, assuming that they are safe because they are "natural." The main ingredient in citrus solvents is d-limonene.

> The American Industrial Hygiene Association (AIHA) set a Workplace Environmental Exposure Level (WEEL) guide for d-limonene at 30 parts per million (ppm). WEELs are similar to PELs. The AIHA's WEEL for d-limonene is lower (more restrictive) than the PELs set by OSHA for turpentine (100 ppm), toluene (50 ppm), n-hexane (50 ppm), and other very toxic solvents. . . . Users of d-limonene can assume its vapor is more toxic than that of petroleum distillates or turpentine. Its slightly lower volatility will result in less exposure by inhalation during use. However, home users should remember that it will all evaporate in time. D-limonene should be used with the same precautions taken with other very toxic solvents with particular care to avoid skin contact (some glove companies recommend nitrile gloves). Children should never use it and it should be kept out of their reach. (*Acts Facts* #Update of Vol. 4, No. 7, 5/20/94.)

To begin with, the buyer of products containing solvents should contact the EPA, OSHA, and the U.S. Department of Health and Human Services, to determine which solvents are considered the most dangerous and eliminate products containing those solvents from the available choices. Given the profound health effects of chlorinated hydrocarbons, solvents containing chlorinated hydrocarbons, such as those commonly found in waxes and degreasers, shouldn't even be considered. After that, the buyer should contact independent groups such as Washington Toxics, Green Seal, and Scientific Certification Systems, to find out if the solvents contained in the remaining choice of products are considered by them, to be hazardous. Once the field is limited to a few products, then consideration should be given to how they are used, if the solvents evaporate quickly, if ventilation will be possible, and if the variables present in connection with each specific product do not cause toxicity. Using this information, the determination can be made about which solvent-based product will have the least amount of effect on indoor air.

Choosing when to use solvent-based products is crucial to the health of indoor air. Ideally all school cleaning jobs requiring the use of solvents, such as stripping and waxing floors, should be done at the beginning of the summer vacation. If floors need to be waxed a number of times a year waxing should always be done in conjunction with vacations. In my opinion, solvent-based products shouldn't be used at all in the winter when the building can't be aired properly—not even during holiday times.

Solvents should be viewed with the utmost caution and only used when absolutely necessary. The use of solvent-based products should be analyzed for possible alternatives.

Disinfectants

The EPA has strict guidelines for approved disinfectants, products intended to destroy germs that cause disease. Disinfectant cleaning products are listed as pesticides, i.e., they are designed to kill. Though allowed to be used in schools, they should not be considered harmless, and they can be significant contributors to indoor air pollution. Product development needs to be furthered in this field to provide safer products.

With the fear of germs heightened because of the AIDS epidemic, many people are overusing disinfectants, with the best of intentions. The U.S. General Accounting Office (GAO) has made a devastating indictment of the EPA's ability to determine that the disinfectants on the market actually work. So significant is the statement that I quote it in its entirety:

> The human eye cannot see whether disinfectants actually kill bacteria, fungi, and viruses. As a result, health professionals and consumers alike rely on the EPA to ensure that disinfectants on the market actually work. Ineffective disinfectants, however, are more than just a waste of money—they pose a threat to public health. GAO found that up to 20 percent of the disinfectants being sold today may be ineffective. Disinfectant claims about germ killing are questionable for several reasons. First, although scientific controversy has raged for a decade over the validity of the methods and performance standards used to assess the efficacy of disinfectants, EPA does not independently test disinfectants before registering them and lacks criteria to assess the validity of test methods and modifications proposed by manufacturers. Second, EPA has made little progress in resolving these matters because of budget constraints and inadequate research management. Third, EPA lacks sufficient internal controls to ensure the quality and integrity of the data that registrants submit on disinfectant quality. Fourth, EPA lacks an enforcement strategy to ensure that, once registered, disinfectants sold and

distributed in the marketplace work as claimed. (General Accounting Office, October, 1990, Reports and Testimony.)

Until less toxic and environmentally safer products are available and approved, the most prudent choice of disinfectant is a 3% solution of household bleach. As to its effect on the environment, existing studies imply that bleach (sodium hypochlorite) does not cause complex or-ganochlorines to develop in the wastewater stream, but the evidence is not conclusive. It should always be used with adequate ventilation, and the warning on the label must be heeded: "Do not use or mix with household chemicals such as toilet bowl cleaners, rust removers, acid or products containing ammonia. To do so will release hazardous gases."

Good ol' soap and water shouldn't be forgotten, either. The EPA recom-mends soap and water as a disinfectant, even for cutting-boards. Use the Integrated Cleaning Management checklist (see *Figure 8-1*) to determine if the need of a disinfectant is justified.

WHEN YOU CAN CHOOSE NONTOXIC PRODUCTS

You may be surprised to learn that many modern synthetic cleaning products often mimic the old folk recipes that have been handed down through generations because they worked so well. The best folk recipes almost always turn out to be based on good science. If cleaning brass requires an acid to eat the tarnish away, the folk recipe makes effective use of the acid in lemon juice or vinegar. Although today's counterpart would also contain an acid, it would be synthetic.

THE TOP FOUR NATURAL INGREDIENT CHOICES FOR CLEANING

The following four ingredients are those I find safest, most effective, and useful for cleaning. I have added some details about why and how they work. I think it is realistic for schools to implement some uses for these ingredients.

Baking Soda

This multi-dimensional mineral, sodium bicarbonate, has more uses than almost any other product I can think of. It is mildly abrasive and can be used as a gentle cleaner. It is also a good scouring powder for sinks and bathtubs, and it can be used on fiberglass. It is slightly alkaline, with a natural pH around 8.1, and it can neutralize acids in water. It will eliminate many odors, making it an ideal nontoxic "malodor counteractant" for carpets. Even in the open air, baking soda adsorbs odors, making it as useful an air freshener in the classroom as it is in the refrigerator.

Washing Soda

Washing soda is sodium carbonate, the chemical neighbor of baking soda. It is mined and processed much like baking soda, but because of the chemical difference (one carbon atom instead of two), washing soda is more strongly alkaline, its natural pH being around 11. Traditionally used (and very effective) as a laundry detergent booster, washing soda is a real find for natural cleaning because it is a powerful heavy-duty cleaner. Since it is slightly caustic, it cannot be called nontoxic, and you should wear rubber gloves when using it, but it releases no harmful fumes and is far safer than a commercial solvent formula. It cuts grease, cleans petroleum oils and dirt, removes wax or lipstick, and softens water. If you have a petroleum spill on the floor, washing soda is the cleaner of choice. If you have wax or lipstick stains, or even a car radiator that needs to be cleaned, look to washing soda. It neutralizes odors in the same way as baking soda, and helps remove stains. One word of caution: washing soda is too caustic to use on fiberglass or aluminum, and don't use it on waxed floors unless you intend to remove the wax!

Vinegar

Vinegar is very useful because it is highly acidic and can neutralize alkaline substances. There are many cleaning uses for natural acids. If you have hard water and have trouble with mineral buildup (scale), soak a cloth in vinegar and rest it on the scale for a few hours. The acid will break down the minerals and they can be wiped away. Acids cut grease, dissolve gummy buildup, and eat away tarnish. Vinegar is good for removing dirt from wooden surfaces, so it is very effective as part of a recipe to clean floors and furniture.

Vegetable-Oil-Based Detergents and Soaps

The fourth ingredient is a good vegetable oil-based detergent or soap. (Always keep in mind that a detergent is distinct from a soap.) Detergents are synthetic, and are considered an improvement over plain soap because they do not form as much soap scum when combined with the minerals in hard water. For cleaning purposes, the suds in soaps and detergents are helpful in cutting grease and oils. Add a little vegetable-based detergent to vinegar and water for an excellent window cleaner, mix detergent with baking soda for a home-made soft scrub that needs almost no rinsing, or use it straight with water for cleaning floors and walls.

POOR MANAGEMENT OF CHEMICALS IN SCHOOLS—LEGAL RECOURSES

Under the Occupational Safety and Health Administration's (OSHA) Hazard Communication Standard "Right to Know" law, anybody working with a cleaning product must be able to tell you what the chemicals are in the product he or she is using at any given time, how hazardous those chemicals are, and what safe procedures should be followed in case of an accident. The employee must also have been given this information in writing. It is up to the Director of Facilities to educate his or her employees in these matters, and it is also up to him or her to buy products that fit within safe guidelines for toxicity in order to safeguard the school from toxic compounds. If the Director of Facilities fails to comply with any of the Hazard Communication Standard guidelines, whether out of ignorance or through neglect, the school may be liable. Any student, parent, or employee can demand to see the Material Safety Data Sheet (MSDS) on any chemical used in the school. If the school doesn't have the appropriate papers for the product, then that person has a right under the law to sue. The Director of Facilities must be well educated in the field, because he or she is responsible for the choice and safe use of cleaning products in the schools. In addition, if a building custodian doesn't follow the directions on the label of a chemical product used for cleaning or other maintenance of a school, the public has a right to sue.

Specifically, the Hazard Communication Standard and "Right to Know" law means, for schools, that:

■ Manufacturers of products sold to the schools must know the safety hazards of every product they sell, and must make that information available on an MSDS and on labels that provide pre-defined and regulated signal words.

■ Every product brought into the school must have an MSDS.

- Every school must provide anyone using chemicals with written specifics concurring with the "Right to Know" laws.

- The school custodian must educate his or her staff about all safety concerns relating to hazardous materials, including how to read an MSDS, and the signal words on product labels.

- All maintenance staff members are required by law to follow the directions and warnings on MSDSs and product labels.

- All maintenance staff must, by law, be instructed about precautions for safe handling of toxic substances.

- All cleaning products must be labeled.

- All school administrators must be able to provide information about where to find an MSDS and any other relevant information on how to handle toxic chemicals safely.

If a teacher or parent thinks chemicals are being mismanaged in a school, the ability to sue gives leverage to bring a change against the school authorities. It seems much better to protect the health of the children in the first place by ensuring that a qualified person is in charge as Director of Facilities.

COMPLYING WITH REGULATIONS

Helping a school choose less toxic cleaning materials is far from simple, because of the myriad state and federal regulations that must be met. A perfect example of the difficulty is presented by the selection of floor waxes. A person investigating safer solvents and drying times in floor waxes may find two less toxic, quickly drying products. Due to the Americans with Disabilities Act (PL101-336), however, by law floors in schools must pass a stringent slip-resistance test. There is no question that the needs of people on crutches and those with other disabilities must be met, and, hence, that the question of slip-resistance of the safer chemical product must be answered satisfactorily. Since it is essential that "greener" products meet every regulation involving their use, it is recommended that all aspects of the laws regarding cleaning products be known to maintenance staffs.

TAKING A PRO-ACTIVE POSITION ON INDOOR AIR

On March 25, 1994, OSHA announced a proposed rule that would regulate indoor air quality in America's non-industrial workplaces, which would include schools. Among other things regarding the recommended use of cleaning and maintenance chemicals the proposal states:

> The employer shall inform employees working in areas to be treated with potentially hazardous chemicals, at least within 24 hours prior to application, of the type of chemicals intended to be applied. . . . The employer shall provide training for maintenance workers . . . which shall include at least the following. . . . Training on how to maintain adequate ventilation of air contaminants generated during building cleaning and maintenance; and training of maintenance personnel on how to minimize adverse effects on indoor air quality during the use and disposal of chemicals and other agents. (OSHA, March 25, 1994, Indoor Air Quality, p. 5)

In the past, less toxic products were often used only because an employee or student complained. If the new OSHA proposal (#1910.1033, Indoor Air Quality) is approved, it will represent a refreshing change in the government's approach to indoor air quality as a national health concern. I recommend that schools obtain copies of the proposed new rule and follow the many excellent recommendations it includes. One suggestion every school should implement is the 24-hour notice of use of toxic compounds. This information is vital for people at risk from exposure to chemicals and is a tool anyone can use for self-protection.

CONTRACT VERSUS IN- HOUSE IN HOUSE CLEANING

Contract cleaning (hiring outside services to do the cleaning) does not usually result in effective cleaning management, because cleaning is then isolated from the functioning of the entire facility system. An independent contract company may come in and clean up the dirt very well, but its employees will probably have little interest in preventing more dirt from accumulating. Most importantly, a contracted cleaning service takes control of the quality of indoor air away from the Director of Facilities: since it isn't ultimately responsible for the indoor air of the school building, the independent cleaning service may not go to the lengths a Director of Facilities would to choose less toxic cleaning products. Therefore, an in-house cleaning staff is preferable to a contract service.

DEVELOPING A DIRECTORS-OF-FACILITIES NETWORK

Networks are a vital source of current information. New York State is lucky enough to have a Board of Cooperative Educational Services

(BOCES). The primary purpose of BOCES is to provide assistance to schools that may not be equipped to handle special needs students, such as those who are blind. But BOCES also provides help in facilities management. All Directors of Facilities in New York State can avail themselves of BOCES as a source of support and help in problem solving. Best of all for cleaning purposes, BOCES provides for the pooling of equipment. With budget cuts a reality in most districts, efficient equipment that improves indoor air quality—floor Auto Scrubbers and the like—may be beyond the means of some schools. With a networking system such as BOCES in place, a district can have access to this equipment by scheduling in advance. If a schools Facilities Director doesn't have a network available, it is highly recommended that one be developed, even if informally. Valuable insights and news can be passed back and forth through a network of same-field professionals. In addition, with such a resource group, mistakes can be avoided and valuable time will not be wasted in reinventing the wheel.

EXISTING GUIDELINES FOR LESS TOXIC PRODUCT PROCUREMENT

Currently, the buyer of cleaning materials relies on information from his or her vendors, trade publications, and the MSDS. Vendors are far from unbiased, and the professional publications are supported mainly by the advertising of manufacturers and vendors of traditional product lines. Until "green" products become mainstream enough to advertise in the trade magazines, these potential sources of information cannot be considered reliable and unbiased.

The MSDS is the most reliable existing source of guidance for procurement of less toxic cleaning products available to most schools. Choosing products with the lowest hazard number (four being the most toxic, flammable, or reactive, and zero being the least) is prudent. But many MSDS sheets do not list ingredients, because the manufacturers do not wish to disclose trade secrets. And the MSDSs do not reveal data about the long-term toxicology of chemicals in a given product, nor how those chemicals may combine with others in the environment to compound exposure risks.

The existing means of determining the ability of a product to meet criteria for environmental health are entirely inadequate. There is no clearinghouse of information on the subject available to maintenance staff, and there is no national standard of safe cleaning products for them to rely on. Developing a clearinghouse for information about cleaning products and determining safe standards for their use are the highest and most crucial priorities for those trying to establish and maintain systems using less toxic cleaning products in the schools.

The large chemical companies that manufacture cleaning products are not looking to tougher indoor air standards with pleasure. These companies have a lot of money at stake and heavy investments in their product formulas, whether they contain toxic materials or not. Nonetheless, healthier standards must be defined for cleaning products, despite legal and public-relations pressures from large manufacturers to keep standards ill-defined. Fortunately there are a number of corporations that are formulating less toxic products, but they, too, need dependable guidelines. Until guidelines and standards for safer products are developed, there will be continuing confusion, misinformation, and mistaken assumptions as to what constitutes a safer product and what doesn't.

DEVELOPING A NETWORK FOR CREDIBLE INFORMATION

Another network the school custodian must enter, or must be helped to enter if he or she hopes to have a truly healthy school is that of the experts searching for criteria with which to choose products that are less toxic and environmentally preferable. Until national standards have been developed, such a network is an essential source of reliable information for the development of criteria and guidelines. The field is changing almost every day, and new studies reveal new dangers almost every other day, so to be up to date requires access to the latest research.

The four organizations listed below develop criteria for safer cleaning products. Custodians are advised to contact each group for access to their current research and for the most up-to-date information on product lines that successfully meet their requirements.

Philip Dickey, Ph.D.
Washington Toxics Coalition
4516 University Way NE
Seattle, WA 98105
206/632-1545

Dr. Dickey has established criteria for products by finding the names of chemicals on the MSDS, and researching the effects of these chemicals on health and the environment. His sources include government and private research organizations. When applicable, he runs his own tests, and combines his results with the research data of others to rate the product in a range from green to black. Green is least toxic, red causes a significant impact on health and the environment, gray indicates lack of enough information to make an educated decision, and black is not recommended.

Green Seal
1250 23rd St. NW
Washington, DC 20037
202/331-7337

Green Seal standards are based on four main considerations:
1. *Protect the Earth:* reduce air and water pollution, reduce the waste of energy and resources, protect wildlife and habitats.
2. *Public Review:* all standards are published for review by business, government, environmental and consumer organizations, and the public.
3. *Reduce Packaging Waste:* Green Seal requires the minimal use of packaging. Also, toxic metals (often found in inks on packaging) cannot be added to packaging materials.
4. *Quality Performance:* to ensure that "environmental" products perform as well as or better than mainstream consumer products.

Scientific Certification Systems
1611 Telegraph Ave., Suite 1111
Oakland, CA 94612-2113
510/832-1415

Scientific Certification System (SCS), formerly Green Cross, provides the public with the Environmental Report Card, a life-cycle analysis of products. The report card lists the resources depleted, energy consumed, pollutants released into the air and water, and the solid wastes generated throughout the life-cycle of the product. SCS-certified products are reported on a consumer hotline, 800/ECO-FACTS.

Ronald Robbins, Environmental Compliance Coordinator
United States Postal Service
6 Griffin Road North
Windsor, CT 06006-7030
203/285-7197

Ronald F. Robbins has prepared the Environmental Compliance Model Vehicle Maintenance Facility for vehicle maintenance and plant maintenance staff. What is interesting about the criteria for environmental acceptability Ronald Robbins has chosen, is that he has scoured government agencies for existing red flags on chemicals, and has eliminated them from his field of choice. Specifically, the criteria include:
1. No Class I or Class II Ozone Depleting Substances.
2. No presence of any of the 17 chemicals targeted for reduction by U.S. EPA.
3. The product needed to be evaluated as to performance, and needed to achieve at least a good or better performance rating from a field of poor, fair, good, very good, and outstanding.
4. The product needs to be free from environmental health and safety liabilities as listed by RCRA Hazardous Waste, CERCLA/SARA Hazardous Substances, OSHA Hazardous Materials, and CAA Hazardous Air Pollutants.
5. The product needs to be cost effective.

VENDORS AND PRODUCT PROCUREMENT

Playing the vendor game well is one of the jobs of the Director of Facilities or whoever else purchases cleaning products for the school system. National sales representatives of every cleaning product company in the country will try to convince the school district buyer to select to buy their products. And the bidding war is fierce.

The buyer of cleaning products should state clearly to vendors, right from the first, that he or she is only interested in "green" products. If the buyer can give brand names he or she is interested in buying, culled from networking with criteria experts, so much the better. The more buyers who stipulate "green" products, the faster the entire industry will change. Further, once large manufacturers develop "green" products, the more quickly manufacturers themselves, because of competition, will begin to set higher standards for the industry.

SUMMARY OF RECOMMENDATIONS FOR INTEGRATED CLEANING MANAGEMENT

State authorities should:

■ Establish a program to certify Directors of Facilities or equivalent positions, and all persons aspiring to such positions should be required to pass through the certification program.

■ Help local school districts develop a clearinghouse for information about cleaning-product safety.

School district authorities should:

■ Make sure that all those responsible for building maintenance are knowledgeable about the management of chemicals.

■ Obtain copies of the new OSHA proposed rule on Indoor Air Quality (#1910.1033).

■ Make sure that 24-hour notice is given to all persons in or near the area where toxic compounds are to be administered.

■ Employ an in-house cleaning staff in preference to a contract cleaning service.

School Custodians and their staffs should:

■ Contact organizations that monitor cleaning products for environmental safety and nontoxicity and become as familiar as possible with information about toxic substances that might be used in a school.

■ Stipulate "green" products when buying cleaning supplies.

■ Contact EPA, OSHA, and HHS to determine which solvents are considered most dangerous, and eliminate them from use in the school.

■ Use a 3% solution of household bleach as a disinfectant rather than a toxic chemical disinfectant.

Teachers and all other staff members should:

■ Try to work directly with the Director of Facilities, or the equivalent person, to develop a cleaning program using less toxic products that benefits students and staff.

8

RADON AND ASBESTOS

by Mary Oetzel

In this chapter, Ms. Oetzel defines and discusses the health effects of radon followed by an exploration of the topic of asbestos. She points out that these two known contaminants are present in school buildings across the country and discusses practical ways for school districts to manage both hazardous materials. Ms. Oetzel advises school districts to develop a thorough understanding of both radon and asbestos, become familiar with the EPA guidelines and regulations on both substances, and learn how both can be controlled to protect the health of students and school staff. This chapter gives practical answers to these questions:

□ *What are the best devices or methods for detecting radon in schools?*

□ *Why is a high level of radon present in many existing school buildings?*

□ *How may new schools be constructed to minimize the hazard of radon exposure?*

□ *Why is asbestos more dangerous to children than to adults?*

□ *Why is it sometimes safer to leave asbestos in place, rather than remove it?*

□ *How should asbestos best be managed if left in place?*

The health effects of radon and asbestos can be devastating to individuals who have been exposed to elevated levels of either substance over many years. These silent killers cause thousands of lung disorders and cancer deaths annually, and studies conducted on miners exposed to radon underground and on workers in a number of asbestos industries confirm the risks. The United States Environmental Protection Agency (EPA) has formulated guidelines to minimize radon exposures in schools and has developed comprehensive regulations to manage and control asbestos. Every school district should develop a thorough understanding of both radon and asbestos, should become familiar with the EPA guidelines and regulations relative to each, and should learn how both can be controlled to protect the health of their students, teachers, and other school staff.

RADON: WHAT IS IT AND WHERE IS IT FOUND?

Radon is a tasteless, odorless, and colorless radioactive gas that occurs naturally. It is found in varying amounts in rocks, in soil, and in underground water throughout the United States and other parts of the world. It results from the natural breakdown or decay of uranium into radioactive particles. Present in low levels in the air outdoors, radon can and does accumulate to much higher levels when it is trapped in schools and other buildings. When inhaled into the lungs, it can damage lung tissue, especially if the levels are excessive and the exposure takes place over many years. *Figure 8-1* is a map indicating the geologic radon potential in each of the 3,141 counties in the United States. This map was prepared by the EPA after an examination of available data on indoor radon measurements, geology, aerial radioactivity, soil parameters, and foundation types.

The EPA and other major health organizations have determined that radon is a serious environmental health problem. Although not mandated to do so, since 1989, the EPA has recommended that schools nationwide test for the presence of radon, and, if elevated levels are found, schools are advised to take measures to remediate the problem.

HEALTH CONCERNS AND RISKS

Radon is a known human carcinogen. The EPA estimates that 7,000 to 30,000 lung-cancer deaths annually can be attributed to radon exposure, making it the second largest cause of lung cancer. While the precise number of deaths due to radon is disputed by some scientists, the Centers for Disease Control, the American Lung Association, the American Medical Association, and other major health organizations agree that radon causes thousands of preventable lung-cancer deaths each year. *Figure 8-2* compares the estimated deaths due to radon exposure to the number of deaths from other causes.

Of course, not everyone who breathes excessive levels of radon will develop lung cancer. The risk of developing lung cancer as a result of radon exposure depends upon the susceptibility of the individual, the

EPA Map of Radon Zones

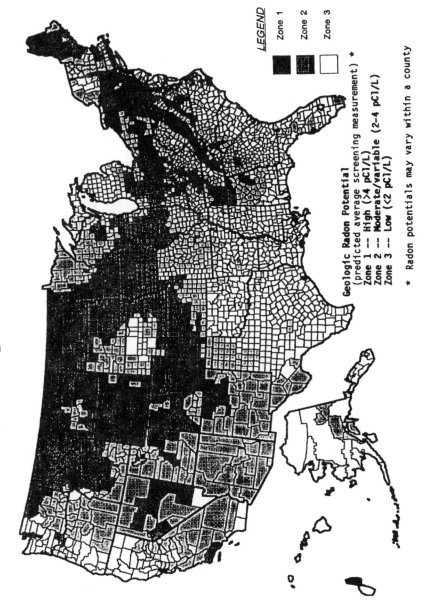

LEGEND

Zone 1

Zone 2

Zone 3

Geologic Radon Potential
(predicted average screening measurement) *
Zone 1 -- High (>4 pCi/L)
Zone 2 -- Moderate/variable (2-4 pCi/L)
Zone 3 -- Low (<2 pCi/L)

*   Radon potentials may vary within a county

This map indicates the geologic radon potential in each of the 3,141 counties in the U.S. The purpose of this map is to assist National, State and local governments and organizations to target their radon program activities and resources.

Figure 8-1.
This map indicates the geologic radon potential in each of the 3,141 counties in the U.S. Its purpose is to assist federal, state, and local governments and private organizations to target their radon program activities and resources..

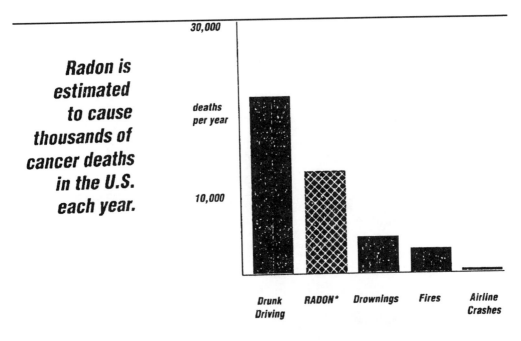

Radon is estimated to cause thousands of cancer deaths in the U.S. each year.

Radon is estimated to cause about 14,000 deaths per year—however, this number could range from 7,000 to 30,000 deaths per year The numbers of deaths from other causes are taken from 1990 National Safety Council reports

Figure 8-2.
Estimated radon-caused deaths in the U.S. each year. This graph was reproduced from the U.S. Environmental Protection Agency's Publication, *A Citizen's Guide to Radon: The Guide to Protecting Yourself and Your Family from Radon*, 2nd Edition, #402-K92-001, May 1992.

level and duration of the radon exposure, and the individual's smoking habits. Although exposure to environmental tobacco smoke in a school is minimal, smoking is still permitted in some faculty lounges. In addition, school staff members who smoke or students who smoke should be aware that the risk of developing lung cancer is significantly higher when smoking is combined with radon exposure. *Figure 8-3* indicates an individual's risk of developing lung cancer from long-term exposures to various levels of radon. It also compares the risk of cancer from radon to other causes of death.

On May 23, 1990, Vernon Houk, M.D., Director of the Center for Environmental Health and Injury Control of the Centers for Disease Control, testified on indoor radon before the U.S. Senate Committee on Environment and Public Works. According to Dr. Houk, children are

RADON RISK EVALUATION CHART

Annual Radon level	If a community of 100 people were exposed to this level:	This risk of dying from lung cancer compares to:
100 pCi/L	About 35 people in the community may die from Radon	Having 10,000 chest x-rays each year
40 pCi/L	About 17 people in the community may die from Radon	Smoking 2 packs of cigarettes each day
20 pCi/L	About 9 people in the community may die from Radon	Smoking 1 pack of cigarettes each day
10 pCi/L	About 5 people in the community may die from Radon	Having 1,000 chest x-rays each year
4 pCi/L	About 2 people in the community may die from Radon	Smoking about 4 cigarettes each day
Levels as high as 3500 pCi/L have been found in some homes. The average Radon level outdoors is around .2 pCi/L or less.		
The risks shown in this chart are for the general population, including men and women of all ages as well as smokers and non-smokers. Children may be at higher risk.		

Figure 8-3.
The risks of developing lung cancer from long-term exposures to various levels of radon.

particularly sensitive to the effects of exposure to radon. He further stated that estimates indicate that children's lungs receive a higher radiation dose than do those of adults for the same level of exposure to radon. The example he gave was that of a child ten years of age who receives twice the lung dose of an adult's when exposed to the same radon level.

THE PROBABILITY OF RADON IN OUR NATION'S SCHOOLS

Exposure to radon in our nation's schools is a recognized problem which was confirmed by a National School Radon Survey conducted by the EPA during the 1990-1991 school year. The study, based upon radon measurements taken from more than 900 schools in 16 states, gives an accurate representation of the radon problem at the national level. The results indicate that radon contamination in schools is widespread. According to the survey, 19.3% of U.S. schools, or nearly one in five, have at least one frequently occupied room with short-term radon levels above the level at which the EPA recommends mitigation. In addition, at the time of the survey 10% of the nation's schools with elevated levels of radon were actually located in areas of low radon potential.

All states have maps based upon information provided by the EPA, which indicate the radon potential on a county-to-county basis. *Figure 8-4* shows the radon probability in the state of Minnesota. School districts should be able to obtain a similar map and other current radon information by contacting the radiation department in their state. (See the **Resources** chapter at the back of this book.)

Contributing Factors

Although levels of radon are present in outdoor air, radon levels frequently accumulate and build up to much higher levels inside buildings. Factors that contribute to the entry of radon gas into a school building include:

- The radon levels present in the soil gas under the school.
- The permeability of the soil. Radon gas is more mobile if the soil is permeable.
- The type of structure and the procedures used during construction. Expansion joints in concrete slabs, basements, crawl spaces, utility tunnels, subslab ductwork, and cracks or other penetration points in a concrete slab frequently provide an access for radon-containing soil gas to enter the building.
- The heating, ventilating, and air conditioning (HVAC) system, depending upon its design and how it is operated and maintained.

TESTING FOR RADON

Radon gas in the air is generally measured in picocuries per liter of air (pCi/L). EPA studies have determined that the radon levels in the outdoor air average about 0.4 picocuries per liter (0.4 pCi/L). Although no level of radon is considered safe, the EPA recommends that, since there is no threshold level for radon, levels be reduced as much as possible. The EPA's long-term goal is to lower indoor radon levels to the ambient levels in the air surrounding each building.

While radon tests are not mandatory, the EPA recommends that all schools test for radon, especially those schools in areas with a greater

MINNESOTA - Map of Radon

This map is not intended to determine if a home in a given zone should be tested for radon.
Homes with elevated levels of radon have been found in all three zones. **All homes should be tested,
regardless of geographic location.**

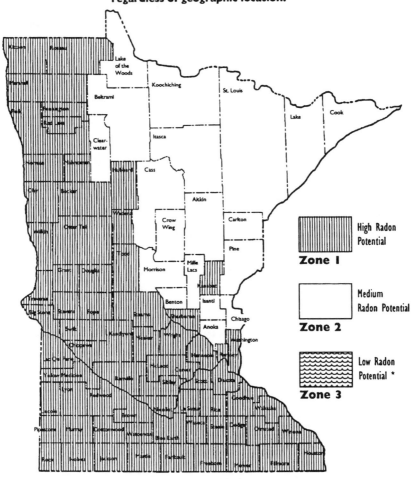

High Radon Potential **Zone 1**	Medium Radon Potential **Zone 2**	Low Radon Potential * **Zone 3**

IMPORTANT: This map is based upon information provided from the U.S. Environmental Protection Agency (EPA). Consult the publication entitled "Radon Potential of Minnesota" before using this map. EPA also recommends that this map be supplemented with any available local data in order to further understand and predict the radon potential of a specific area.

* Minnesota **does not** have any low radon potential areas.   Minnesota Department of Health 6-93

Figure 8-4.

Radon potential in one state, Minnesota, that has no areas of low radon potential. This map is based on information provided by the EPA. The Minnesota Department of Health urges that the publication entitled *Radon in Minnesota* be consulted before this map is used. The EPA also recommends that this map be supplemented with available local data, in order that the radon potential of a specific area be understood fully and predicted accurately.

radon potential. Radon levels are normally higher in basements and in first floor rooms than they are in upper-level rooms. Also, radon concentrations can vary from room to room within a school and from one school (or home) to another in a given area. For these reasons, measurements in schools should be taken in all frequently-occupied rooms in basements and on the first floor if they have substantial ground contact. This includes rooms over crawl spaces.

The first step in testing is to use a screening device to determine quickly if there is a potential radon problem. Three of the most commonly available passive detectors used for screening purposes are charcoal canisters, alpha track detectors, and electret ion chambers.

Two-day *charcoal canisters* are inexpensive, yield quick results, and can be used on weekends under controlled conditions. After the canisters are exposed, they are sealed and returned to the laboratory for analysis. The disadvantage of two-day measurements is that they may differ by a factor of two to three when made in the same classroom on different weekends. This is due to the dramatic fluctuations in radon concentrations. Also, radon concentrations are affected by extremes in temperatures and rapid changes in atmospheric pressure.

Alpha track detectors are used over a three month period. They are better integrating devices than the charcoal canisters and they are not as affected by fluctuating radon levels. Thus, they give a better estimate of the average radon concentration. A disadvantage of the alpha track detector is that it can be tampered with easily because it must be used when school is in session. Also alpha track detectors cost more than charcoal canisters and more time is required for completion of the measurement.

The *electret ion chamber* registers radon concentration by means of an electrostatic charge. When radiation strikes the device, the resulting charge can be read on a voltage meter, and the concentration of radon in the room is also shown on a percentage meter. The electret ion chamber appeals to many users because it gives an accurate and immediate reading, it can be used over and over, and school personnel can use it easily after a period of training. Although the initial cost of the electret ion chamber is higher than that of other devices, the cost per measurement is competitive with the per-measurement cost of other devices.

Ensuring the Accuracy of Radon Measurements

Regardless of the device used, the tests should be conducted during the colder months (ideally October through March) when the windows and doors are likely to be closed. Additionally, the HVAC system should be operating throughout the testing period so that conditions are typical of those on regular school days.

The accuracy of the testing instruments can be determined by placing two detectors side by side in the same location during the measurement period. To confirm further the accuracy of the detectors, a third detector that is unopened (blank) may be placed in some areas to act as a control. These unopened blanks are to be returned to the laboratory for analysis along with the used detectors. All blanks should have a reading of zero. If any have a reading above zero, it is an indication of a defective device or an inaccurate laboratory analysis.

Regardless of which screening device is used, confirmatory measurement should be taken if elevated levels of radon are found. This is important because of the risk of laboratory or clerical error and the possibility that a measurement may be faulty or that the measurement was taken during an unusual peak in the radon concentration. Confirmatory measurements should be carried out under weather and ventilation conditions as close as possible to the original screening tests. *Figure 8-5* indicates the appropriate action recommended by the EPA if the screening test results show elevated levels of radon.

Screening Test Results	Action
Over 20 pCi/L	School officials should take confirmatory measurements that last 2 days to 4 weeks. If screening measurement is above 100 pCi/L, school officials may wish to relocate children.
4 pCi/L–20 pCi/L	School officials should take 9-12 month confirmatory measurements.
less than 4 pCi/L	School officials should decide whether confirmatory measurements are necessary.

Figure 8-5.
Action based on screening test results.

DEVELOPING AN ACTION PLAN

For Existing Schools

When confirmatory measurements have determined the presence of elevated levels of radon in a school building, steps should be taken to understand the problem fully and to develop a mitigation strategy. The following procedures are an aid to guide you through this process:

■ Review all radon test data, placing the emphasis on the confirmatory measurements.

■ Contact your state and regional EPA radiation departments to determine the resources available to your school. This could include some funding, especially for low-income school districts. (See the **Resources** chapter at the back of this book.)

■ Consult experienced radon mitigation firms. Check the EPA list for mitigators that have met the requirements of the Radon Contractor Proficiency Program.

■ Conduct a walk-through audit of the building. Look for radon entry routes such as foundation cracks and points of entry for utility lines.

■ Evaluate the HVAC system. Check for different types of systems as well as differences in pressure.

■ Review building specifications, and study foundation plans. Determine the soil conditions or type of aggregate beneath the concrete slab and look for the presence of subslab ductwork.

■ Plan a strategy for mitigation. It is generally best to proceed in phases. Begin with the simplest and most effective system. Test after each phase.

For New School Construction

In new construction, technology is now available to achieve indoor radon levels near the levels in the ambient air. Further, it is always easier and much more cost-effective to mitigate radon in a school building when radon reduction techniques are implemented during the design and construction of the building. The decision to incorporate these procedures during construction should be determined by research regarding the probability of radon in the area and by radon tests in local school buildings and nearby residences.

Also, school districts may conduct soil tests on the building site to measure radon concentrations in the soil gas. Soil testing, however, is not always productive because the radon measurements derived from soil testing may vary and are not necessarily an indication of what the radon levels will be within the school once construction is completed.

School districts preparing for new construction may wish to contact the radiation department at the national level, as well as state and regional offices. Assistance on a one-to-one basis is available along with a considerable amount of information. (See the **Resources** chapter at the back of this book.)

SPECIFIC RADON MITIGATION TECHNIQUES

Because the design, construction and operational patterns of schools vary greatly, it is impossible to recommend specific mitigation techniques that will apply to all schools. The basic approaches for mitigating radon discussed below are prudent and reasonable. They are of a general nature, however, and will need to be adapted to fit specific situations.

Subslab Depressurization

Radon is generally drawn into the building by pressure differentials between the soil surrounding the substructure and the building interior. Thus the most successful technique to mitigate radon is to depressurize the area directly beneath the slab. This is known as subslab depressurization (SSD) and is appropriate for slab-on-grade schools (slab-on-grade accounts for nearly 75% of all existing schools) and schools with basements. Simply stated, the procedure involves inserting pipes through the concrete slab to access the crushed rock or soil beneath. A fan is then used to suck the soil gases from beneath the slab, releasing them outdoors. The number of suction points depends upon the permeability of the subslab material, as well as the number of subslab barriers and the size of the fans and suction pipes used.

If the soil beneath an existing slab/basement is not permeable enough to allow air movement, an alternative mitigation approach may be necessary.

Subslab depressurization is frequently more effective in new construction because the foundation can be designed with a minimum of subslab barriers. Also, the proper size aggregate can be used and covered with a well-sealed polyethylene membrane prior to pouring the concrete slab. This is explained in EPA's Technical Guidance Manual entitled *Radon Prevention in the Design and Construction of Schools and Other Large Buildings*. (See the RECOMMENDED READING section at the end of this chapter.)

HVAC System

The HVAC system should be designed to operate with adequate ventilation. If it is operating with less than the recommended amount of outside air, the school can expect to have higher levels of radon.

When the HVAC system is functioning so that a positive pressure is maintained, the inflow of radon is reduced. This simply means that the density of outside air coming into the building should be equal to or slightly greater than the air being exhausted from the building through the numerous exhaust fans. On the other hand, when the HVAC system operates with a negative pressure, the potential for radon entry increases. When radon is controlled with a positive air pressure, it is critical that the operation and maintenance of the system be monitored carefully. Further, schools in very cold climates should be aware that this procedure may increase the risk of moisture and condensation problems.

Radon Entry Routes

Seal all cracks and penetration points in the foundation with an appropriate sealant or caulking. The effectiveness of this technique in existing buildings is limited because it is nearly impossible to access and seal all radon entry routes. Subslab return air ducts, subslab utility tunnels, and uncapped block walls provide entry routes for radon. Because each poses a specific problem, they must be dealt with on an individual basis.

It is easier to control the radon entry routes in new construction than in older buildings. The foundation can be designed to minimize cracks, and remaining cracks and other penetration points in contact with the soil can be sealed during the construction process.

Ventilation

An increase in building ventilation rates will reduce radon levels. Although this can be accomplished by opening vents, doors, and lower level windows, it is not a practical approach in most cases and should be considered a temporary measure.

Schools with Unique Situations

A small percentage of existing schools have been built with crawl spaces. Further, many schools have utility tunnels under the buildings. In these and other unique situations, the best approach to mitigate radon is to follow procedures recommended by the radiation department in your state.

THE COST FACTOR

It is always less expensive to incorporate the appropriate radon mitigation components into a school during construction than it is to mitigate radon in an existing school. Radon mitigation techniques have been applied successfully to buildings during construction at a cost of under 10 cents per square foot.

In contrast to this, based upon one EPA survey of seven experienced radon mitigators, the estimated cost to mitigate radon in a typical existing school building would be roughly 50 cents per square foot. The cost would be even higher for schools with extensive subslab walls and poor subslab communication.

According to Alfred B. Craig, Senior Physical Scientist at the EPA's Air and Energy Engineering Research Laboratory in Research Triangle Park, North Carolina, it is far more expensive to mitigate radon in an existing building than to apply the appropriate mitigation techniques to a building during construction.

For existing buildings, as well as for new construction, technology is available to mitigate radon. Schools—especially those in high risk areas—should make every effort to conduct the necessary tests and implement remediation procedures if radon levels are excessive. This is one important step that can be taken to reduce the health risks facing our nation's children.

ASBESTOS: WHAT IS IT AND WHERE IS IT FOUND?

Asbestos is the term used to describe six naturally occurring fibrous minerals present in certain rock formations. When mined and processed, asbestos takes the form of very thin fibers that can be positively identified only with a special microscope. Because these fibers are so light, they can remain suspended in the air for many hours, even for days, when released from asbestos-containing material (ACM).

In the 1920s, asbestos was hailed as a miracle product because of its strength and its fireproofing, insulating, decorating, and soundproofing qualities. It was widely used for 40 or more years until a number of ACMs were banned from the market in the 1970s due to a growing concern about their health effects. The use of asbestos continued to decline, and the EPA's 1989 Asbestos Ban and Phase-out was intended to discontinue all use of asbestos by 1997. Unfortunately, the Asbestos Ban was challenged in the courts, and, at the time of this writing, a final decision still has not been reached.

HEALTH CONCERNS AND RISKS

Information available regarding the adverse health effects associated with asbestos is the result of studies of workers who had long-term exposures in the various asbestos industries. These studies indicate that the risk of developing an asbestos disease appears to be related to an individual's susceptibility, as well as to the physical and chemical properties of the asbestos and to the concentration of fibers in the air. It is estimated that only a small proportion of people exposed to low levels of the fibers will develop an asbestos-related illness. The specific illnesses associated with exposures to asbestos are:

■ Cancers of the lungs, esophagus, stomach, colon, and other organs.

■ Cancer of the lining of the chest and abdominal cavity known as mesothelioma.

■ Asbestosis, a condition that occurs when the lung becomes scarred with fibrous tissues.

As with radon, a smoker's risk of developing lung disease from exposure to asbestos fibers is greater than either the risk from smoking or asbestos exposure alone. Further, the risks to children are increased because they breathe through the mouth more than adults do, and have higher levels of activity, and because asbestos particles remain in their bodies longer than do those inhaled by adults.

EXPOSURES IN OUR SCHOOLS

The EPA estimates that ACM is present in most of the nation's approximately 107,000 primary and secondary schools. The most frequently found sources are:

- Insulation on pipes, boilers, and ductwork.

- Surface materials such as acoustical plaster that have been troweled on or sprayed on for the purpose of fireproofing or insulating.

- Ceiling tiles, floor tiles, and wallboard.

The amount of asbestos present in these products may vary from 1% to 100%, depending upon the product and its use. An analysis of samples by a qualified laboratory is necessary to identify asbestos positively and to determine the precise amount present in a product.

The mere presence of asbestos does not constitute a hazard. The hazard occurs when asbestos becomes friable, meaning that it crumbles or can be reduced to powder by hand pressure. Some ACMs are more friable than others, and all can be reduced to a friable state if they become damaged or are allowed to deteriorate. Note the section of ductwork in *Figure 8-6*. The 100% pure asbestos duct tape is friable and deteriorating in a school building less than 20 years old. Asbestos fibers from wallboard and floor and ceiling tiles may become friable when the materials are sawed, sanded, or otherwise disturbed during building repair and renovation projects. The water damaged lay-in ceiling panel in *Figure 8*-7 contains asbestos. Due to the extensive water damage, the panel may crumble easily and be reduced to a friable state.

Vinyl floor tiles 15 years old and older are likely to contain asbestos. In addition to advising that appropriate action be taken during removal of asbestos tiles, the EPA strongly suggests that its recommended guidelines be followed when vinyl asbestos tiles are stripped of old wax in preparation for rewaxing.

PROTECTING CHILDREN FROM ASBESTOS EXPOSURES

On October 22, 1986, the Asbestos Hazard Emergency Response Act (AHERA) was signed into law. The act required the EPA to develop comprehensive regulations for dealing with asbestos in public and nonprofit private elementary and secondary schools. The regulations

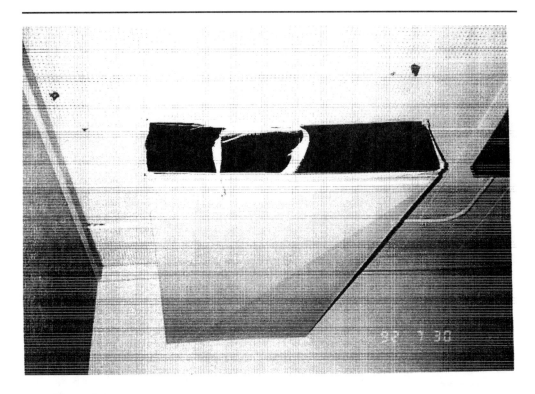

Figure 8-6.
The 100% pure asbestos duct tape used on this section of ductwork is friable and has deteriorated in less than 20 years.. (Picture courtesy of the Texas State Health Department.)

were published on October 30, 1987. Local Education Agencies (LEAs) were then given one year to submit a management plan for review and approval to the designated agency within each of their states. Although some LEAs were given extra time to complete their management plans, all schools were required to begin putting their plans into action no later than July 9, 1989. LEAs were required to develop a management plan that included the following actions with regard to asbestos-related activities:

- Designate and train an individual to oversee all asbestos-related activities in the school system.

- Prepare a plan for managing asbestos and controlling the exposures in each school.

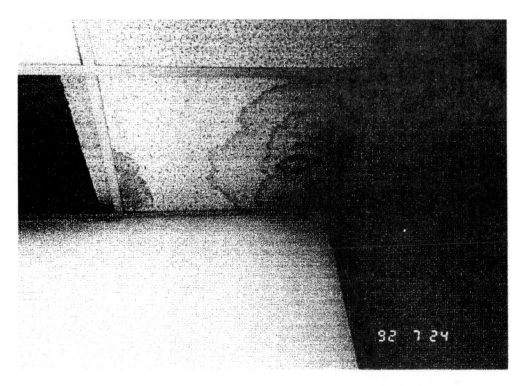

Figure 8-7.
Due to severe water damage, this asbestos-containing ceiling panel has been changed from a nonfriable to a friable asbestos that will crumble easily. (Picture courtesy of the Texas State Health Department)

- Conduct a thorough inspection of every school building for ACMs and determine if they are friable or nonfriable. As a follow-up, at least once every six months, the LEA must conduct a periodic surveillance in its buildings, and at least once every three years it should reinspect each school building known to have asbestos-containing material.

- Consult accredited inspection and management professionals to ensure that all required inspections are performed by qualified personnel. These professionals should also carry out the appropriate response actions to protect the building occupants and the environment. All actions are to be documented in the management plan.

- Notify the public at least once a year about the asbestos activities in each school and the availability of the management plan for review. Notification should be given to all teachers, parents, and school employee organizations.

- Maintain accurate records of all asbestos-related activities in the management plan and make the records available for public review.

RESPONSE ACTIONS FOR MANAGING ASBESTOS

Current information published by the EPA emphasizes *managing asbestos in place*, which is the subject of one of its publications. (See the RECOMMENDED READING section at the end of this chapter.) Managing asbestos does not mean doing nothing. It means, rather, having an operation and maintenance program to ensure that the day-to-day management procedures are carried out in a manner that minimizes the release of asbestos fibers into the air. Minimizing asbestos release can be accomplished through:

- *Maintenance*---Developing and carrying out a maintenance plan to ensure that ACM is kept in good condition.

- *Repair*—Assuring that damaged thermal insulation on pipes and boilers is repaired as soon as possible after damage occurs.

- *Encapsulation*—Spraying sealants on ACMs to prevent the release of fibers.

- *Enclosure*---Placing a barrier around the ACM is a way to manage asbestos in some cases.

These procedures may be sufficient to control the release of asbestos fibers until the ACM in a school is scheduled to be disturbed by renovation or demolition activities, at which point removal may be necessary to protect the health of students and staff. The value of managing asbestos in place can be supported by the following facts published in the EPA guidelines:

- The risk of asbestos-related disease depends upon exposure to airborne asbestos fibers.

- Current data indicate that the average airborne asbestos level in a building seems to be very low.

- Removal may not be the best course of action. In fact, an improper removal can create a dangerous situation where none previously existed.

The EPA recommends a pro-active in-place management program whenever ACM is discovered.

As a result of EPA efforts and the AHERA, asbestos is one of the more recognized and managed hazards found indoors. Yet there are still many instances in which asbestos is a hazard due to misinformation, neglect, or improper management. The asbestos crisis that occurred in the New York City Schools at the beginning of the 1993-94 school year is one of the best examples of the results of neglect and improper management. It was discovered that the asbestos tests carried out on more than 1,000 New York City school buildings over a four-year period were seriously flawed. As a result, the start of classes for one million students was delayed. Early in August, 1993, New York City Mayor David Dinkins called for an emergency effort to reinspect every school for friable asbestos before school opened. This was a formidable and nearly impossible task. When classes finally got underway in late September, some facilities still remained closed, so that many students faced extra bus rides and crowded classrooms.

School districts are encouraged to seek assistance from their designated state agency or their regional EPA office to develop programs for managing and controlling asbestos. (See the **Resources** chapter at the back of this book.) These agencies should also be aware of the availability of loans and grants to assist needy public and private schools with serious asbestos problems.

According to conversations with officials from the asbestos division of the Texas State Health Department, school districts are frequently reluctant to contact state or federal agencies for information and assistance regarding procedures for controlling asbestos. This reluctance stems from the concern that the district will be cited and an enforcement action will be forthcoming. Texas officials have stated that districts requesting consultative help do not subject themselves to possible enforcement action. The intent of the law is not to create problems for school districts, and the state encourages districts to ask for assistance when in doubt. The primary concern of all involved should be to protect children from the health risks resulting from exposure to asbestos.

RADON AND ASBESTOS RESOURCES

Radon

Technical information is available from the Air and Energy Engineering Research Lab, USEPA, Research Triangle Park, North Carolina 27711.

■ Contact person: Alfred B. Craig, 919-541-2824.

A technical guidance manual entitled *Radon Prevention in the Design and Construction of Schools and Other Large Buildings* is available from USEPA, EPA/625/R-92/016, Office of Research and Development, Washington, D.C. 20460.

Asbestos

EPA Toxic Substance Control Act (TSCA). This will answer questions about AHERA regulations and about asbestos in general.

■ Hotline: 202-554-1404.

EPAs ombudsman assists citizens with their concerns regarding asbestos-in-schools issues.

■ Hotline: 800-368-5888.

RECOMMENDED READING

Radon

Craig, Alfred B., Kelly W. Leovic, and D. Bruce Harris, April 1991, *Design of Radon Resistant and Easy-to-Mitigate New School Buildings,* United States Environmental Protection Agency, Air and Energy Engineering Research Laboratory, North Carolina. Paper presented at The International Symposium on Radon and Radon Technology, Philadelphia, Pennsylvania.

Houk, Vernon, M.D., May 23, 1990, *Indoor Radon,* Testimony before U.S. Senate Committee on Environmental and Public Works.

Phillips, Jeffery L., and Lisa A. Ratcliff, *Results of EPA's National School Radon Survey,* United States Environmental Protection Agency, Washington, D. C. 20460.

United States Environmental Protection Agency, May 1992, *A Citizen's Guide to Radon* (Second Edition). Air and Radiation (ANR-464), EPA 402-K92-001.

United States Environmental Protection Agency, October 1990, *Environmental Hazards in Your School, A Resource Handbook*, Publication #2DT-2001.

United States Environmental Protection Agency, July 1993, *Radon Measurements in Schools*, Revised Edition, Air and Radiation EPA 402-R-92-014.

United States Environmental Protection Agency, June 1992, *EPA Radon Mitigation Research Update*, EPA/600/N-92-009, Washington, D.C.: Office of Research and Development.

United States Environmental Protection Agency, August 1993, *EPA Radon Mitigation Research Update*, EPA/A/600/N-93/013, Washington, D. C.:Office of Research and Development.

United States Environmental Protection Agency, January 1993, *Radon Prevention in the Design and Construction of Schools and Other Large Buildings*, EPA/625/R-92-016, Washington, D. C.: Office of Research and Development.

United States Environmental Protection Agency, October 1989, *Radon Reduction Techniques in Schools; Interim Technical Guidance*, EPA #520-1-89-020, Center for Environmental Research Information, USEPA, 26 W. Martin Luther King Drive, Cincinnati, Ohio 45268.

Asbestos

Indoor Air Review, October 1993, "Bureaucratic Mishaps Precipitate New York Asbestos Crisis," Volume III, No. 8.

National School Boards Association, September 1989, *Updating School Board Policies, Environmental Policy—A Priority for Schools in the '90s.* Volume 20, Number 8.

Small, Bruce M., and Associates, May 1985, *Recommendations for Action on Pollution and Education in Toronto*. A report prepared for the Pollution and Education Review Group of the Board of Education for the city of Toronto.

United States Environmental Protection Agency, June 1989, *The ABCs of Asbestos in Schools*, TS 799.

United States Environmental Protection Agency, October 1990, *Environmental Hazards in Your School: A Resource Handbook*, Publication #2DT-2001.

United States Environmental Protection Agency, June 1985, *Guidance for Controlling Asbestos-containing Materials in Buildings*, Publication #560/5-85-024.

United States Environmental Protection Agency, July 1990, *Managing Asbestos in Place; A Building Owner's Guide to Operations and Maintenance Programs for Asbestos-Containing Materials*, 20T-2003.

United States Environmental Protection Agency, May 1988, *100 Commonly Asked Questions About the New AHERA Asbestos-in-Schools Rule.*

9

SCHOOL FLOOR COVERINGS

by Mary Oetzel

In this chapter, Ms. Oetzel shows how the selection and maintenance of floor coverings in schools affect the air quality within the school and, consequently, the health of students, teachers, and other school staff. In discussing the health hazards of various carpeting materials, showing the comparative advantages of such floor coverings as terrazzo, ceramic tile, and hardwood, and comparing the long-term maintenance costs of terrazzo and carpeting, she answers important questions about the installation and maintenance of various floor covering materials.

☐ *What floor coverings meet the highest standards of health maintenance and safety?*

☐ *Why is some carpeting material hazardous to the health of students and teachers?*

☐ *What does the labeling of various kinds of carpeting mean?*

☐ *How should carpeting be selected for a school?*

☐ *What are the best floor maintenance procedures, and why is it important for custodial staff to plan them carefully?*

☐ *What factors should school officials take into account when investing in new floor coverings?*

One of the most important decisions in planning, constructing, or renovating a school building is the selection of a floor surface. The vast surface area and heavy traffic common to most schools, has a long-term impact on the quality of the indoor air. Floors are generally categorized as carpeted or hard-surfaced (the latter category includes masonry, hardwood, and resilient floor coverings), and both categories vary in appearance, comfort, cost, durability, and ease of maintenance. Since there are advantages and disadvantages associated with every floor surface, a thorough analysis of each will help schools make the choice that is right for their needs.

HARD-SURFACED FLOORS, GENERALLY

The masonry floor surfaces typically found in schools are concrete, terrazzo, and ceramic tile. Although these surfaces are unyielding under foot, they generally provide a life-time floor. Hardwood, a once popular floor surface is now used primarily in gymnasiums. Vinyl and vinyl tile are the most frequently used resilient floor coverings. Of these, the vinyl composition tile (VCT) is most often found in schools. In addition to durability and ease of maintenance, hard-surface floorings are attractive and healthful for school environments.

CONCRETE, TERRAZZO, CERAMIC TILE, AND HARDWOOD

Finished Concrete

Finished concrete is the most economical choice in a floor surface. Smooth-troweled concrete with the right finish provides excellent wear resistance. Options for finishing include painting or the application of a wax or clear sealant. In addition, pigments can be added directly to the concrete mixture prior to pouring the floor. The raw concrete floor can also be stained after it has been troweled to a smooth finish.

Terrazzo

Terrazzo is made by grinding and polishing a concrete surface that consists of granite or marble chips set into a matrix of colored portland cement or other binding agent. Polishing brings out the color and pattern of the stone chips. A sealer is then applied to enhance the appearance further and reduce staining. Because of their rich texture and varied colors, terrazzo floors are often used where durable and decorative floor patterns are desired. Terrazzo floors can be formed in place or installed from factory-made tiles. Terrazzo is frequently avoided or used minimally in new school construction because of its initial high cost. When amortized over 20 to 40 years, however, terrazzo is a good buy. (See *Figure 9-2* in the COST CONSIDERATIONS IN SCHOOL FLOOR COVERINGS section of this chapter, below.)

Ceramic Tile

Fired clay tiles with either a glazed or an unglazed surface are referred to as ceramic tiles. Available in a wide assortment of colors, textures, and sizes, they provide an attractive and lasting floor surface. Glazed ceramic tile can generally be found in restrooms, locker rooms, and other high-moisture areas of a school. They are ideally suited to these rooms because they are easily maintained and are not affected by dampness, features that make ceramic tile a desirable floor surface for other parts of a school. Like terrazzo, ceramic tile is more expensive than some other floor surfaces, which frequently limits its use to high-visibility areas.

Hardwood

Traditionally, hardwood floors were constructed from tongue and groove oak or maple. These strips were driven tightly together and blind-nailed to a wood subfloor. Although many school buildings still have strip flooring of this type, new schools are rarely built with hardwood flooring because of the initial high cost. It is most often used in gymnasiums or for special applications.

RESILIENT FLOOR COVERINGS

The resilient floor coverings used most extensively in schools today are vinyl composition tile, rubber tile, cushioned rubber, and vinyl flooring.

Vinyl and Vinyl Composition Tile.

Vinyl floor coverings account for approximately 64% of the hard-surfaced flooring sales in the United States. This includes vinyl tiles and sheet vinyls. The major component of the vinyl and VCT floor coverings used today is polyvinyl chloride (PVC). This and other chemicals in vinyl floor coverings emit volatile organic compounds (VOCs) during and after installation. The main source of these emissions is the plasticizer, and since sheet vinyls contain more plasticizers, they are a greater source of emissions than vinyl tiles. According to the *AIA Environmental Resource Guide* published by the American Institute of Architects, however, the emissions decrease substantially after 24 hours if the space is well ventilated.

The resilient floor covering used extensively in schools today is commercial grade vinyl composition tile. VCT is a hard material and less volatile than residential vinyl floor tiles. This lower-cost covering provides an attractive, hygienic, and easily maintained floor surface.

Rubber Tile, Cushioned Rubber, and Vinyl Flooring

Rubber flooring is made from synthetic rubber combined with various fillers, minerals, and pigments. It is available in sheet or tile form. Although appealing and easily cleaned, rubber surfaces are quite expensive.

Cushioned flooring materials, available in varying thicknesses, provide a more buoyant walking surface than other resilient flooring materials. They are often used as sports floors in gymnasiums and other athletic facilities. Cushioned floor coverings of vinyl and synthetic rubber frequently emit chemical fumes for a much longer period than VCT. Parents in one Washington school reported that emissions from a cushioned flooring installed in the school gymnasium persisted for more than a year.

HEALTH RISKS OF HARD-SURFACED FLOORS

The health risks associated with hard-surfaced floorings are minimal. Most of the chemical emissions from these surfaces occur during the preparation, installation, and finishing of the floor. You can minimize exposures to harmful emissions by following recommended procedures for the selection, installation, and ventilation of the space.

Although the presence of asbestos in vinyl floor tiles installed prior to the mid-1980s is a potential health risk in existing schools, the asbestos in floor tiles is a hazard only if asbestos fibers are released into the air. (See Chapter 8.) Exposures to the fibers can occur when a floor is being stripped for rewaxing, when the vinyl flooring begins to crumble and deteriorate, and during renovation or demolition. Whenever possible, it is preferable to contain the asbestos by installing new flooring over the old vinyl tiles. Schools should contact the designated state agency to determine the recommended procedure for their particular situation.

SELECTION OF HARD-SURFACED FLOORING MATERIALS

Masonry flooring materials, hardwood, and VCT are low-emission products. They are of less concern than the waxes, adhesives, surface sealants, and other wet floor preparations used to install and finish flooring. The following guidelines will provide assistance in the selection of these wet materials, as well as in dealing with problems unique to ceramic tile, hardwood, and resilient floor coverings:

Wet Materials

- Request manufacturers' emission data on all products being considered. This should include specific VOCs as well as the total volatile organic compounds (TVOCs).

- Check data to determine emission levels one, two, and four days after application.

- Select adhesives with the lowest levels of VOCs. (Some adhesives are available with virtually no VOCs.)

- Select waxes and sealants with the lowest levels of VOCs.

- Minimize the use of products containing biocides (pesticides) whenever possible.

Glazed Ceramic Tile

- Select ceramic tile with a high-fired glaze to withstand the heavy traffic in a school.

- Contact the manufacturer for data to ensure a lead-free glaze. Keep in mind that lead is more likely to be present, and thus of a greater concern, if the tile is imported.

Hardwood

- Choose solid hardwood strip flooring, instead of laminated strips, to avoid the formaldehyde resins.

- Minimize the use of construction adhesives, foam cushions, and the plywood subflooring commonly used to install flooring.

Resilient Floor Coverings

Of greatest concern are the vinyl and rubber sheet materials and cushioned floor coverings.

- Review emissions data supplied by the manufacturer. Check for both specific VOCs and TVOCs.

- Do a sniff test by placing a sample of the product(s) under consideration in a clean, well-sealed glass jar. Leave it in an area slightly above room temperature overnight. When the jar is opened, the odor it emits should reflect accurately the odor in the room once the flooring material is installed.

INSTALLATION AND MAINTENANCE OF HARD-SURFACED FLOORS

Construction procedures involving the installation of masonry surfaces, hardwood flooring, and resilient floor coverings should take place in unoccupied buildings. Construction dusts, floor preparation adhesives, and, after the floor is in place, the waxes and sealants used for finishing introduce high levels of contaminants into the indoor air. Although emissions from waxes and sealants dissipate rather rapidly, it would be prudent to ventilate the area for up to one week before occupying the space.

The procedures used to wax or seal a new hard-surface floor are similar to those performed annually as part of the maintenance program. Generally, this work is carried out during the summer break and should be scheduled to allow the same amount of airing time as is allowed in new construction.

CARPETING

Carpeting was introduced into schools as a floor covering in the early 1960's. Since that time, the use of carpeting in schools has increased dramatically. It is only in the last five to ten years that public attention has been drawn to the health effects associated with the its use. These health effects result from the chemical fumes emitted by new carpeting, usually during the first few weeks or months after the carpet is installed. Also, as the carpet ages, other contaminants accumulate in it, creating an on-going problem. Carpeting is selected primarily for its aesthetic appeal and acoustical value. It also provides a yielding surface underfoot and may reduce the number of falls and the severity of the injuries resulting from those falls.

Carpeting can be referred to as a system with several components which include floor preparations, adhesives, seam sealers, and possibly a carpet pad. The carpets used in schools are generally manufactured from synthetic fibers with the vast majority being tufted nylon. Typically, the carpet fibers are attached to a primary backing that is stabilized with latex. Depending upon the process used, the carpet may or may not have a secondary backing. *Figure 9-1* is a diagram of tufted carpeting with a secondary backing.

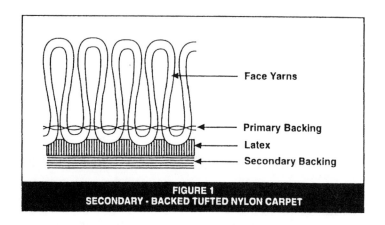

FIGURE 1
SECONDARY - BACKED TUFTED NYLON CARPET

Figure 9-1.

Secondary-backed tufted nylon carpet. (Reprinted from the Technical Bulletin, *Carpet and Indoor Air Quality in Schools,* Maryland State Department of Education.

HEALTH RISKS LINKED TO NEW CARPETING

In recent years, carpeting and carpet-related products have come under scrutiny due to the increasing number of complaints from consumers who have experienced adverse health effects from the chemical emissions common to new carpeting. Many of the chemical fumes emitted from carpeting and carpet systems are toxic, and some are known or suspected to cause cancer. Although there are dozens of volatile organic compounds present in carpeting, 4-phenylcylohexane (4-PC), the chemical that gives carpets their distinctive odor, has been the main focus of many investigations. Other toxic chemicals found in carpeting include toluene, xylene, benzene, and those contained in the pesticides, fungicides, and stain-resistant treatments somtimes introduced when carpets are manufactured. A majority of the chemical fumes from carpet systems dissipate in the first weeks or months after a carpet has been installed. In some instances, however, chemical emissions from new carpeting have persisted for a year or longer. Typical health problems associated with exposure to fumes from new carpet include flu-like symptoms, eye, nose, and throat irritation, headaches, rashes, nausea, fatigue, respiratory problems, asthma, and multiple chemical sensitivity.

Doris Rapp, M.D., a pediatric allergist and one of the country's leading specialists in environmental medicine, made the following statement that sums up the concerns of a number of experts in the field: "From the environmental medical point of view, carpets should not be placed in schools. An ever-expanding group of children and teachers appear to be able to trace the onset of their acute or chronic health, memory, and mood problems directly to the time that new synthetic carpeting was installed." (Rapp 1995)

CARPETING—A CONTROVERSIAL FLOOR COVERING

Public attention was drawn to the carpeting problem in 1988 following the installation of carpeting at the United States Environmental Protection Agency (EPA) headquarters building in Washington, D.C. Approximately 125 of the 2,000 employees became ill after exposure to the chemical fumes emitted from the new carpet. The chemical 4-PC, common to most latex-backed carpeting, was thought to be the primary culprit. The EPA replaced the carpeting with an acceptable carpet that did not contain 4-PC. This did not solve the problem for some employees who continued to experience health problems as a result of the initial exposure.

This incident prompted the National Federation of Federal Employees (NFFE), Local 2050, to petition the EPA, under Section 21 of the Toxic Substance Control Act (TSCA), to initiate proceedings to reduce emissions from new carpet. Although the petition was denied, the EPA recognized the Union's concern and in August of 1990, formed the Carpet Policy Dialogue Group. Among the members of this diverse group were representatives from the NFFE, the EPA, the carpet industry, research laboratories, public interest groups, and the general public.

The primary goals of the Carpet Policy Dialogue Group were to identify the VOCs emitted from carpeting and carpet systems, develop a methodology to test for carpet emissions, and establish controls for reducing these emissions. As a result of a 13-month-long dialogue, representatives from the carpet industry voluntarily agreed to test their products and submit periodic reports. Also, associations representing manufacturers of the various carpet components signed agreements with the EPA to govern the testing of their products. One of the criticisms of the carpet dialogue was that it did not address the health effects associated with new carpeting.

The Green Tag Program

An outcome of the Carpet Policy Dialogue was the controversial "Indoor Air Quality Testing Program," frequently referred to as the Green Tag Program. This was established in July of 1992 by the Carpet and Rug Institute (CRI), the trade association which represents about 95% of the industry. The initial press release by CRI stated that, *"the CRI label will tell consumers that the carpet or rug they buy meets the predetermined indoor air quality testing criteria."* Under this program manufacturers can obtain a Green Tag for an entire product line of carpeting by having one piece of carpet tested each year. The tests conducted on each carpet sample measure styrene, 4-PC, formaldehyde, and the TVOCs emitted from the product. The program has been criticized because it does not include specific tests on all of the toxic chemicals present in carpeting.

Further, because carpets can vary chemically from one production lot to another, testing only one sample per year of an entire product line may not be meaningful. The Attorneys General from New York, Vermont, Connecticut, and Oregon investigated the program and stated the following in a report called *Carpets and Indoor Air: What You Should Know*: "As of this date there is an insufficient scientific basis to set standards for carpet emissions or, by implication, to make safety claims about carpets. Clearly, no certification program, such as the one instituted by CRI, is appropriate until safety standards are proposed and subjected to review and public comment."

An Independent Study

The carpet controversy gained momentum in the summer of 1992, when Anderson Laboratories, Inc., of Dedham, Massachusetts, released the results of its bioassay studies on carpets that had previously produced adverse reactions in humans. Anderson Laboratories reported that mice exposed to emissions from these problem carpets suffered severe neurological impairment, and 15 of the 30 mice in the study died. The study was replicated by Dr. Yves Alarie, a researcher from the University of Pittsburgh. Although the EPA also achieved similar results when they repeated the study at Anderson Laboratories, later EPA studies using different parameters achieved different results. At the time of this writing, further research is being conducted by Anderson Laboratories, Dr. Yves Alarie, and the carpet industry.

The Anderson Laboratories study prompted concerned groups to renew their efforts to warn the public of the health risks associated with carpeting. One such effort was a petition by the Attorneys General from 26 states to the Consumer Products Safety Commission (CPSC) to place warning labels on carpeting. Their request was denied in spite of the fact that the New York Attorney General's office and federal agencies had received over 800 complaints from people who had suffered adverse reactions after carpets were installed in their homes.

The Carpet Industry Takes a Stand

On November 15, 1993, the CRI responded to the public's growing concern about the health problems associated with new carpeting by announcing a consumer information campaign. Effective January 1, 1994, a three-inch by five-inch label was attached to all new carpeting to alert consumers to the health risks associated with the installation, cleaning, and removal of carpeting. Specific information on the label includes:

- Symptoms people might experience, along with a directive to call a physician if any symptoms occur.

- A warning to allergic or sensitive individuals that they should leave the premises when carpeting is being removed or installed.

- Guidelines for carpet installations.

This label and an accompanying manual were developed by CRI with input from the EPA, the CPSC, the Attorneys General from New York, Connecticut, Vermont, and Oregon, members of Congress, and consumer groups. The labeling is recognized as a major step forward for all concerned about reducing the pollutant levels in the indoor air. Although the "Green Tag" program will continue, a spokesperson for CRI stated that the frequency of carpet testing will be increased, and efforts will be made to reduce product emissions.

SELECTION AND INSTALLATION OF CARPETING

While CRI's new labeling program is intended to alert consumers to the risks associated with new carpeting, it still does not guarantee the safety of carpeting. School districts that elect to use carpeting, despite the health risks, should observe recommended guidelines for the selection and installation of carpeting. Although not inclusive, the following recommendations will provide assistance in those efforts:

Selection of Carpeting

■ Obtain the following information from the manufacturer on each product being considered for a carpet system:

1. The specific contents of the product.

2. A list of substances, including amounts:

> a) on the list of chemical carcinogens published
> by the International Agency for Research on Cancer.

> b) on the National Toxicology Program list of carcinogens.

> c) in the catalog of Teratogenic Agents on the
> Reproductive Toxins List.

3. Emissions data for specific VOCs, as well TVOCs.

4. The name of the laboratory that performed the emissions testing and the protocol used.

5. Consultative input from health professionals and scientists.

■ Based upon the manufacturers' emissions data, select the carpet with the lowest emissions of TVOCs and the lowest content of toxic components.

■ Specify only low VOC carpet adhesives.

■ Avoid the anti-microbial (pesticide) treatments often applied to carpeting during the manufacturing process.

■ Do the sniff test (explained on page 167) in the guidelines for resilient floor coverings.

■ Select durable carpeting in order to minimize the emissions from frequent replacements.

■ Review maintenance procedures.

Installing the Carpeting

- Unroll and air the carpeting in a well-ventilated location two to four days prior to installation.

- If the carpet is a replacement, vacuum old carpet before removing it, and vacuum and clean the floor thoroughly prior to installing the new carpeting.

- Operate the building ventilation system at normal temperatures and with the maximum amount of outdoor air during the installation. This should be continued for a minimum of 72 hours after the installation is completed. The State of Washington employs a 30-day airing period after carpeting has been installed in a state building. During this time, the HVAC system, in the unoccupied building, is operated at maximum outdoor air 24 hours a day.

- Air returns should be closed to avoid recirculating air into the HVAC system during the installation. Instead, create a temporary system using fans, open doorways, stairwells, and windows.

- Do not install carpeting when areas of a school are occupied.

- Install floor mats at the entrances to reduce the tracking-in of outdoor contaminants.

MICROBIOLOGICAL, LEAD, AND CHEMICAL CONTAMINANTS

Ongoing Health Risks

In addition to the chemical fumes emitted from new carpeting, biological contamination associated with carpeting in schools is an ongoing concern. Bacteria, viruses, fungi, pollen, molds, animal dander, dust mites, and other insects are biological agents usually invisible and frequently present in indoor air. Carpets provide an ideal environment for these agents to accumulate and multiply. A less recognized problem is the presence of lead, pesticides, and other chemical contaminants tracked into buildings on shoes, which often become lodged in the carpet pile.

Microbiological Concerns

With regard to microbiological concerns, a 1993 book entitled *Indoor Allergens* published by the National Academy Press, reports that:

carpeting can provide niches for both the accumulation and production of allergens and has been characterized by some as a "cultivation medium" for microorganisms when wetted. Carpeting can also serve as a reservoir for pollen and pollen fragments. The magnitude of the potential significance of carpeting as a source and reservoir of indoor allergens indicates that it should be given consideration as a serious problem.

The American Lung Association supports this position and states in an "Indoor Pollution Fact Sheet" entitled *Biological Agents* that bacteria, fungi, and molds find nourishment and can flourish in, among other things, carpets.

Because high humidity increases the risk of biological contamination, carpeting should not be used in areas susceptible to moisture. Further, carpeting that becomes saturated with water may have to be discarded if the water is not removed quickly.

Lead, Pesticides, and Other Chemicals

Information on lead and other chemical contaminants in carpeting was reported by Seattle-based consulting engineer John Roberts and his colleagues in a presentation at the American Society of Heating Refrigeration and Air Conditioning Engineers' Indoor Air '93 conference in Helsinki, Finland. According to their studies, there is a correlation between the levels of lead (Pb), pesticides, and other chemicals found in carpet dust and the concentration present in the soil around the foundation and entryways, or in the yard of a home. In some cases, the indoor levels were significantly higher than those found outdoors. To complicate matters, pollutants found in carpet dust are protected from degradation and can accumulate over years. Similar results were reported in a study done by the EPA and in a survey of hundreds of homes by David E. Camann of the Southwest Research Institute in San Antonio, Texas.

Although most of the research has been conducted in homes, according to my conversations with John Roberts and David Camaan, we can anticipate finding the same or even higher levels of these pollutants in school carpet dust. This is due to the heavy traffic in a school building and the number of people per square foot occupying the building.

OPTIONS

Because of the health concerns associated with carpeting, some school officials are opting to reduce or restrict the use of carpeting. Among them are officials of the Dade County School District in Dade County, Florida. Other schools have elected to use area rugs or, in some cases, especially in the primary grades, rugs for individual children.

Dade County, Florida

The following paragraphs were excerpted from the minutes of the Dade County School District's School Board Meeting of February 17, 1993:

> There has been considerable controversy regarding the use of carpeting in schools. While carpeting does provide certain aesthetic and acoustic advantages when compared to the resilient floor coverings such as vinyl composition or rubber flooring materials, the life cycle cost for installing and maintaining carpeted flooring is significantly higher than such cost for vinyl flooring. Additionally, and of perhaps greater importance, is the growing concern regarding indoor air quality in carpeted areas.

> Carpet harbors allergens and pathogenic organisms such as mildew, dust mite feces, pollens, toxins, and bacteria. Frequent and extensive cleaning can reduce but not eliminate the presence of such undesirable elements; however, the cost is considerably greater than that of vinyl floor surfaces. The Executive Directors of both Facilities Operations and Plant Operations have advised that they strongly favor reduced use of carpet at school sites.

> In general, carpeting should be restricted to media centers, administrative spaces, lounges, and areas which experience minimal traffic when personnel using those spaces strongly desire carpeting.

Area Rugs

Area rugs are an alternative to carpeting in classrooms, especially in the primary grades when children may sit on the floor for some classroom activities. Area rugs allow students and teachers to enjoy some of the benefits of carpeting without the health risks. They eliminate the need for adhesives and they can be removed for a thorough cleaning.

MAINTENANCE

With the decision to use carpet in a school comes a corresponding commitment to implement a preventive and scheduled maintenance program. If this commitment cannot be executed due to budget constraints, inadequately trained staff, or other reasons, carpet should not be used. Without proper maintenance, carpet will have a shortened life span and will become a contaminant source for the indoor air. (Maryland State Department of Education 1993. Technical Bulletin, *Carpet and Indoor Air Quality in Schools*, 6. (See the RECOMMENDED READINGS section at the end of this chapter.)

School districts should follow guidelines for carpet cleaning outlined by experts in the field. The following recommendations for carpet care are basic to all maintenance programs:

- Vacuum heavy traffic areas (which include most of the floor areas in a school) at least once a day. Vacuum cleaners with high-efficiency particulate arresting (HEPA) air filters are necessary to avoid dispensing and suspending allergens and other particulates in the air.

- Clean up all spills as soon as they occur.

- Combine shampooing with hot-water extraction for most effective cleaning. Frequency of shampooing should be determined by the process used and the amount of traffic in the area to be cleaned.

- Select low emission shampoos free of fragrances and antimicrobial agents.

COST CONSIDERATIONS IN SCHOOL FLOOR COVERINGS

A study entitled *Comparative Cost of School Floor Coverings*, presented at the American Academy of Environmental Medicine Conference in Chicago in October of 1992, indicates that hard-surface floorings are considerably more economical than carpeting. (See *Figure 9-2*.)

The information in the study was obtained from the building facilities managers of five major city school districts, representing 282,600 students and 458 schools. These facilities managers were asked to compare the cost of the materials, installation, and maintenance for various school floor coverings when amortized over 20 and 40 years.

Since the vast majority of school districts install either vinyl composition tile or carpeting, the comparative costs focus on these two surfaces. Also, the study covers only the day-to-day costs for a 36-week school year. It does not include maintenance costs typically incurred during summer break when carpeting is shampooed thoroughly and VCT floors are stripped and waxed.

COMPARATIVE COST OF SCHOOL FLOOR COVERINGS

Study Based on a School of 50,000 Square Feet

MATERIAL COSTS (INC. INSTALLATION)--FREQ.OF REPLACEMENT

Floor Covering	Cost per Square foot	Frequency of Replacement	40 year cost of materials
VCT	$1.32	33 years	$ 49,315.80
Carpeting	$1.83	8 years	$389,938.40
Terrazzo	$6.00	never	$300,000.00

MAINTENANCE COSTS
Day-to-Day Cleaning--School Year of 36 Weeks

Floor Covering	Per Year	20 Years
VCT	$113,249.00	$2,264,980.00
Carpeting	$204,394.00	$4,087,880.00
Terrazzo	$113,249.00	$2,264,980.00

TOTAL COST OF SCHOOL FLOOR COVERINGS
Materials--Installation--Maintenance

Floor Covering	20 Years	40 Years
VCT	$2,655,091.00	$ 5,105,539.00
Carpeting	$5,290,976.00	$10,581,952.00
Savings w/VCT	**$2,635,885.00**	**$ 5,476,413.00**
Terrazzo	$2,564,980.00	$ 4,829,960.00
Savings w/Terrazzo	**$2,725,996.00**	**$ 5,751,922.00**

Environmental Education and Health Services, Inc. 1992.
"Comparative Cost of School Floor Coverings".
(See resources at the end of the chapter)

Figure 9-2.

Comparative cost of school floor coverings: vinyl composition tile (VCT), carpeting, and terrazzo. (Reproduced from Environmental Education and Health Services, Inc., "Comparative Cost of School Floor Coverings," 1992, updated March 1994.)

COMPARATIVE COST OF SCHOOL FLOOR COVERINGS
STUDY BASED ON 250,000 SQUARE FEET

MATERIAL COSTS (INC. INSTALLATION) -- FREQ. OF REPLACEMENT

Floor Covering	Cost per Square Foot	Frequency of Replacement	Cost of Materials
VCT	$ 1.412	33 years	$ 353,000.00
Carpeting	$ 1.932	8 years	$ 483,000.00
Terrazzo	$ 6.00	never	$1,500,000.00

MAINTENANCE COSTS
Day-to-Day Cleaning -- School Year of 36 Weeks

Floor Covering	Per Year	20 Years
VCT	$ 114,582.78	$ 2,291,655.60
Carpeting	$ 206,425.48	$ 4,128,509.60
Terrazzo	$ 114,582.78	$ 2,291,655.60

TOTAL COST OF SCHOOL FLOOR COVERINGS
Materials--Installation--Maintenance (Inc. Replacement Costs not shown above)

Floor Covering	20 Years	40 Years
VCT	$ 2,699,655.60	$ 5,168,168.34
Carpeting	$ 5,401,366.64	$ 10,802,733.40
Savings w/VCT	**$ 2,701,711.04**	**$ 5,634,565.06**
Terrazzo	$ 3,791,655.60	$ 6,083,311.20
Savings w/Terrazzo	**$ 1,609,711.04**	**$ 4,719,422.20**

Environmental Education and Health Services, Inc. 1992. Updated March, 1994. "Comparative Cost of School Floor Coverings." (See resources at the end of the chapter.)

In addition, managers were asked to compare the maintenance time spent on terrazzo floors with that required for vinyl composition tile floors. Responses ranged from slightly less time to slightly more time. Thus the figures on terrazzo represent the original cost of terrazzo plus the same maintenance costs as vinyl composition tile. It is interesting to note that terrazzo, with its high initial cost, is still a better buy than carpeting when amortized over 20 and 40 years.

CONCLUSION

Today we are fortunate to have an abundance of information regarding the impact environment has on health. When a decision seemingly unrelated to health, such as the choice of a school floor covering, can have such a tremendous effect on our children's well-being, school officials have a responsibility to address the issue adequately. If the number one priority of a school system is the health of the students and staff, the decision will be to install hard-surfaced floors. Fortunately, this decision does not compromise the common priorities of a lower cost, and a durable and easily maintained floor surface.

RECOMMENDED READINGS

Floor Coverings in Schools

Carpet and Indoor Air Quality in Schools, Technical Bulletin available from the Maryland State Dept. of Education, School Facilities Branch, 200 West Baltimore Street, Baltimore, Maryland 21201. Phone No. 410-333-2508.

Comparative Cost of School Floor Coverings, Environmental Education and Health Services, Inc., P.O. Box 92004, Austin, Texas 78709. Phone No. 512-288-2369.

Floor Coverings, General

"Abrams Announces Carpet Industry Agreement to Place Health Information Labels on New Carpets," November 1993, News from Attorney General Robert Abrams, Albany: Department of Law, The State Capitol.

Abrams, Robert, New York Attorney General; Jeffrey L. Amestoy, Vermont Attorney General; Richard Blumenthal, Connecticut Attorney General;

and Theodore R. Kulongoski, Oregon Attorney General, June 1993, *Carpets and Indoor Air: What you Should Know,* pp. 18-19.

Allen, Edward, 1985, *The Professional Handbook of Building Construction, New York, NY,* New York: John Wiley and Sons.

American Institute of Architects, July 1992, *AIA Environmental Resource Guide,* Washington, DC: American Institute of Architects.

American Lung Association, 1990, "Biological Agents," *Indoor Air Pollution Fact Sheet.*

Analyzing Carpet Chemicals, Indoor Air Quality Update, October 1990, Arlington, MA: Cutter Information Corp., vol. 3, no. 10, pp. 7-11.

Ashford, Nicholas A., and Claudia S. Miller, 1991, *Chemical Exposures, Low Levels and High Stakes,* New York: Van Nostrand Reinhold.

Bayer, Charlene, March 1991, "Carpet Policy Dialogue," *Progressive Architecture,* Stamford, CT: Penton Publishing, pp. 127-128.

Carpet and Indoor Air Quality in Schools, October 1993, Technical Bulletin, Baltimore: Maryland State Department of Education, Division of Business Services.

Carpet Emissions and Indoor Air, December, 1989, Indoor Air Quality Update, vol. 2, no. 12, Arlington, MA: Cutter Information Corp., pp. 1-6.

"Carpet Industry Program Steps Out Front on Indoor Air Quality: Labeling for Consumers Now Underway," July 1992, News Release, Dalton, GA: The Carpet and Rug Institute.

Carpeting in Schools, 1993, School Board meeting, Dade County School District, Dade County, Florida.

Carpets and Indoor Air, Indoor Air Bulletin, vol. 2, no. 6., Santa Cruz, CA.

Chemicals in New Carpets Pose Potential Health Hazard, April 1991, Consumer Alert, New York: Attorney General's Environmental Protection and Consumer Protection Bureaus and the Office of Public Information,.

Construction Details from Architectural Graphic Standards, Eighth edition, 1992, New York: John Wiley and Sons,.

Ellison, Donald C., W. C. Huntington, and Robert E. Mickodict, 1987, *Building Construction Materials and Type of Construction*. New York: John Wiley and Sons, Edition C.

EPA Carpet Dialogue Concludes, Indoor Air Bulletin 7-9, Santa Cruz, CA.

"Home Carpets: Shoeing in Toxic Pollution," August 11, 1990, *Science News*, vol. 138, no. 6, Washington, D.C.: Science Service, p. 86.

Installing Carpet Safely, December 1990, Indoor Air Quality Update, vol. 3, no 12, Arlington, MA: Cutter Information Corp., pp. 11-14.

Institute of Medicine, 1993, *Indoor Allergens, Assessing and Controlling Adverse Health Effects*, Washington, D. C.: National Academy Press.

Oetzel, Mary, October 1992, Updated March 1994, *"Comparative Cost of School Floor Coverings,"* Paper presented at the American Academy of Environmental Medicine Conference, Chicago.

"Problem Carpets Spur Calls for Action, EP Research Program," February 1993, Indoor Air Quality Update, vol. 6, no. 2, Arlington, MA: Cutter Information Corp., pp.1-6.

Progress on Carpets, May 1991, Indoor Air Quality Update, vol. 4, no. 5, Arlington, MA: Cutter Information Corp., pp. 1-5.

Rapp, Doris J., M.D., 1995, *Is Your School Safe for Students and Teachers?* Buffalo: Practical Allergy Research Foundation.

Roberts, John W., William T. Budd, Jane Chuang, and Robert G. Lewis, 1993, *Chemical Contaminants in House Dust: Occurences and Sources*, vol.2, Proceedings of the International Conference on Indoor Air Quality, Helsinki, Finland.

Taylor, Steven T., December 1993, "Carpet Industry Announces New Consumer IAQ Label Program," Bethesda, MD: *Indoor Air Review*, vol. III, no. 10, pp. 1, 13.

Taylor, Steven T., December 1993, "CRI President Explains 'Consumer Information' Carpet Label," Bethesda, MD: *Indoor Air Review*, vol. III, no. 10, p. 10.

Testimony Covering Carpet Studies Presented to the United States Senate Committee on Governmental Affairs, October 1, 1992, Dedham, MA: Anderson Laboratories, Inc.

10

ENLIGHTENED CLASSROOMS:
The Potential Adverse Effects of Artificial Lighting on Learning and Behavior in Children

by Irene Ruth Wilkenfeld

Although natural light has long been recognized as a powerful stimulus to learning, many schools have been built without adequate windows, and many students are still forced to carry on their learning activities in artificial light. In this chapter, Ms. Wilkenfeld presents a number of arguments for a more informed and positive approach to lighting in schools, and she answers questions teachers, administrators, and parents ask about the importance of light to children's learning.

☐ *How do we know that natural light is more conducive to learning than standard bulbs or fluorescent tubes?*

☐ *What are the symptoms of light deprivation?*

☐ *What effect does daylight have on hyperactivity?*

☐ *What is the effect of ultraviolet light in the classroom?*

☐ *How common is Seasonal Affective Disorder (SAD), and how does it hamper teaching and learning?*

Light is a powerful, but often overlooked, ally in the learning process. Regrettably, most of us have been kept in the dark about light deprivation, despite almost a century of compelling research on the subject. Indeed, it is troubling how little attention is being paid to something as basic as lighting in our nation's schools.

In the preface to his book, *The Influence of Ocular Light Perception on Metabolism in Man and in Animals*, Fritz Hollwich, M.D. writes, "Light is a primal element of life. Artificial light may be an optic substitute but it is by no means equivalent to nature's light in physiological terms." (Hollwich 1979) There is growing evidence in the scientific literature that living things react to natural light in unexpected ways and that artificial lighting can upset a host of delicate natural balances. By ignoring this primal role of natural light in our classroom environments, we just may be diminishing the effectiveness of all our other best educational efforts.

Many ancient cultures worshiped the sun as a supreme god, ascribing numerous healing properties to its full spectrum of light. Throughout history, most people have lived and worked primarily *outdoors* in natural, balanced sunlight. But in our urban, developed world, life has become an *indoor event.* We now spend our days under artificial light that bears little resemblance to the natural source. This dramatic lifestyle change is having subtle but significant effects on health and learning.

Most of us realize the benefits of a balanced diet, regular exercise, and adequate sleep. But few are aware of our daily requirement for natural light. People, like plants, need sunlight to thrive. Light, "the sunshine vitamin," is an essential nutrient, as important to our health as whole-some food, clean water, and fresh, unpolluted air. Without a balanced diet of light in our daily menu, we risk "malillumination," (a term coined by photobiologist, John Ott) just as we subject ourselves to malnutrition when we continue to indulge in an unbalanced diet. "When trace amounts of certain wavelengths of light are missing from your 'light diet' this can have a staggering effect on your health," says John Ott. (Liberman 1991)

Light synchronizes most body functions, and its absence or imbalance can cause a reduction in our physiological, emotional, and intellectual functioning. Light not only permits us to see, but through its stimulation of the pineal and hypothalamus glands, it also affects virtually every function of the body. The spectral properties of sunlight are fundamental to the endocrine system, biological clock, immune system, circulatory system, respiratory system, and sexual development; to the ability to control stress and fatigue; and to the healthy functioning of the nervous system. Prolonged exposure to artificial lighting has been associated with: irritability, eyestrain, headaches, fatigue, hyperactivity, allergies, frequent minor illnesses, inability to concentrate, vision problems, sus-ceptibility to osteoporosis and rickets, increased incidence of dental cavities, changes in heart rate, changes in blood pressure, changes in electrical brain wave patterns, changes in hormonal secretions and body rhythms, depression, alcoholism, suicide, weight gain, anxiety, and insomnia. Even just this partial list should raise our curiosity about the importance of light to optimum health, to disease prevention, and to the learning process.

Artificial light is very different from the natural light of the sun. It does not provide the stimulation needed for healthy functioning of the mind and body. Natural outdoor light is variable and subtle. It includes the whole range of visible colors: violet, indigo, blue, green, yellow, orange, red, as well as wavelengths invisible to the eye at either end of the spectrum (ultraviolet and infrared waves). Compare this subtle, balanced light to the harsh, glaring, piercing, flickering (60 times per second) light that overwhelms the senses of children bathed in artificial fluorescent light in classrooms across the country.

Artificial sources of light attempt but fail badly to duplicate the full spectrum of natural sunlight, which casts a broad, continuous rainbow of colors. Most indoor, artificial light tends to be weak in strength and density and *distorted* in terms of color. Most of us spend the majority of our waking hours drenched in light whose spectral characteristics differ markedly from those of sunlight.

Energy- and money-saving concerns have created classroom lighting conditions that foster the "sunlight starvation syndrome." The light distribution in our schools tends to be so deficient in most parts of the natural spectrum that we may just be fighting an uphill battle, attempting to teach students in "the twilight zone." It's time to acknowledge that light is a *cooperating teacher* in every classroom.

According to Richard J. Wurtman, M.D., *16 hours of artificial lighting provides less physical and emotional benefit than one hour of natural lighting!* Traditional indoor lighting supplies 50 to 100 footcandles of light. This accounts for less than 10% of the light normally found in the shade of an oak tree on a bright, sunny day. (Full sunlight on a clear day yields 10,000 footcandles.)

Not only does the incandescent bulb lack the intensity of sunlight, but also most of its light is in the yellow, orange, and red range. Conventional incandescent bulbs operate at relatively high temperatures and can cause problems for people suffering from allergies and asthma. The heat generated by the bulb can literally stir up and fry dust particles and other airborne contaminants, producing irritating particles and gases. In 1967, a full-spectrum "incandescent" bulb (Chromolux) was commissioned and developed by the Finnish government for vision improvement in schools, nursing homes, and hospitals. It claims to distribute a more balanced light that more closely simulates natural sunlight.

Fluorescent lights were first introduced commercially at the Worlds Fairs of 1938/39 in San Francisco and 1939/40 in New York. They were promptly accepted with enthusiasm and rapidly found their way into schools, factories, hospitals, and homes. Today the ubiquitous, institutional fluorescent light is the primary artificial light source in our nation's schools. It is cheaper and more efficient (yielding more light while consuming less energy) than incandescent bulbs which generate undue amounts of heat. But there's much more to this comparison than initially meets the eye.

Standard fluorescent lights, prevalent in our schools, provide a rather distorted spectrum of light that contains only a limited portion of the total spectrum. They can be made to give off virtually any color or mix of colors by blending different phosphors. These lights tend to concentrate energy in the blue, green, or yellow range, depending on the brand or variety. Many people attribute numerous unwelcome symptoms to the flicker, hum, and glare produced by these ever-present lights.

Full-spectrum fluorescent lights boast the closest solar match in commercially available tube lighting. Numerous researchers have called for their widespread use in schools. In some circles, they are credited with lowering bodily stress and improving health, mood, behavior, and learning.

The Color Rendering Index or CRI is a measurement of how closely a light duplicates the visible spectrum of sunlight. The CRI for sunlight is 100; 99 for a Chromolux full-spectrum incandescent bulb; 91 for the most popular brand of full-spectrum fluorescent lights (about which we will have much more to say); 90 for incandescent bulbs; 68 for cool-white fluorescent lights; and 52 for warm-white fluorescents.

LIGHT AND LEARNING

Jacob Liberman, O.D., Ph.D., in his book *Light: Medicine of the Future*, describes the groundbreaking work of Dr. Darell Boyd Harmon and his 1951 publication, *The Coordinated Classroom*, as "the most comprehensive, yet least known, study on the effects of lighting on human functioning and development." Harmon was a specialist in the growth and development of school children with an emphasis on the environmentally- and visually-centered aspects of learning. He served as Director of the Division of School Services for the Texas State Department of Health for 10 years. Under his supervision, in January 1938, the Department launched a long-range project in child development as part of its services for protecting and promoting the health of school children. A network of professionals including the Committee on Child Health of the Texas State Teachers Association, the State Medical Association of Texas, the Texas State Dental Society, the Illuminating Engineering Society, and the Texas Society of Architects, formed the Texas Inter-Professional Commission on Child Development. (Liberman 1991)

This project involved the screening of 160,000 children in 4,000 schools in the state. During the first three years of the program, an inventory was assembled of the physical, psychological, and educational difficulties afflicting Texas school children. Classroom factors that might be related to those difficulties were reviewed. An initial analysis of the resulting data revealed that by the time children graduated from grade school, over 50% of them had an average of two recognizable but preventable deficiencies. *Many of these deficiencies, including distorted writing and drawing and problems of educational performance, were found to be light-related.* When lighting was adjusted, many of the observed educational problems were drastically reduced both in number and severity.

Harmon's study implicated improper classroom lighting as a potent bodily *stressor* that forces the child to expend undue energy in his/her attempts to adapt to the classroom environment. For example, Harmon reported that attempts to adapt to or overcome glare, stressed the back and head; rendered bodies out of balance; disturbed proper eye-hand coordination; and squandered energy that should be devoted to classwork and diverted it from the task at hand, merely to compensate for some of the adverse factors in the classroom environment.

In the fall of 1942, under Harmon's administration, an experimental center was set up at the Becker School in Austin, Texas, for the purpose of determining the ideal lighting, seating, and decor that would maximize school performance. The children involved in the project were given thorough pediatric, dental, and psychological examinations. Nutritional, visual, and educational tests were administered. Medical, dietary, and social histories were collected. And physical characteristics of the classrooms were manipulated in detail.

Twenty-one classrooms in the building were rearranged and redecorated to free them from *light stress*. A group of matched control students in a comparable building but with no lighting or seating changes, was selected for the experiment. And in May 1943, six months after the remodeling, the children were retested. The noteworthy results can be seen in *Figure 10-1*. Notice the dramatic reductions in every category, with an astounding decrease of 65% in visual difficulties leading the list.

Problem	% 11/42	% 5/43	% Change
Visual Difficulties	55.3	18.6	-65.0
Nutritional Problems	71.3	37.2	-47.8
Chronic Problems	75.2	42.6	-43.3
Posture Problems	30.2	22.4	-25.6
Chronic Fatigue	20.9	9.3	-55.6

Figure 10-1.

Comparison of some health problems observed by D. B. Harmon at the beginning and end of the six-month experimental period (November 1942 through May 1943) at the Becker School in Austin, Texas.

Comparable changes were seen in educational achievement as well. After functioning in the improved classrooms for six months, the children in the Becker school advanced a mean average of 10.2 months in educational age. Seventy-six percent of the children grew educationally more than six months of educational age in the six-calendar-month interval. In the control classrooms, the mean educational growth was 6.8 months of educational age. Only 33.4% of the children in the control group grew educationally more than six months of educational age. Harmon's "Coordinated Classroom" experiment demonstrated *the undeniable relationship between the lighting in a child's classroom environment and his or her health and learning.*

The field of photobiology in the classroom was further expanded at this time by the work of Dr. T. A. Brombach, a respected vision researcher who found that 69% of children with reading disabilities had a measurable enlargement of the *blind spot*, a portion of the optic nerve at the retina. Brombach's work was corroborated by the efforts of Thomas Eames, M.D., of Boston University, who studied constricted fields of vision in school children. He found that 9% of the students in his study had this vision disorder. And of that 9%, a disproportionate 83% were failing in their schoolwork. He discovered also that children with learning disabilities consistently had smaller visual fields than their peers. And he explained this disparity by observing that visual field constrictions significantly limited the speed of visual perception or reading. He noted that the chief complaints among these educationally challenged youths were poor reading ability, poor spelling, poor writing, and generally poor schoolwork. After treatment, which included remedial education measures in the form of flashcard drills requiring recognition of progressively larger and larger flashed units, there appeared to be a correlation between an increase in the visual field and improved school performance.

The work of both these researchers (Brombach and Eames) is closely connected because it is now accepted that a visual field constriction is often associated with an enlargement of the blind spot. And both scientists used visual field size as a major diagnostic and prognostic indicator of problems affecting classroom performance. In 1954, Virginia I. Shipman, presented her paper entitled "A Constriction of the Perceptual Field Under Stress" at the Eastern Psychological Association in Philadelphia, saying that stress causes constriction of the perceptual field, forcing a patient to "observe less, see less, remember less, learn less, and become generally less efficient." Anyone struggling with this deficit is likely to have the feeling of *being lost in space*, a description educators often apply to their learning-disabled children. And this all relates to the classroom when we are reminded that *inadequate classroom lighting is a potent stressor*. (See *Figure 10-2*.)

Jacob Liberman designed a controlled study of his own which was published in the *Journal of Optometric Vision Development*, in June of 1986. In "The Effect of Syntonic Colored Light Stimulation on Certain Visual and Cognitive Functions," he demonstrated that, using light therapy, the visual field, visual attention, visual memory, and auditory memory of students facing academic difficulty could be dramatically

PHOTOBIOLOGY IN THE CLASSROOM

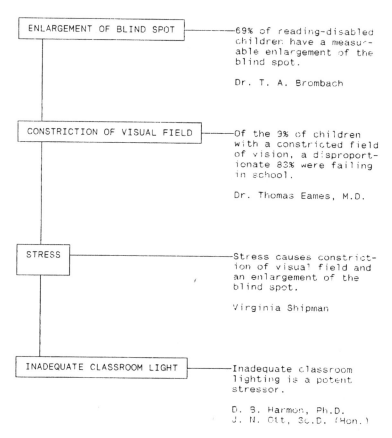

ENLARGEMENT OF BLIND SPOT ——————69% of reading-disabled children have a measurable enlargement of the blind spot.

Dr. T. A. Brombach

CONSTRICTION OF VISUAL FIELD ——————Of the 9% of children with a constricted field of vision, a disproportionate 83% were failing in school.

Dr. Thomas Eames, M.D.

STRESS ——————Stress causes constriction of visual field and an enlargement of the blind spot.

Virginia Shipman

INADEQUATE CLASSROOM LIGHT ——————Inadequate classroom lighting is a potent stressor.

D. B. Harmon, Ph.D.
J. N. Ott, Sc.D. (Hon.)

Figure 10-2.
Photobiology in the classroom.

improved. Withdrawn children came out of their shells, hyperkinetic ones calmed down, weaning themselves from Ritalin in the process, and there was an overall 75% improvement in academic achievement.

This concept was further elaborated in 1989 by Mark Anderson, Ph.D. of Beloit College and Jean Williams, Ph.D. of the University of Arizona. Their work confirmed that stress directly impacts the peripheral field of vision, thus reducing how much we see. And they identified schoolwork, in general, and reading, in particular, as the most visually demanding and stressful tasks with which we have to contend.

Given all this compelling evidence, it makes no sense to invite standard fluorescent lights, a known stressor, into the classroom to undermine the learning process. Growing numbers of experts tell us that full-spectrum lights exert significantly less stress on the nervous system, enhance productivity, and even reduce the number of absences due to illness.

THE PIONEERING WORK OF JOHN OTT

John Nash Ott, Sc.D. (Hon.), a self-made photobiologist and trailblazing researcher, has given us an enormous fund of knowledge in the field of malillumination. While doing time-lapse photography for the Disney Studios, Ott noticed that the spectral quality of light is critical to plants, to animals, and to humans. One unifying thread links all his diverse experiments together: *light is a vital nutrient.* The kinds and intensities of light to which a living organism is exposed, have a great deal to do with its health and behavior.

Dr. Ott believes that "humans are photosynthetic." He postulates that full-spectrum light acts as the ignition switch for all human biological functions. "The light-mediated process known as photosynthesis in plants is, in my opinion, the same thing as METABOLISM in humans." (Liberman 1991) Ott's experiments indicate the life-altering effects of specific wavelengths of light on the cells of plants and animals. He observed that:

- Pumpkin seedlings would not mature fully under fluorescent lights.

- Plant cells (Elodea) can be made to move in different, random directions by exposing them to different colored lights. Is this comparable to hyperactivity and/or anxiety in humans?

- The plant cell wall weakens under adverse lighting conditions. Is this comparable to a breakdown of the immune system in humans?

- Male rodents kept under standard fluorescent lights tended to be irritable and to cannibalize their young. When kept in natural sunlight, they were docile and friendly, and were actually seen to care for the litter.

- Rats placed in front of a TV set initially became hyperactive and aggressive. Eventually, lethargy set in and they ALL died. Rats placed in front of a lead-shielded TV all remained normal.

- There was a dramatic difference in the life spans of his experimental animals. Mice living under pink fluorescents lived an average of 7.5 months. Those exposed to natural sunlight survived for 16.1 months, on average.

Furthermore, Ott believes that:

- Light determines the sex of plants, fish, and some animals (for example, chinchillas).

- Light can impact life span, demeanor, and tumor development in laboratory mice.

John Ott theorizes that these and other altered growth and behavioral responses may be due to the *absence* of wavelengths in artificial light; that the lack of a specific wavelength causes a biochemical or hormonal deficiency. If we remember that Ott considers light an essential nutrient, it follows that malillumination is similar to malnutrition, which occurs when there is a specific deficiency in the diet.

OTT'S CLASSROOM EXPERIMENT

In 1960, Ott was instrumental in the development of commercially available full-spectrum fluorescent lights—Vita-Lite for the Duro-Test Corporation—that more closely duplicate the spectral qualities of natural daylight. He attempted to evaluate the impact of these lights on health and classroom performance, when in 1973, under the auspices of the Environmental Health and Light Research Institute, he engaged in a five-month-long study involving four first-grade classes at the Gocio School in Sarasota, Florida. He installed full-spectrum, radiation-shielded, fluorescent light fixtures in two windowless classrooms, each containing 49 students. Standard cool-white tubes (Westinghouse F40CW, 40 watt—4 bulbs per fixture) were installed in two other identical rooms, which served as controls. Box shelters were constructed to conceal hidden time-lapse cameras. Some five times throughout the semester, from January through June 1973, 16mm cameras photographed the activity in the classroom in random sequence. Neither students nor teachers were aware of being photographed .

Dr. Lewis Mayron, a biochemist with the Veterans Administration Hospital in Hines, Illinois, analyzed the study and attributed the improvements achieved to the installation of the alternative lights. Under the full-spectrum lights, and without the use of any prescribed mood-altering drugs, behavior, performance, and academic achievement improved markedly within one month. Likewise, disciplinary referrals and absenteeism diminished. Several learning-disabled children, previously labeled hyperactive, calmed down noticeably, and seemed to overcome their learning and reading problems. Those children in the control room, under standard cool-white fluorescent lighting demonstrated nervous fatigue, irritability, lapses in attention, and hyperactive behavior (fidgeting, leaping from seats, flailing arms). Ott's Gocio School Experiment clearly indicated *a correlation between light and educational performance*.

An unexpected benefit of full-spectrum lighting was reported by the Sarasota County Dental Society. The children in the test group at the Gocio School developed only one-third the number of cavities in their teeth compared to the control group. And the severity of the decay found was 10 times worse in those children under cool-white fluorescent lights. Similar findings were disclosed by a group of Canadian researchers at the University of Alberta in Edmonton. They speculate that *sunshine favorably affects dental health* by:

■ Increasing the availability of vitamin D, which is essential for normal calcification of teeth.

■ Increasing saliva, which helps wash away food particles in the mouth, thereby reducing plaque.

Results similar to those obtained from the Gocio School experiment have been reported in other studies conducted in two schools in California (1975) and later in Washington state. Burnis Lyons, a teacher of autistic and emotionally disturbed youngsters at Green Acres Elementary School in Santa Cruz, California, turned off the fluorescent lights in her classroom and substituted incandescent lights. *Hyperactive behavior* (including jumping, inappropriate walking around the room, standing on chairs, yelling, clapping, hitting, grabbing another's possessions, and disruptive behavior eliciting a reprimand) *decreased by 32.3%*. Originally there had been 297 hyperactive incidents recorded. When the fluorescent lights were extinguished, only 201 incidents were observed. One extremely hyperactive child, usually unable to control his behavior, calmed down and sat for six minutes, giving his full attention to his teacher! Again in Santa Cruz, teachers at the Bonnie Doon Elementary School noticed positive results when two classes were transferred to an older portion of the facility with incandescent lights. Students exhibited fewer instances of headaches, nausea, and irritability, compared with the previous year when they were assigned to rooms lit by standard fluorescent lights.

Judith Bartholomew Raiter and Judy Thut, teachers in an elementary school in Longview, Washington (1976) engaged in a small research project on the effects of fluorescent lighting versus natural window lighting on the behavior of second-grade students. They concluded that the "students spent a statistically significant greater amount of time in attentive behavior during the time the fluorescent lights were shut off." (Ott 1986)

Despite all this compelling evidence about the light-learning link, John Ott is troubled that educators have not heeded the obvious implications. In a personal telephone conversation, on February 17, 1992 he said, "Educators are unbelievably resistant to the benefits of light in the classroom."

STANDARD FLUORESCENT LIGHTS, X-RAYS, AND HYPERACTIVITY

In his book *Light, Radiation and You*, John Ott strongly urges us to pay closer attention to the importance of trace amounts of radiation as a significant environmental exposure. It is Ott's hypothesis that *conventional fluorescent lights give off stressful X-rays capable of triggering hyperactivity*. He feels that electrical stresses caused by ordinary fluorescent lights can decrease muscle strength, suppress the immune system, and adversely affect the brain and its ability to function at full capacity.

Ott's assumption that radio waves emanating from standard fluorescent lights might contribute to hyperactivity is based, in part, on research by Allan Frey, a biophysicist with Randomline, Inc., Willow Grove, Pennsylvania. Frey observed that animals experienced changes in behavior and transient shifts in their central nervous systems after they were exposed to radio and television frequencies. This issue of low-grade radiation toxicity of neurological tissue was further explored by Gordon in a paper in *Science* and by Korbel and Thompson in *Psychological Reports*. Gordon found that radio fields caused an accumulation of acetylcholine (an important neurotransmitter in the brain) along nerve fibers. A build-up of acetylcholine can lead to hyperactivity. (Gordon 1961; Korbel and Thompson 1965)

Ott's contention connecting X-rays (from conventional fluorescent lights) and hyperactivity, also resulted from personal observations made during his filming of geraniums for the Barbra Streisand film, *On A Clear Day You Can See Forever*. He noticed that the flowers grown near the cathode ends of the fluorescent lights did poorly when compared to those located at the center of the tubes. He also observed stunted, irregular growth patterns in bean seedlings exposed to X-rays and increased aggression in laboratory animals nurtured under unshielded fluorescent lights. As part of his rodent experiments, Ott made slides of brain tissue taken from the unprotected animals. They showed evidence of multiple lesions of the thalamus and possible demyelination of nerves. (Myelin is a fatlike substance that forms a protective cover around certain brain structures.)

Because of his concerns about X-ray exposure from fluorescent lights, Ott further modified the full-spectrum Vita-Lite (without the support of the Duro-Test Corporation) by adding lead shielding to screen out harmful radiation from the cathode ends of his tubes. (Similar results can be obtained by wrapping two inches of a lead-foil tape around each end of the cathodes of a full-spectrum tube. The tape, which is available from the 3M Corporation, *should not touch* the metal.) Ott's adapted tube, on the market since 1983, is sold under the name Ott-Lite. It also contains an auxiliary black light tube, as a source of ultraviolet light.

THE ULTRAVIOLET CONTROVERSY

It is widely accepted that too much ultraviolet light (UV) is harmful. It has been implicated in sunburn; dry, wrinkled, leathery skin; skin cancer; and cataracts. This is especially true of the *short-wavelength UV* (sometimes referred to as *far UV*), those wavelengths next to X-rays. The vast majority of this kind of ultraviolet light is typically filtered out of sunlight by the atmosphere, by the upper ozone layer, and by ordinary glass. But John Ott believes we've gone overboard in our efforts to protect ourselves from the hazards of ultraviolet light. In *Light, Radiation and You*, he writes:

> When it was discovered that the little extra oxygen given to premature babies in their incubators caused blindness, brain tissue damage, deafness, and other abnormalities, the practice was discontinued. Fortunately, no one jumped to the conclusion that this proved oxygen hazardous to one's health, therefore, henceforth everyone should learn to live without oxygen. As ridiculous as this sounds, it is, nevertheless, exactly what is happening with

regards [sic] to ultraviolet light. There is no doubt that too much ultraviolet can be harmful, but in so completely protecting ourselves from any trace of it, I believe we are creating a deficiency of important life-supporting energy. (Ott 1982, p. 173)

John Ott advocates the inclusion of modest amounts of *near UV* or *long-wavelength UV,* in a visually balanced solar-like spectrum. These wavelengths can be found right next to the violet part of visible light. Zane R. Kime, M.D., in his book *Sunlight* wrote, "The most 'biologically active' part of sunlight is the ultraviolet. It is absolutely critical for optimal health." And Jacob Liberman, O.D., Ph.D. takes it a step farther when he writes, "There should be a recommended daily allowance (RDA) for UV light just as there is for Vitamin C!" (Kime 1980; Liberman 1991)

Ultraviolet light is a biologically crucial component of sunlight, but we rarely receive any of it indoors. It is virtually absent from incandescent lighting, shielded in standard fluorescent tubes, and blocked by normal window-pane glass and eyeglass lenses. In *Light, Color, and Environment*, Faber Birren (1982) credits UV light with stimulating blood circulation, lowering blood pressure, preventing rickets, increasing protein metabolism, decreasing fatigue, stimulating glandular activity, stimulating white blood cell activity, increasing the release of endorphins, and enhancing the production of Vitamin D, thereby increasing absorption of calcium and phosphorus.

In *Health and Light*, John Ott's report on a serious outbreak of the Hong Kong flu that swept the United States in 1968-1969, giving credence to the benefits of UV light, the Florida Health Department reveals that some 6,000 people----5% of the population of Sarasota County—were affected by the flu. Many businesses had to close temporarily, due to employee illness. Obrig Laboratories, a large manufacturer of contact lenses, employing 100 workers, was the exception. *Throughout the flu epidemic, not a single employee missed a day of work due to flu-related problems.* Shortly before the flu outbreak, Obrig Labs had designed a new building using full-spectrum lighting and ultraviolet-transmitting plastic window panes throughout their facility. At this same time, worker productivity was reported to be up by at least 25%. And it was the general consensus that everyone was much more cheerful and in better spirits after the newly constructed building was put into operation.

UV light is beneficial to children as well. In *Healing Environments*, Carol Venolia writes, "Youngsters who receive the UV light, so often missing indoors, tend to have fewer colds, grow faster, and have better mental and physical development than those who don't." (Venolia 1988)

In a paper entitled "Effect of Irradiation by Ultraviolet Erythema Lamps on the Working Ability of School Children" by M. A. Zamkova and E. I. Krivitskaya, of the Department of Psychoneurology and Hygiene at the Pedagogical Institute of Leningrad, the Soviet scientists reported that UV light had a favorable effect on the health and physical development of school children. They concluded that UV light raised the level of the students' academic ability and increased resistance to fatigue. (Zamova and Krivitskaya 1966)

Professor Harry Wohlfarth of the University of Alberta, under the auspices of the Alberta Education System, published the report "Colour and Light Effects on Students' Achievement, Behaviour and Physiology" in May of 1986. It compared the rate of school absences in two groups of students. The control group of 19 students, exposed to standard fluorescent light, registered *311 absences* over the school year. By comparison, the 20 students exposed to supplemental UV light, experienced only *138 absences* over that same period.

Also in the 1980's, Jerome Werlin, director of The Living Light Center at the Overbrook School for the Blind in Philadelphia noticed a measurable calming effect on his hyperactive students from the ultraviolet light, making it possible to reduce their dependence on prescription medication. If as reported by John Ott and others, the inclusion of healthful amounts of UV light in a classroom environment can stimulate the immune system; can reduce fatigue, headache, hyperactivity, and absenteeism; and can increase productivity and performance, I think we need to advocate aggressively the use of UV light therapeutically in our nation's classrooms. The evidence to support these claims is very compelling.

CORROBORATING RESEARCH

In a pioneering study at Cornell University, published in 1974, psychologist James B. Maas and his associates, compared the fatigue levels of student volunteers who studied for four hours under standard cool-white fluorescent lights with those who used full-spectrum lights. While the students seemed unable to detect any significant differences between the lighting conditions, objective measurements revealed less fatigue and better visual acuity in the full-spectrum group. Dr. H. Richard

Blackwell, professor emeritus of Ohio State University, supported Maas' findings by doing studies of his own. They showed that worker productivity increased by 11.7% under full-spectrum lighting. (Maas and Kleiber 1974)

In her book, *The Healing Environment*, Cristina Ismael reports that standard fluorescent lights made students self-conscious and less than receptive to instruction. By turning off these lights, her students seemed more willing to interact with one another, and more cooperative in a meaningful way.

In 1978, H. Ertel found that using bright, warm colors like yellow and orange on the walls of classrooms significantly improved the IQ and academic performance of school children. Dr. Harry Wohlfarth, considered one of the world's leading color researchers, decided to build on Ertel's work, by conducting a series of experiments to evaluate the effects of light and color in the classroom. In 1981, he studied the effects of color and full-spectrum lighting on the behavior and performance of a group of handicapped youngsters at the Elves Memorial Child Development Centre in Edmonton, Alberta, Canada. He revealed that blood pressure dropped and aggressive behavior diminished dramatically. In yet another study (1982-83), conducted at four matched elementary schools in Wetaskiwin, Alberta, Canada, Wohlfarth confirmed his earlier observations of the impact of color and light. In the school outfitted with both full-spectrum lights and warm colors, he found the students to be less stressed, quieter, and less moody. These students had the best results on IQ and achievement tests and were absent due to illness only one-third as often as their peers in the other schools. (For permission to use Dr. Wohlfarth's recommended classroom paint colors, you are invited to contact him at: Colorpsychodynamic Design, Ltd., 11025-82nd. Ave., Edmonton, Alberta, Canada T6G 0T1.)

In 1980, Dr. Fritz Hollwich, an international authority on the influence of light on the human body, demonstrated that *cool-white fluorescent lights cause a significant biological disturbance of the body's stress hormones which can result in behavioral difficulties.* In a study comparing the impact of exposure to either cool-white or full-spectrum lights, Hollwich found increased levels of ACTH and cortisol (the stress hormones) in individuals sitting under cool-white lights. No such changes were registered in those in the full-spectrum test group. Hollwich's research confirms the work of John Ott and others categorizing standard fluorescent lights as a stress factor leading to agitated hyperactivity, fatigue, and reduced classroom performance. It is important to note that, based on Hollwich's work, cool-white tubes were legally banned in German hospitals and medical facilities.

Richard J. Wurtman, M.D., director of the neuroendocrine laboratory at the Massachusetts Institute of Technology, and Robert Neer, a medical researcher at the Massachusetts General Hospital, issued an important report in 1981 suggesting that light is vastly more important than food as a source of vitamin D, so critical in bone mineralization. It is widely accepted that the body's ability to absorb calcium and phosphorus is necessary for the proper development and maintenance of healthy bones and teeth. Full-spectrum light reaching the skin acts as a catalyst for a series of reactions in the body, leading to the production of Vitamin D, a prerequisite for the absorption and utilization of calcium. (This type of Vitamin D, synthesized by the skin on exposure to light, is nontoxic, unlike that found in dietary Vitamin D supplements, which can accumulate in the body fat.) And it should be pointed out that a Vitamin D deficiency (responsible for osteoporosis and osteomalacia, a softening of bone in adults) can cause rickets, dental cavities, and plaque build-up, in children.

In her book, *Do You Really Need Glasses,* self-published in 1985, Marilyn B. Rosanes-Berrett, Ph.D. writes, "There is a very close relationship between our emotional state and visual acuity. Vision will tend to be relatively poor at the end of a tiring day, keener in the morning when we feel refreshed."

This mimics the much earlier work of behavioral ophthalmologist, William H. Bates, M.D. (1860-1931) who identified the correlation of tension and reduced visual acuity. As we've seen repeatedly, fluorescent lights cause both stress and fatigue. As such, they have no place in the classroom, where much of the learning is dependent on healthy vision.

The November 21, 1987, issue of *The Lancet* reported on a study in an elementary school in Brattleboro, Vermont, conducted by Dr. Wayne London. It suggested that full-spectrum lighting may reduce sickness and absenteeism. The students at this particular school exhibited a 24% reduction in sick days, after the installation of full spectrum lights.

SEASONAL AFFECTIVE DISORDER (SAD)

In 1962, the Ingmar Bergman film *Winter Light* depicted a character plunged into the doldrums during a bleak Scandinavian winter. More than 10 million Americans suffer from a related affliction, called *Seasonal Affective Disorder* or *SAD*, according to Dr. Norman E. Rosenthal, chief psychiatric researcher at the National Institute of Mental Health (NIMH) in Bethesda, Maryland. This debilitating syndrome is directly related to *light*.

It is believed that winter's feeble light rays, some 70% weaker in intensity and duration than summer sunlight, are responsible for the deep depression experienced by 5% of the population and for the less serious *winter blahs* familiar to some 30% to 40% of us. SAD patients complain of sleep disorders, fatigue, headaches, digestive problems, food cravings, weight gain, an uncharacteristic desire to withdraw from social interactions, a general malaise, severe depression, and even suicidal feelings.

Photobiologists attribute SAD to disturbances in light cycles that interrupt the body's circadian rhythms. These rhythms are synchronized by exposure to the daily intervals of light and dark. Did you ever wonder how a bear knows when to hibernate or when to wake up? All animal behavior—feeding, sleeping, breeding—is controlled by the rotation of the earth around the sun and the resulting solar light fluctuations. Artificial or inadequate lighting literally confuses nature's body clock, disrupts the pre-established harmonious patterns, and thrusts many into deep despair. This form of *light stress* can cause biochemical changes in the human body identical to those caused by physical stress.

The issue of SAD is pertinent to any discussion about school children because of a very disturbing emerging observation. Teen depression is more prevalent than ever before. Teenagers are being admitted to psychiatric hospitals in record numbers. More than 5,000 young Americans kill themselves every year, making suicide the third leading cause of death for young adults. This rate has tripled in the last 30 years. And all this may, in some part, be a function of the SAD syndrome, a problem too often overlooked by medical specialists when treating dysfunctional youngsters in distress.

Dr. Thomas A. Wehr of NIMH believes that SAD has "a tremendous impact on children's ability to function in school. They start out the school year fairly strong, thinking they will enjoy it. In November, it starts to fall apart. They sleep 12 hours a day. They're not creative. They've lost the spark. Those with winter depression are slowed down. Their behaviors include overeating, oversleeping and sluggishness." (Ubell 1991.)

Others report an increased incidence of anxiety and irritability, an inability to tolerate stress, difficulty getting started in the morning, crying spells, and an overall decrease in activity levels, specifically during the fall semester. *Why is this happening?*

For the answers, we need to take a look at the pineal gland, the light meter and conductor that orchestrates our body clocks. This little known, pea-sized master gland, shaped like a pine-cone, is located deep in the center of the brain between the two hemispheres and behind and above the pituitary gland. It is our internal clock, coordinating our entire physiological relationship with the external environment. This gland's hormonal messages have a profound impact on mind, mood, and body. It plays a vital role in virtually every aspect of human function, regulating reproduction, growth, body temperature, blood pressure, motor activity, sleep, tumor growth, mood, immune function, and even longevity. And interestingly, *the activity of the pineal gland is governed by environmental light.*

The pineal gland is responsible for the night-time production of the hormone *melatonin*. Increasingly longer hours of darkness during the winter months trigger its increased output. As daylight diminishes, the pineal gland signals for more melatonin, which works like the substances that tell the bear when to hibernate. It induces sleep, modifies the secretions of other glands, and acts on the neuroendocrine control centers in the brain, producing sluggishness and an emotional downturn. *Light exposure----2,500 lux of light intensity---is required to **stop** the oversupply of melatonin.* (A bright sunny day supplies 100,000 lux.) Conventional light at standard indoor levels is interpreted by the pineal as *darkness* and is often inadequate to suppress melatonin production.

What is the prescribed treatment for SAD? *Full-spectrum lights* have been proven capable of deactivating the melatonin-induced melancholia of this debilitating illness, giving the patients a natural high. In 1985, Dr. Norman E. Rosenthal, mentioned earlier as a SAD researcher at NIMH, reported at the American Psychiatric Association convention in Dallas on school children who appear to be suffering from SAD. He treated four boys and two girls, ages 6 through 14, who were having school achievement problems and troubling fatigue during the fall semester. He exposed the children to a daily regimen of full-spectrum light in the early morning and evening. Five of the six patients exhibited a favorable response to the light therapy.

It should be clear now, that artificial light is capable of disrupting hormonal levels, which may have serious implications for our mental health. Indeed, MIT psychologist Harris Lieberman found that larger than normal doses of melatonin could produce drowsiness and significant reductions in reaction time in healthy young volunteers. He concluded that melatonin has "significant sedative-like properties." (Smith 1986) Due to our indoor-oriented lifestyles and our reliance on inferior sources of classroom lighting, it's safe to say that even if the majority of our students are not suffering from Seasonal Affective Disorder, many of them just may be living in "a melatonin haze." In any case, the evidence of the SAD researchers indicates that educators, counselors, clinicians, and parents must actively consider the possibility of SAD whenever diagnosing and treating youngsters for school-related problems.

COST EFFECTIVENESS OF FULL-SPECTRUM LIGHTS

The issue of *cost effectiveness* undoubtedly emerges when the subject of the installation of full-spectrum lights in a school is raised. In personal conversation with Edward Remington, a representative of the Duro-Test Corporation, I was pleased to learn that, on average, the cheaper, standard fluorescent tube will need to be replaced more than seven times before its full-spectrum counterpart. So, while initial installation costs are admittedly quite high, the bulbs are very cost-effective long-term. How do you put a price tag on a student body that feels better, is more alert and more relaxed, has better visual acuity and less eyestrain, and is more productive? Why, if you advertised these qualities and told school officials that such a product were readily available in a box in their local hardware store, I'll bet you couldn't keep full-spectrum lights on the shelves.

IN CONCLUSION

Very little has been done to protect citizens in general and students in particular from the potentially harmful effects of inadequate lighting. Richard J. Wurtman, M.D., Ph.D addressed this issue in his article, "The Effects of Light on the Human Body." He wrote, "Both government and industry have been satisfied to allow people who buy electric lamps, to serve as unwitting subjects in a long-term experiment on the effects of artificial lighting environments on human health. One hopes that this casual attitude will change. *Light is potentially too useful an agency of human health not to be more effectively examined and exploited*." (Wurtman 1975)

The 14th Amendment guarantees the right of an optimal education to every child according to his or her ability. It makes no sense to spend billions of dollars on education and then stack the cards against educational success by ignoring the issue of polluted light. With our increased interest in ecology, we need to add another priority to our growing list of concerns----*environmental light deprivation*. You wouldn't expect an undernourished child to excel in school any more than you would bet on the child hopping on one foot to win the 50-yard dash. And likewise, we can't presume that an unbalanced, light-deprived school environment can sustain educational excellence. Light deprivation in the classroom, in a very real sense, denies our students the pursuit of happiness.

Clearly, no comprehensive plan for educational reform can be complete without assessing light distribution in our schools. "Only by a blinding prejudice of an inexcusable egoism can man ignore the overpowering influences of sunlight and skylight." (Luckish 1946)

A WORD OF CAUTION

Hazards from exposure to harmful insulating materials in older buildings are a widely recognized problem. The National Institute of Occupational Safety and Health (NIOSH) has recently identified a previously unrecognized danger related to fluorescent lights in the classroom. In fluorescent lamp ballasts----the electronic devices that start the lamp and protect the fixture from variations in electrical voltage----manufactured before 1978, the capacitor contains an insulating fluid made of PCBs (polychlorinated biphenyls). During a ballast burnout, when an electrical malfunction dramatically increases the temperature within the ballast, PCBs may leak from the fixture. After a burnout, PCBs can remain in the air and on room surfaces at unhealthful concentrations for months under normal ventilation conditions. PCBs are considered potential carcinogens. And NIOSH recommends that exposures be controlled to the lowest feasible level (LFL) or 1 ug/m3.

The best way to reduce PCB contamination in schools is to prevent exposure before it happens. *NIOSH recommends that schools routinely replace old ballasts with PCB-free varieties manufactured after 1978.* (The average lifespan of a ballast is 12 years, but burnout is not uncommon earlier.) Some local power companies offer incentives for the installation of the newer, energy-efficient, PCB-free ballasts. For identification purposes, the EPA requires that PCB-safe fluorescent light ballasts be imprinted with the words, "NO PCBs."

Possible health effects from PCB exposure include acute symptoms: headache, eye irritation, sore throat, nasal congestion, and nausea. Undetected chronic exposure can result in neurotoxic and carcinogenic disorders. From 1981 to the present, surveys of schools in Cincinnati, Seattle, and Cross Lanes, West Virginia, have discovered PCB contamination in classrooms where these older ballasts had burned out. In Stanton, Delaware and in Detroit, Michigan, teachers and students experienced acute eye, nose, and throat irritation from PCBs leaking out of tubes subject to ballast burnout.

It is critical that school officials familiarize themselves with the proper procedures to follow should a ballast fail in a classroom. *Turn the lights off and evacuate immediately.* No one should return to the classroom until remediation has been achieved, under professional supervision. For complete information on PCBs in ballasts contact:

NIOSH
Hazard Evaluation & Technical Assistance Branch
4676 Columbia Parkway
Cincinnati, OH 47226
1-800-35NIOSH

REFERENCES

Arehart-Treichel, J., 1974, "School Lights & Problem Pupils (Hyperactivity may be stimulated by certain kinds of fluorescent lights in schools)," *Science News,* 105: 258-259.

Birren, F. 1982, *Light, Color & Environment*, New York: Van Nostrand Reinhold Company.

Buffington, P., 1987, "Lighten Up!" *Sky,* Atlanta, GA: Delta Airlines, no. 7: 38-41.

Crandall, M., L. Elliott, A. Votaw, 1990, "PCBs—Ballast Burnout in Schools," *Applied Occupational & Environmental Hygiene* 5, no. 9: 580-82.

Eames, T. H., 1936, "Restrictions of the Visual Field as Handicaps to Learning," *Journal of Educational Research*, no. 2: 460-63.

Fishman, G., 1986, "Ocular Phototoxicity: Guidelines for Selecting Sunglasses," *Survey of Ophthalmology* 31, no. 2.

Harmon, D. B., 1951, *The Coordinated Classroom*, Grand Rapids, MI: American Seating Company.

Hollwich, F. 1979, *The Influence of Ocular Light Perception on Metabolism in Man and in Animals*, New York: Springer-Verlag.

Ismael, Cristina, 1976, *The Healing Environment*, Millbrae, CA: Celestial Arts.

Kime, Z., 1980, *Sunlight,* Penryn, CA: World Health Publications.

Kosta, L., 1989, "Sunlight & You," *The Human Ecologist*, no. 43: 10-13.

Kotzsch, R., 1989, "Bringing the Sun Indoors," *East/West Journal*, no. 3: 48-52, 75-78.

Liberman, J., 1991, *LIGHT: Medicine of the Future*, Santa Fe, NM: Bear & Company Publishing.

Liebmann-Smith, R., 1985, "The Man Who Patented Sunlight," *American Health*, no. 12: 32-35.

Luckiesh, M. 1946, *Applications of Germicidal Erythema & Infrared Energy*, New York: Van Nostrand Reinhold Company.

Maas, J. B., and D. Kleiber, 1974, "Effects of Spectral Differences in Illumination on Fatigue," *Journal of Applied Psychology* 59, no. 4: 525-26.

Mayron, L., 1978, "Ecological Factors in Learning Disabilities," *Journal of Learning Disabilities* 11, no. 8: 40-47.

Ott, J. N., 1973, *Health and Light*, Greenwich, CT: Devin-Adair.

Ott, J. N., 1982, *Light, Radiation and You*, Greenwich, CT: Devin-Adair.

Ott, J. N., 1985, "Color & Light: Their Effects on Plants, Animals and People (part 1)," *International Journal of Biosocial Research*, no.7.

Ott, J. N., 1986, "Color & Light: Their Effects on Plants, Animals and People (part 2)," *International Journal of Biosocial Research*, no. 8.

Ott, J. N., 1987, "Color & Light: Their Effects on Plants, Animals and People (part 3)," *International Journal of Biosocial Research*, no. 9.

Ott, J. N., 1988, "Color & Light: Their Effects on Plants, Animals and People (part 4)," *International Journal of Biosocial Research*, no. 10.

Ott, J. N., 1989, "Color & Light: Their Effects on Plants, Animals and People (part 5)," *International Journal of Biosocial Research*, no. 11.

Ott, J. N., 1990, "Color & Light: Their Effects on Plants, Animals and People (part 6)," *International Journal of Biosocial Research*, no. 12.

Ott, J. N., 1991, "Color, Light & Low Level Electromagnetic Radiation and their Effects on Plants, Animals and People," *International Journal of Biosocial Research*, no. 13.

Ott, J. N., and L. Mayron, 1974, "Light, Radiation & Academic Behavior (Initial Studies on the Effects of Full-Spectrum Lighting and Radiation," *Academic Therapy* 10, no. 1.

Pearson, D., 1989, *The Natural House Book (Creating a healthy, harmonious, and ecologically-sound home environment)*, New York, NY: Simon & Schuster.

Ponte, L., 1981, "How Artificial Light Affects Your Health," *Reader's Digest*, no. 2: 131-134.

Randegger, Z., 1985, "Focus on Light," *Environ*, no. 3: 14-20.

Smith, R.D., 1986, "Light & Health: A Broad Overview," *Lighting Design & Application*, no. 2: 32-40.

Thorington, L., L. Parascandola, and L. Cunningham, 1971, "Visual & Biologic Aspects of an Artificial Sunlight Illuminant," *Journal of Illuminating Engineering Society*, no. 10: 33-41.

Trexler, G. E., 1986, Proof of attempts by G.E. to discredit Ott's work," *Townsend Letter for Doctors*, no. 34: 23, 25.

Ubell, E., 1991, "Lighten Up Winter Sadness," *Parade Magazine*, Nov. 3, p. 14.

Venolia, C., 1988, *Healing Environment,*. Berkeley, CA: Celestial Arts.

Walker, M., 1992, "The Therapeutic Power of Color—Part II," *Townsend Letter for Doctors*, no. 102: 26-30.

Waslerand, M., and V. M. Hitchins, 1986, *Optical Radiation & Visual Health*, Boca Raton, FL: CRC Press.

Weisbord, M., 1991, "Let There Be Light," *Healthy Home & Workplace* 1, no. 2: 1-4.

Wurtman, R. J., 1975, "The Effects of Light on the Human Body," *Scientific American* 233: 68-77.

Zamkova, M. A., and E. I. Krivitskaya, 1966, "Effects of Irradiation by Ultraviolet Erythema Lamps on the Working Ability of School Children" (in Russian) *Gig. i Sanit* 31: 41-44.

11

ELECTROMAGNETIC FIELDS IN THE CLASSROOM

by Andrew A. Marino, Ph.D.

> *Electromagnetic fields (EMFs) are present in every area of our environment, including the classroom and the home. Dr. Marino shows that although they cannot be seen, EMFs may have a powerful effect on those exposed to high doses of them over a period of time. In describing EMF sources outside the school, as well as inside the classroom, he answers questions that teachers and other school staff members often ask about the hazards of computers and other classroom equipment.*
>
> ☐ *Why are EMFs a problem in the school and workplace?*
>
> ☐ *How do EMFs affect individuals at various ranges from their source?*
>
> ☐ *How much influence should powerlines, television towers, and other power transmitters have on the location of new school buildings?*
>
> ☐ *How does wiring in the walls of a school affect teachers and children in nearby classrooms?*
>
> ☐ *What shielding devices are available to protect individuals from EMFs?*

Many of the factors capable of affecting the school environment adversely, such as radon and lead, can also degrade the environments of homes, offices, and factories. The electromagnetic field (EMF) is another example of a potential hazard that is not unique to the teaching environment, but that also affects society generally. Our science and general outlook have matured to the point where we can begin to understand and confront the problems associated with all these factors. There was a time when the concept of risk to health was associated with what could be seen, for example, a wild animal, a speeding automobile, or the edge of a precipice. Subsequently, the concept was expanded to include

221

unanticipated consequences of something otherwise innocent: cancer due to smoking, birth defects caused by a morning-sickness drug, or heart disease caused by fats in the diet. Now the possible consequences of something unseen, such as benzene in drinking water or asbestos particles in the air, are also recognized to be within the meaning of risk.

EMFs must be included with this latter group of factors, not because the evidence is overwhelming or crystal clear, but because it would be foolish to do otherwise. Unfortunately, the notion of an EMF is somewhat counter-intuitive, and this presents difficulties in obtaining a realistic understanding of the nature and extent of the inherent risks. Nevertheless, it would be profitable to learn to identify the principal sources of classroom EMFs, and to avoid them, because such efforts provide the best protection against the possibility that EMFs could trigger reactions in the body leading to symptoms and disease.

WHAT TEACHERS SHOULD KNOW ABOUT EMFs

Numerous technical descriptions of EMFs are available, but from the viewpoint of the classroom teacher interested in obtaining a reasonable knowledge of the issue to permit a rational response within the teaching environment, I think that there are only seven facts that must be appreciated to gain a basic understanding of the possible hazards associated with field exposure.

First, EMFs are real in the sense that they can be directly measured by the proper instruments. Just as we might measure distance in meters, time in seconds, temperature in degrees centigrade, or speed in miles per hour, the various kinds of EMFs can similarly be expressed in appropriate units. These units are likely to be unfamiliar to the lay person, but their peculiar names should not obscure the fact that EMFs are real and measurable, and, hence, that there is an objective basis for evaluating the strengths of EMFs at particular locations.

Second, although EMFs are real, they are not composed of atoms, and hence do not have many familiar properties such as weight or shape. An EMF is simply a form of energy, like light. An important difference between light and other kinds of EMFs (*Figure 11-1*) is that the means by which the body detects light—the eye---- is known, but the means whereby the other kinds of EMFs are detected by the body are not precisely known.

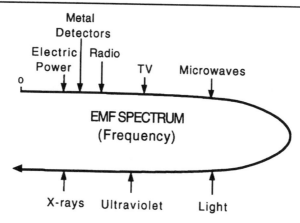

Figure 11-1.

Electromagnetic fields form an infinite spectrum of frequencies. This chart shows the relative location within this spectrum of various familiar uses of EMFs.

Third, since EMFs consist of energy, not matter, they can do things that seem strange if one limits one's thinking to characteristics of material objects. For example, if Johnny adds one apple plus one apple, he winds up with two apples, but if he adds one EMF plus one EMF, he may wind up with two EMFs, a third EMF that is distinct from either of the two original EMFs, or no EMFs at all, depending on the type of EMFs he started with. Such addition and cancellation are basic properties of EMFs.

Fourth, EMFs are created by every electrical device—that is, every device that operates either by battery or by plugging into a wall outlet. For this reason, EMFs in the classroom are not unusual, and it is therefore not their existence that is the object of concern, but rather their cumulative strength and the duration of exposure to them. EMFs are a signature of modern society because, for the most part, they simply did not exist in the everyday human environment prior to the 20th century. It is not possible or desirable to avoid artificial EMFs completely because exposure to them is the price of the myriad benefits made possible by the electrification of society. The focus, therefore, ought to be on the sources of fields in the classroom that are unusual, excessive, or in other ways different from those that exist elsewhere.

Fifth, although EMFs originate from devices powered by electricity, they are not strictly localized to the device itself, but rather spread throughout the surrounding space, becoming progressively weaker as the distance from the device increases. In some instances the spreading of the EMF is an important part of the way the electrical device works. For example, a television signal that is emitted from an antenna is intended to spread so that it can be received by a viewer located many miles from the antenna. On the other hand, the EMF from a computer monitor, fluorescent light, tape player, or electric pencil sharpener is not intended to spread from the respective device; it merely does so as a necessary consequence of the way the device functions, just as exhaust gases are unintended consequences of operating an automobile. The distinction between intended and unintended EMFs is useful for understanding why EMFs may be present in particular environments, but it is irrelevant to a consideration of potential health risks. It would be unwise for a school, for example, to be located near a television tower because of the strong EMFs produced there, and it simply doesn't matter that those EMFs were directly intended to occur as a necessary aspect of the operation of the antenna. The rate at which EMFs become weaker as one moves progressively farther from the source depends on various technical factors, particularly the design of the source. The characteristic distance within which the EMF weakens to the point of vanishing may be one mile from a television antenna, 1,000 feet from a radar, 500 feet from a high-voltage powerline, 100 feet from a telephone communications tower, 50 feet from a building transformer, 10 feet from an electric motor, 5 feet from a computer screen, 1 foot from a light bulb, and 3 inches from an electric clock.

Sixth, the progressive widespread exposure to manufactured EMFs that occurred beginning with this century was based on an assumption of safety, not on affirmative scientific evidence that this was the case. For example, there is no published scientific study showing that children in a school located next to a powerline do not, thereby, undergo an increased health risk. Similarly, there is no scientific evidence suggesting that it would be safe for a child to spend many hours in front of a computer monitor. It would be reassuring if there existed a scientific study that could be reasonably interpreted as showing that being exposed repeatedly to even one kind of EMF was not a health risk. Unfortunately, there is no such evidence. Consequently, the question to be asked is whether the evidence suggesting the existence of risk is credible or not. Much of the remaining portion of this chapter is based on my judgment that the existing state of the scientific evidence warrants the inference that EMFs can be a health risk and, for this reason, that steps ought to be taken to avoid exposure.

There is one final point that everyone should know about health risks such as those due to EMFs: *risk* is an inextricable mixture of value judgment and scientific fact. Risk can sometimes be expressed in a scientific study as a number (see the *Appendix* to this chapter), but this does not indicate that risk is a quantitative measurement in the sense that a minute measures an interval of time or an inch an interval of distance. In contrast, the concept of risk contains a markedly important subjective component contributed by the person making the judgment. Suppose, for example, that Dr. X expresses a judgment of safety under a particular set of EMF exposure conditions. Obviously, such a judgment might be discounted if it were true that Dr. X didn't know anything about EMFs, or had a commercial interest in promoting the electrical device that created them. Although it is less obvious, it is equally true that Dr. X's value system is also a pertinent factor in evaluating the opinion. Suppose, for example, Dr. X believed that it was more important to protect the free and unlimited use of EMFs, rather than burdening such free use for the purpose of providing an added margin of protection to a certain group of device users. The amount of evidence needed to convince Dr. X of risk would then be considerably greater than would otherwise be needed, and the interest of such a Dr. X in an exposed subject not getting sick would simply be a lot less than the exposed subject's would be.

WHY EMFs ARE A PROBLEM

Animal studies are frequently used to evaluate the side-effects of potentially harmful substances. The substances are administered to animals, and from observing the levels at which no important effects are produced, judgments may be made concerning the risks to human beings by employing suitable safety factors. Despite the expenditure of large sums of money on bioeffects research by various industries and governmental agencies, safe doses of EMFs have not been established, because animal studies have not disclosed field levels at which no important effects occur. On the other hand, many studies by independent scientists have shown that EMFs of the type and strength typically found in classrooms can cause diverse and significant effects in animals, including effects on growth, healing, and development. (Rivas, Oroza, and Delgado 1987; Hansson 1981; Grissett, Cupper, Kessler, Brown, Prettyman, Cook, and Griner 1977; Marino, Reichmanis, and Becker, *et al.* 1979; 1980) They can also produce potentially dangerous changes in tissues. (Goodman, Henderson 1988; Bawin, Adey 1976) One of the most important characteristics of EMF-induced effects that was discovered in the animal studies is that not every animal responds to EMFs in the same way. For example, when the effects of EMFs on brain electrical activity in rabbits was measured, the results depended on which rabbit was measured. (Becker, Marino 1982) The field caused increased electrical activity in 14 rabbits, decreased activity in 6, and caused no change in 4. (*Figure 11-2*) Similarly, the effects of EMFs on human brain electrical activity were not the same in each subject. (Bell, Marino, Chesson, and Struve 1991) Laboratory studies involving exposure of human beings also suggest that EMFs can be hazardous. The findings include: alterations in blood-fat levels from a one-day exposure (Beischer, Grissett, and Mitchell 1973), in performance on various psychological tests (Gibson, Moroney 1974) and body rhythms. (Wever 1970)

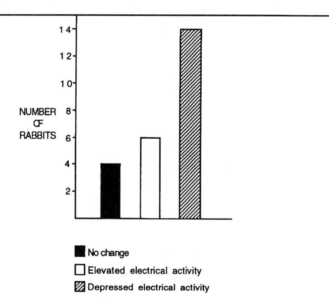

NUMBER OF RABBITS

■ No change
□ Elevated electrical activity
▨ Depressed electrical activity

Figure 11-2.
Effect of EMFs on brain electrical activity in rabbits (8). Brain activity was measured in each rabbit before and after a brief exposure to EMFs. The results showed that the effect of the field varied from animal to animal.

Some people are exposed to higher levels of EMFs because of where they live or work. Many studies of such persons have been performed to determine whether the observed levels of disease were similar to those that would ordinarily be expected irrespective of the fields. (Marino 1993) In such studies (called epidemiological studies), the investigators did not apply or control the fields experienced by the subjects; rather, those subjects who had been exposed because of where they lived or worked were identified and evaluated, thereby permitting estimation of the amount of risk associated with field exposure. The first important epidemiological study appeared in 1979; since then, many studies have demonstrated a positive association between exposure to fields and disease (usually cancer). Pertinent details regarding these studies are summarized in the *Appendix* to this chapter. Not all studies report an association, but there have been enough reports of associations to implicate exposure to fields as a significant factor in human disease.

Fields do not cause disease in the sense that illness results every time individuals receive a specific dose. The usual observation is that the incidence of cancer is greater among subjects who are exposed to EMFs, compared with those who are not exposed, but not all subjects who are exposed develop cancer, and cancer occurs in some who are not exposed. Thus, exposure to EMFs increases the risk for developing cancer, but does not necessarily cause cancer. Some persons, particularly the old or the young, may be particularly susceptible to field exposure, as is frequently the case with toxic agents.

The health risks due to EMFs go far beyond their role in causing cancer. They extend to other diseases, and also have a role in causing various symptoms that do not fit easily into specific diagnostic categories. It is probably the case that EMFs combine with other noxious stimuli and risk factors, thereby taxing the body's overall resistance to disease. (*Figure 11-3*) According to this theory, symptoms of disease develop when an individual's resistance has been exceeded. The particular manifestations that develop depend on the exact mix of adverse factors, which varies from person to person.

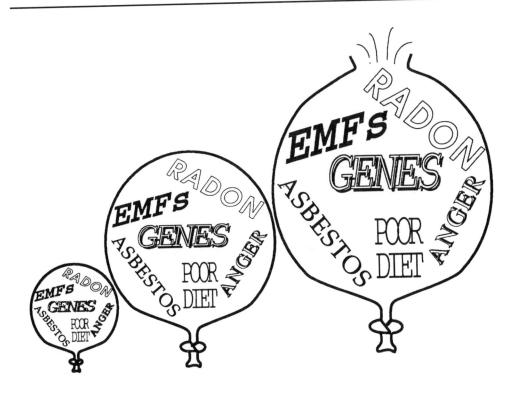

Figure 11-3.
Illustration of the role of EMFs in the total-body-load theory of human disease. No single factor is a complete cause of disease. Each factor adds a burden to the body's adaptive capacity, and disease develops when the body's ability to adapt has been exceeded.

Our present understanding of EMF risks is inadequate in many regards, but perhaps the most glaring shortcoming is the absence of knowledge regarding the effects of EMFs on women. Almost all studies performed to date—both laboratory and epidemiological—have used men as subjects. The most egregious example of this imbalance in the presently available data is that the link between EMFs and breast cancer has been studied in males (see the *Appendix* to this chapter) but not in females. Consequently, judgments of risk to women due to electromagnetic fields must be based solely on extrapolation from animal studies, and from human studies involving children or male subjects.

ELECTROMAGNETIC FIELDS IN THE CLASSROOM

Sources Outside the School

Sources outside of the school building may result in elevated levels of EMFs inside the school, and the continuous and long-term nature of the exposure they produce is a particularly serious concern. For example, *Figure 11-4* depicts a plot of land that is traversed by a 115,000-volt powerline; three possible locations for a school are shown. Location A is near the powerline and consequently would result in continuous exposure to EMFs stronger than 10 milligauss, Location B would result in exposure above 2 but below 10 milligauss, and Location C would result in less than 2 milligauss. Location C would be the optimal choice for the location of the school based on an intention to limit exposure to EMFs, and there is ample reason to do so because studies have indicated that the long-term addition of about 2 milligauss approximately doubles a child's risk of developing leukemia (see the *Appendix* to this chapter). But C may not be the optimal choice from other viewpoints such as cost or convenience. This example illustrates both the importance of choice of location in relation to existing sources of EMFs in reducing EMF levels inside the school, and the financial or other consequences that may be attendant on the choice to provide such protection.

Radio and television towers, as well as microwave communications antennas also emit EMFs that may burden the school environment. For example, the U.S. Environmental Protection Agency (EPA) measured EMFs in McFarland, California at the request of state officials who were investigating a childhood cancer cluster. (Mantiply, Hankin 1989) The EPA had previously determined the median exposure level in U.S. urban areas due to EMFs originating from television and radio signals. The levels measured at School K were more than twice the median level, and additional EMFs from Voice of America transmitters located about six miles away were also detected. (*Figure 11-5*) The EMF levels at School B were three times the median U.S. urban level (and also contained contributions from VOA transmitters). Unfortunately, the final report is not easily read by the lay person, and the significance of the elevated readings is not discussed in relation to health concerns. Nevertheless, the EPA reports are important because they are the public's only present source of reliable information regarding environmental levels of broadcast EMFs.

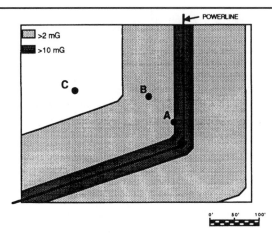

Figure 11-4.
EMF produced by a typical powerline. A 115,000-volt powerline is shown, and the resulting field was calculated under the assumption that the powerline was operating at a normal level. The dark shading indicates the region of strongest field (more than 10 milligauss). The light shading indicates the region where the field is between 2 and 10 milligauss. A, B, and C are possible locations of a new school.

Radio and television towers radiate intense levels of EMFs, and therefore they should not be located near schools. The appropriate separation distance will vary from case to case, but it is difficult to imagine a situation in which it would be appropriate for the distance to be less than 1,000 to 2,000 feet. Communication antennas, such as those used by telephone companies, typically emit significantly lower levels of EMFs, and do so in a particular direction (in contrast to radio and television towers, which emit EMFs in all directions). Consequently, depending on the direction in which the EMFs are emitted, it might be appropriate for the distance between a communications antenna and a school to be 100 to 1,000 feet (less, if the EMFs were radiated in a direction away from the school). Once a choice is made to locate a school near a source of EMFs, or to locate a source of EMFs near a school, there are few practical steps that can be taken to shield or otherwise protect the teachers and students.

Sources Within the School

The school itself is a consumer of electric power, which it uses to operate elevators, lights, computers, and many other electrical devices. The conduit for the power is an overhead or underground electrical cable

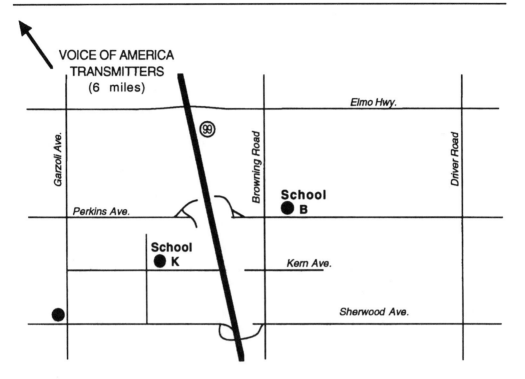

Figure 11-5.
Location of two schools in McFarland, California in relation to Voice of America transmitters. The EMFs from radio and television antennas were found to be much greater
than those arising from the Voice of America transmitters. The radio and television
EMFs at both schools, however, were significantly higher than typical urban background levels.

originating from the local electric power grid, and ending in an electrical
distribution station within the school at which the power is transformed
into ordinary line voltage, and then distributed via the school wiring
system. The school electrical system itself is sometimes located adjacent
to classrooms, thereby resulting in high levels of EMFs within the nearby
classrooms. To reduce this exposure, the feed from the power grid
should be underground, and the transformers and switching circuitry
should be located away from classrooms or offices. If the desirability of
such a separation is appreciated prior to construction of the school, it is
frequently possible to effect reduction in exposure to EMFs from this
source at relatively low cost. The situation is more complicated if an
attempt is made to mitigate exposure as a remedial step.

A further source of significant EMFs in the classroom is the school wiring itself. Whatever electric power is consumed in a classroom will inevitably result in EMFs, and thus the exposure to the EMFs arising from that source is a necessary consequence of enjoyment of the benefits provided by electricity. On the other hand, if classrooms are wired in sequence, then all of the electricity consumed in the classroom at the end of a line of wiring must first pass through the wiring in the walls of the upstream classrooms. The result is that the fields produced in the end-of-the-line classroom arise only from the electricity used in that classroom, whereas the fields in the upstream classrooms receive an additional contribution from all of the electricity flowing through the wires in the wall on the way to the downstream classrooms. In a four-classroom sequence, for example, the fields in the classroom closest the to source would receive EMFs about four times as great as the classroom furthest away. Proper attention to the type and configuration of classroom wiring can reduce the fields, and, hence, the resulting exposure.

A measurement of classroom exposure to EMFs produced by the electrical power system are shown in *Figure 11-6*. (Ungichian 1990) To obtain the data shown in *Figure 11-6*, the teachers each wore a small device that measured the EMFs to which they were exposed, and stored the measured values for later analysis; the average value over one school day is shown. For example, the third-grade teacher in School No. 1 was exposed to an average EMF of the type produced by the electrical power system (and the various devices that are operated by being plugged into an electrical outlet) of about 1.3 milligauss. In contrast, on the same day the teacher at School No. 2 was exposed to an EMF more than twice as strong, but the teacher at School No. 4 experienced an EMF that was approximately equal to the typical U.S. mean background level.

The average EMF exposure levels such as those shown in *Figure 11-6*, are highly dependent on the activities of the individual teacher, which electrical devices are used by the teacher and the length of time of their use, as well as the distribution of EMF sources at or near the school. Thus, it could not be concluded from *Figure 11-6A* that the EMFs at School Nos. 3 and 4 were less than those present in the other schools. This is clearly demonstrated in *Figure 11-6B*, which depicts data obtained during four successive weeks at School No. 3: all of the measured exposure levels were significantly greater than the levels initially measured in the 5th-grade classroom. An insight into the typical exposure pattern of an individual teacher can be obtained from *Figure 11-7*. The

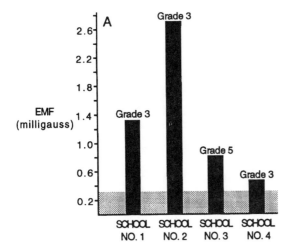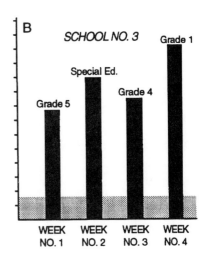

Figure 11-6.
EMFs in typical elementary schools in Florida. The measurements were made using a recording device worn by classroom teachers throughout the school day. Graph A shows the average results of measurements made on the same day in four different schools. Graph B shows average measurements made at weekly intervals in School No. 3. The shading indicates the overall average background EMF of the type measured.

teacher was in one classroom except for 12:20 to 12:40 p.m. when she was in the school lunchroom, and after 1:50 p.m. when she was on car duty in front of the school and then in the school office.

Specific Sources of EMFs

If an electrical device operates by means of batteries (for example, a cellular telephone) or plugs into a wall outlet, it is a source of EMFs and merits consideration with regard to the conditions under which it is

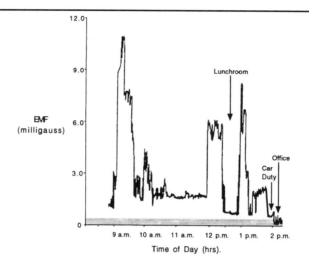

Figure 11-7.

The EMF experienced by a third grade teacher at School No. 2 during the course of the school day. The teacher was in one classroom, except where otherwise indicated. Shading shows the overall average background EMF of the type measured.

used, with the viewpoint of minimizing or eliminating exposure to the resulting EMFs. Computer screens and TV monitors are a significant source of EMFs (*Figure 11-8*), and this fact should be considered in a decision regarding when and how the device is to be located and used. Many companies now market devices that reduce EMF exposure from computer screens and monitors, but none of the devices provides complete protection. Moreover, the federal government has not set standards by which a consumer could determine the nature and extent of the protection provided. Nevertheless, some objective testing procedures do exist, and have been adhered to by various manufacturers. These devices should be standard equipment on all computer screens and video monitors in the school room, not because the protection they provide is perfect, but because it would be imprudent to do otherwise.

All cellular telephones on the market today produce extraordinarily high levels of EMFs, compared with the levels present when the device is not operating. (*Figure 11-9*) From the point of view of the welfare of a passively exposed child, it is difficult to rationalize permitting repeated exposure for the benefit of the user of the cellular telephone.

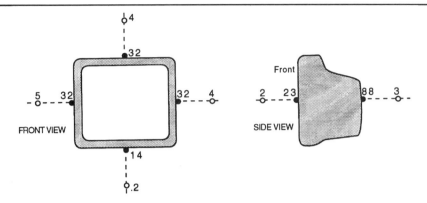

Figure 11-8.
EMF (in milligauss) produced at the surface (solid dot) and at one foot in each direction (open dot) by a Macintosh SE computer (data from Electrical Power Research Center, Iowa State University). Because of the type of measuring instrument that was used, only a portion of the EMF produced by the computer was measured. The fields were reduced an average of 71% following installation of a magnetic-field shield inside the computer (Fairfield Engineering, Fairfield, IA).

SUMMARY AND RECOMMENDATIONS

Electromagnetic fields of the type produced by common and familiar devices may result in relatively high doses of field exposure, and can produce a significant risk to health. High EMF doses can come about as a result of either short exposure to high-strength EMFs, or long-term exposure to low-strength EMFs. Presently, there is no reasonable evidence suggesting what might be regarded as a safe dose of any type of EMFs, but considerable evidence exists indicating that EMFs have profound effects on animal and human physiology, and are associated with the occurrence of disease in human subjects (cancer has been studied most). Taken as a whole, this evidence indicates that one's personal risk comes into being when the dose of EMFs received is greater than the average background exposure that is a necessary consequence of the extent of the electrification of modern society. Therefore, for the individual, the goal is to identify the sources of EMFs in one's personal environment, and to minimize the resulting exposure by modifying the extent or nature of the use of the device with the ultimate aim of achieving a kind of parity in EMF dose received with that of other members of society. Then, an individual's risk of EMF-related disease would be no greater than that of others, and it is not possible to improve

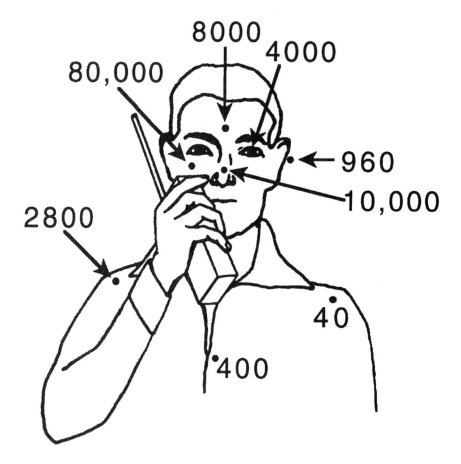

Figure 11-9.
EMF exposure in the vicinity of the face and head of a user of a cellular telephone. The illustration is based on measurements by the EPA and has been scaled to represent a typical cellular telephone. The data is expressed with reference to the median U.S. exposure levels to broadcast EMFs, as determined by the EPA. For example, the typical shoulder-level EMF exposure (right side) is 2,800 times greater than the median U.S. exposure level.

on this degree of risk while still enjoying the benefits of modern society. Further, as is true of smoking, not everyone exposed to EMFs develops disease, and not all disease is attributable to EMFs; consequently, it's clear that other factors must function as co-causes in bringing about any particular symptom or disease. The total-body-load theory of disease (*Figure 11-3*) provides a rational basis for self-protection even when EMF exposure is unavoidable. Consequently, it is prudent to survey one's environment, work habits, and the activities of others that potentially impact on one's work environment, and to eliminate gratuitous or otherwise avoidable EMF exposure.

EMF audits ought to be conducted in each classroom by competent and independent engineers for the purpose of identifying the devices, activities, and outside sources of EMFs that result in significant classroom exposure of teachers and students. Such an audit should include both the type of EMFs associated with the electrical power system, and broadcast EMFs such as those from television and radio towers, and cellular telephones. Much of the present exposure experienced by teachers and pupils is unnecessary in the sense that it could easily be reduced or eliminated. Other sources of EMF exposure such as the nearby powerline or television antenna cannot be easily moved, and, where they are concerned, the question of what, if anything, ought to be done to reduce EMF exposure should be a joint decision involving both those responsible for producing the EMFs, and those who are subjected to it. Only when the interests of both groups are represented can an appropriate balance between risks and benefits be struck.

Some devices—cellular telephones, for example—simply should not be operated routinely around children because they result in very high EMF levels in the vicinity of the user.

Shielding devices of various kinds are presently on the market, and they should be considered in the construction of schools and the operation of equipment within schools. For example, glasses, windows, and glazed panels that pass light but block other EMFs such as those from radio and television antennas are available and could be used to lessen significantly the levels of such EMFs in individual classrooms. Similarly, shields that provide some protection against EMFs from computer monitors are available. Presently, such devices do not provide complete protection, but the amount of EMF exposure reduction that they can bring about warrants their routine use in the classroom to minimize exposure of teachers and students. It is likely that the extensive use of even the present generation of imperfect devices would lead both to better devices, and to appropriate redesigns of computer equipment and monitors, thereby eliminating the problem at its source.

REFERENCES

Bawin, S. M., and W. R. Adey, 1976, "Sensitivity of calcium binding in cerebral tissue to weak environmental electric fields oscillating at low frequency." *Proceedings of the National Academy of Science*, 73:1999-2003.

Becker, R. O., and A. A. Marino, 1982, *Electromagnetism & Life*, Albany, NY: State University of New York Press, p. 99

Beischer, D. C., J. D. Grissett, and R. E. Mitchell, 1973, *Exposure of Man to Magnetic Fields Alternating at Extremely Low Frequency*, Pensacola, FLA, Naval Aerospace Medical Research Laboratory.

Bell, G., A. A. Marino, A. Chesson, and F. Struve, 1991, "Human sensitivity to weak magnetic fields, *The Lancet*, 338: 1521-1522.

Gibson, R. S., and W. F. Moroney, 1974, *The Effects of Extremely Low Frequency Magnetic Fields on Human Performance*, Pensacola, FLA, Aerospace Medical Research Laboratory.

Goodman, R., and A. S. Henderson, 1988, "Exposure of salivary gland cells to low-frequency electromagnetic fields alters peptide syntheses," *Proceedings of the National Academy of Science*, 85:3928-3932.

Grissett, J. D., J. L. Cupper, M. J. Kessler, R. J. Brown, G. D. Prettyman, L. L. Cook, and T. A. Griner, 1977, *Exposure of Primates for One Year to Electric and Magnetic Fields Associated with ELF Communications Systems*, Pensacola, FLA: Naval Aerospace Medical Research Laboratory.

Hansson, H.-A., 1981, "Lamellar bodies in Purkinje nerve cells induced by electric field," *Brain Research* 216: 187-191.

Lambdin, D. L., 1979, *An Investigation of Energy Densities in the Vicinity of Vehicles with Mobile Communications Equipment and Near a Hand-Held Walkie Talkie*, ORP/EAD 79-2, Las Vegas NV, U.S. Environmental Protection Agency.

Mantiply, E. D., and N. N. Hankin, 1989, *Radiofrequency Radiation Survey in the McFarland California Area*, U.S. Environmental Protection Agency, EPA/520/6-89/022.

Marino, A. A., 1993, "Electromagnetic fields, cancer, and the theory of neuroendocrine-related promotion," *Bioelectrochemistry & Bioenergetics* 29: 255-276.

Marino, A. A., M. Reichmanis, and R. O. Becker, 1979, "Fracture healing in rats exposed to extremely-low-frequency electric fields," *Clinical Orthopedics & Related Research*, 145: 239-244.

Marino, A. A., M. Reichmanis, R. O. Becker, B. Ullrich, and J. M. Cullen, 1980, "Power frequency electric field induces biological changes in successive generations of mice," *Experientia* 36: 309.

Rivas, L., M. A. Oroza, and J. M. R. Delgado, 1987, "Influence of electromagnetic fields on body weight and serum chemistry in second generation mice," *Medical Sci. Research* 15: 1041-1042.

Ungichian, V., 1990, *Sandpiper Shores 60-Hertz Magnetic Field Project*, Florida Atlantic University.

Wever, R., 1970, "The effects of electric fields on circadian rhythms in man," *Life Sci. Space Research* 8: 177-187.

APPENDIX

Summary Of The Peer-reviewed Scientific Literature Dealing With The Link Between Exposure To Electromagnetic Fields And Cancer

The studies listed establish that exposure to electromagnetic fields, regardless of frequency, has been consistently linked with increased risk for cancer. For further details and a complete citation of the references cited in this table see *Marino 1993* listed in the REFERENCES section of this chapter.

Reference from Marino 1993	Place and time	Parameter evaluated	Increased risk due to EMF
69	Denver, CO 1950-73	Childhood cancer	*130%
70	Denver, CO 1976-83	Childhood cancer	*50%
71	Seattle, WA 1981-84	Leukemia	50%
73	Rhode Island, 1964-78	Childhood leukemia	10%
74	Los Angeles, CA, 1980-87	Childhood leukemia	*70%
75	Stockholm, 1958-73	Childhood tumors	*110%
76	England, 1971-83	Cancer Lung cancer (female)	0 *80%
77	Sweden, 1960-73	Cancer (males) Cancer (females)	*15% *8%
80	Polish military, 1971-80	Cancer Leukemia & lymphoma	*200% *590%
81	New Hampshire, 1952-77	Leukemia	*240%
83	Canada, 1965-73	Leukemia	*250%
84	Sweden, 1961-73	Leukemia	0
85	Washington, California, 1979-84	Leukemia	*80%

Reference from Marino 1993	Place and time	Parameter evaluated	Increased risk due to EMF
86	Sweden, 1977-82	Leukemia	*280%
87	USA, 1983-87	Male breast cancer	*80%
88	Montreal, 1976-83	Melanoma	*170%
95	Greater Denver, CO, 1967-77	Cancer	*30%
96	England, 1983-85	Leukemia Lymphoma	20% 20%
97	London, 1965-80	Leukemia	20%
98	USA	Leukemia	*150%
99	France, 1984-88	Leukemia	*300%
100	New Zealand, 1980-84	Leukemia	*60%
101	England & Wales, 1973	Leukemia	*130%
102	USA, 1985-86	Brain cancer	*40%
91	Maryland, 1969-82	Brain cancer	*120%
103	USA 1978-81	Brain cancer	*130%
104	East Texas, 1969-78	Brain cancer	*360%
105	Washington, 1950-79	Leukemia	*40%
106	Washington state, California, 1971-83	Leukemia	*90%
107	London, 1961-79	Leukemia	*20%
108	Los Angeles, 1972-79	Leukemia	30%
109	Wisconsin, 1963-78	Leukemia	0
101	England & Wales, 1970-72	Leukemia	0
110	Finland	Leukemia	20%

*Statistically significant increase (P < 0.05)

12

JARED'S STORY:
Least Toxic Approaches To Managing Pests In Schools

by William Forbes

Chemical pesticides can be a major source of some children's health and behavior problems. In this chapter, Mr. Forbes describes the plight of Jared, a disruptive student whose sensitivity to chemicals resulted from his mother's exposure to a pesticide before his birth. Discussing the health hazards of chemical pesticides, and showing how schools can deal with pest problems by using the Integrated Pest Management (IPM) system now mandated in Texas, Mr. Forbes answers questions of vital importance to school custodial staff, as well as to administrators.

- ☐ *What are the health risks of exposure to chemical pesticides?*

- ☐ *How can pesticides be managed most effectively in the school setting?*

- ☐ *What is an Integrated Pest Management (IPM) program?*

- ☐ *What are least-toxic alternatives to chemical pesticides?*

- ☐ *How can good pest-management practice be included in the curriculum?*

Jared's story isn't a complicated one. As a bright, active ten-year-old, Jared appears to be much like any other child his age. His love of soccer, reading, and video games probably typifies many of his former classmates.

Unfortunately, however, Jared suffers from what has often been considered an unusual syndrome. Though he would prefer to be in the classroom, he has been forced into the sheltered world of home-instruction because of a sensitivity to chemicals.

This syndrome causes Jared to act irrationally both at home and in the classroom. His disruptive behavior is characterized by periods of depression interspersed with aggressiveness towards his brother and sister as well as other students in school. His performance on his classwork is poor, his handwriting resembles scrawled pictures, and, at best, his attention span is limited to a few minutes, which frequently causes him to be sent to the principal's office for discipline.

Jared's problem results from exposure to an unidentified toxic chemical during his development in the womb, and both his doctor and his parents believe that a "bug bomb" used to kill cockroaches may have been the culprit. While he was in the early grades, Jared's unique needs were regarded by many within the school system as the result of either attention deficit syndrome (ADS) or over-protective parents. It wasn't until he was taken to a new pediatrician that his parents discovered that the cause of his problem might lie in an area they had not explored so far.

Jared's parents have battled long and hard to gain their son a seat in a classroom in the nearby elementary school. And for Jared it has often been a true challenge to face school personnel, who, for whatever reason, have refused to honor the requests of both his parents and his doctor that he not be exposed to any chemical substances, from pesticides to perfumes. Of course, pesticides have been deadly substances in Jared's short life, ones that might already have robbed him of his tomorrow.

Although the pesticide issue that affects Jared may sound far-fetched, it has a serious impact on many students across America. Because a classroom is treated with "bug-spray," students exposed to toxins in the pesticide may be in jeopardy of losing a lifetime of normal activity. Of course, not all students or adults react in the same way when exposed to a pesticide, nor do they readily react on initial exposure. Chronic effects from pesticides have yet to be measured adequately, and data about such effects are not generally included in statements about the results of product testing. Furthermore, the effects of the interaction of pesticides with children's biochemistry have not been assessed adequately either, and this ignorance of the results of pesticide use causes a serious breach of safety standards in our schools nationwide.

CLASSROOM ENVIRONMENTS

Classroom environments can be extremely volatile sites, constantly offgassing pesticides that have been applied repeatedly for years in the same routine fashion. The general application of pesticides fails to address those micro-environments where insects actually live. Instead, poisons are placed within the confines of the classroom, making it possibly the most toxic place a child will spend time in during his or her entire life.

Those very areas and objects that provide cockroaches a safe haven, unfortunately, also allow children to be exposed unnecessarily to toxins. The earliest signs of toxic exposure in children may be those of behavioral disorders and learning disabilities, problems seen with increasing frequency in today's children.

RISK OF EXPOSURE

Studies from the University of North Carolina provide a grim picture of how pesticides move within the confines of a structure. One study showed that use of the pesticide diazinon in a 1% formulation was detected four rooms away from the original site of application. The study also indicated that the active ingredient was present for a little more than 21 days. Neurotoxins such as diazinon have not been tested for their toxic effects on children, and it is this class of pesticides that could very well be responsible for behaviors related to learning disabilities.

Pesticides are not harmless; they are intended to kill target organisms. Although the government may require testing of these substances for sale, very little is actually known about the effects of their properties. Many people think tests imply that a safe standard has been met by a product, but a statement on a container that a product has been tested by the government is not a guarantee of safety nor should it be confused with a seal of approval. In fact, trust in such statements seems pervasive among school personnel. I often hear people say, "Oh, that stuff can't be that dangerous. Why it's approved by the government!" My personal favorite is, "Well, they stock the stuff on the grocery store shelves, don't they? It must be okay."

Every year the Centers for Disease Control (CDC) receive thousands of reports of children being poisoned. The numbers are growing dramatically as we take aim at insects that have developed genetic resistance to a large number of pesticides. In 1991, the CDC received reports of 83,325 pesticide exposures; of those, at least 67% involved children under the age of 18. These are phenomenal numbers representing a broad spectrum of children who have been exposed unnecessarily. Children are at greater risk pound for pound than adults, because they consume oxygen, food, and water at a much greater rate than adults. Their exposure to pesticides is also increased simply because they are more readily in contact with pesticide residues. Just the simple act of playing on a carpet treated for fleas greatly increases the risk to a child of being exposed to a toxic substance.

Registration of a pesticide involves analysis of its active ingredients only and not of its inert properties. Though manufacturers often classify inert ingredients as "trade secrets," these ingredients can be just as toxic if not moreso than active ingredients. Many inert ingredients post serious health threats to those exposed to them; indeed a number of them are considered possible cancer-causing agents. Several of the testing requirements imposed by Congress through the enactment of the Federal Insecticide, Fungicide, Rodenticide Act (FIFRA) still fail to provide sufficient data about toxic effects.

On October 27, 1992, the Westchester County, New York, Department of Public Health closed down the Eastchester High School for three weeks, after students and staff complained of headaches, nausea, eye irritation, and respiratory problems. The school had been treated the day before with resmethrin, chlorpyrifos, and diazinon. This is by no means an isolated incident. In fact, incidents of this nature are reported regularly nationwide.

POLICIES FOR MANAGING PESTICIDES IN SCHOOL SETTINGS

Clear statements of policy are necessary to establish firm guidelines for any organization. Any agency involved in providing indoor air programs is likely to have a written policy directing that the activities of the agency be performed only under certain conditions.

Public schools in particular have the burdensome responsibility of adhering to policies they may not be able to carry out without assistance from outside the school. They may be forced to rely either on a contractor or an agency well enough equipped to assist the school administration in implementing its policy.

Most school systems don't have a policy that specifically addresses those issues surrounding pesticide use. The State of Texas does have a policy, however, and by 1995, every school system in Texas will be required to have a functioning Integrated Pest Management (IPM) program. Dallas, Texas will be the first large city in the country to have such a program. When it is fully operative, the state law, which also contains a list of those pesticides that may be used within a school structure, will require that a coordinator oversee the IPM program in order that it function exactly as it should. Clearly stated regulations are an extremely important part of the program, because they help each school comply with the policies and procedures set forth in the legislation.

Policy adoption should not be limited to pesticide use, but should also cover a broad base of activities involved in school maintenance. Any chemical oversight policy should include the following:

- Establishment of specific contractual amendments that will attract vendors capable of delivering services to contract specification. Policies that have allowed for low-bid acceptance as the norm should be modified. A stringent policy of bid acceptance that emphasizes value for dollars spent based on a 60% technical and 40% value standard will better serve both the contractor and the school system.

- Discontinuance of the practice of routine spraying.

- Reduction of pesticide use, targeting specific amounts (percentages) over a given period of time. Not many school systems are equipped to move from one approach to another overnight. It is important, therefore, that time constraints be imposed, and that appropriate scheduling be followed when the practice of routine spraying is discontinued.

- Determining that staff members understand the pesticide regulations and the reasons for them. Staff members who apply pesticides either should be state-certified or should practice under the guidance of a certified applicator. Anyone who violates pesticide regulations during the application of a pesticide, especially by applying a pesticide prohibited by the policies of the system or state, should face disciplinary action. Contractors who send in workers without proper documentation should be dismissed.

- Notification of all concerned when pesticide application is scheduled.

- Documentation of all chemically sensitive students, teachers, and other persons who are involved in the daily function of the building.

- Provision on request of full disclosure of the materials used by both the school system and its contractors.

- Establishment of standards for pesticide use. It should be determined which pesticide will have the least negative impact on human beings and which areas will be acceptable for the application of the pesticide.

Keeping track of and communicating policy changes will be necessary to assure a smooth transition of essential services in a given system. No two systems are alike, nor do they operate under the same directives. Policy changes should be expected to help school officials maintain a continuing dialogue with staff, students, and parents.

INTEGRATED PEST MANAGEMENT (IPM)

The purpose of integrating management practices is twofold. First, IPM recognizes that several different ingredients are necessary for the success of a program. Secondly, this approach can reduce reliance on the use of pesticides, especially the routine practice of pesticide application. Although the reduction of pesticides can be considered paramount in diminishing undesirable exposure to toxic chemicals, it should not be considered an environmental-impact statement.

On occasion chemical pesticides will not only be necessary, but will be the first choice in managing a pest problem. The use of pesticides should not be considered, however, unless biologically-targeted practices have failed to solve the problem. For instance, if foodstuffs are readily available for cockroaches to feed on, success in controlling them cannot be guaranteed. Removal of foodstuffs, water, and harborage is extremely important if management practices are to permit a noticeable reduction in the cockroach population. Without proper precautions, pesticides will again become a necessary evil.

Managing structural pests can be extremely difficult when there are open invitations such as improper sanitation controls, structural problems that allow pests to gain access to a structure, or human behavioral problems that encourage the presence of pests. Often the greatest difficulty in managing structural pests is not the pests themselves, but rather the people who create an environment conducive to pest reproduction.

Much of the practice of IPM has to do with prior planning to combat the pest problem. In order to construct a sound plan, data must be collected to determine where pests are hiding, breeding, or feeding. This is done by monitoring the facility, or observing the structure in its entirety. The practice of data collection helps to determine species, population, and the site of infestation. Unfortunately, I have discovered that very often human observation alone, without systematic data collection, produces deceptive data and encourages poor planning. If I rely only on the complaints made by school staff or administrators, without the backup of scientific data collection, I may develop an inaccurate sense of the nature and scope of a pest problem.

Trapping devices coupled with visual inspection can best determine what exactly is going on within the confines of the school structure. Traps are set about the building to collect data critical in determining the actions necessary to control the target organism. Though various species of insects look alike, and, hence, may be confused with each other, their biological characteristics may cause them to behave in differing fashions. (For example, brown-banded cockroaches look very much like other cockroaches, but they behave in very different ways.) Their dietary needs and their habitats are quite different from those of other species such as German cockroaches. Depending on the area being monitored, *action levels* are set to measure certain types of activity that occur when pest numbers exceed predetermined tolerance levels. Such monitoring devices will also help school personnel plan pesticide applications in advance, permitting ample time for them to notify staff and students about the application schedule.

The determination of threshold levels helps to minimize the repeated use of pesticides, especially when school personnel manage the microenvironment of the target organism. Again, such management can be achieved by applying sanitation controls, modifying the structure (i.e., caulking, sealing doors, replacing broken windows), or modifying the behavior of staff and students (i.e., removing foodstuffs from lockers at the end of each day, storing foodstuffs securely in home-economics rooms and lounges, etc.).

Actions that may be taken by the pest management specialist (PMS) can be determined when sufficient data have been collected, and they may range from setting additional trapping devices to the actual application of a pesticide. All such activities can be implemented only when sufficient data have been collected. Although least toxic approaches should be utilized whenever possible, when all other avenues have failed or have proven ineffective in the past, it may be necessary to employ toxins to control a particular pest.

Another component of the IPM process should include a step-by-step review procedure that allows for evaluation of collected data. A review will enable the coordinator to determine whether pest control has been successful, and it will also help the pest management team to plot future strategies for intervention. Since the activity of several pests is seasonal and may be managed most effectively before they become a serious problem, planning the management of target organisms is certainly preferable to attacking them on an emergency basis. In the case of stinging insects, scouting early nest construction will save a great deal of time, money, and the potential for stings or the exposure to pesticides.

ALTERNATIVES TO PESTICIDES

Alternatives to pesticides allow for greater versatility at the same time that they remove the possibility of human exposure to toxic substances. From parasites that would normally attack target organisms, to lite beer for the control of Norway rats, alternative management materials offer control with a least-toxic approach. Mechanical trapping devices, biological trapping devices, and light traps, are all highly successful when integrated in the management of target organisms. Other means of control might include vacuum cleaners that remove cockroaches, their cast skins, and their fecal matter, and thick liquid soaps that block the respiratory passages of pests or prevent their flight. Alternatives are generally target-specific means that have been proven successful because they address particular mechanisms that support or protect the existence of target organisms.

Least Toxic Chemical Pesticides

Least-toxic chemical pesticide choices can be made with the understanding that other pesticides may be necessary. Very often these least-toxic choices are based on the LD-50 formula: lethal dose response for 50% of test organism. This isn't the only rule of thumb that should characterize least-toxic pesticide choices, however, and the mode of action (how the pesticide kills its target) and the formulation (the form in which the pesticide is applied; i.e., dust, bait, liquid, or gas), should play an important part in determining choice. As a general rule, choice should be based on the least disruptive material containing the fewest properties toxic to human beings, their immediate environment, and the surrounding environment. If I decide that I'm going to kill grubs with Formula XYZ, it is vital that no children come in contact with the site of application and that all label precautions be followed. Since I live next to a pond, if I am not careful, I may in fact kill all the fish in the pond and the birds that might feed on the grubs.

Pesticides should be target- and site-specific. This means that a pesticide will only kill the intended target in its given environment. Many pesticide materials are stomach poisons in bait formulations, dusts, or insect growth regulators (IGR's). Realizing that insects, like people, have to eat, scientists have developed baits that will also integrate materials that ensure their acceptance by the pests.

Applications of pesticides other than those deemed least-toxic should be announced in writing well ahead of their use. Notification allows those with long-standing health problems the time to consult with doctors or make arrangements suitable to avoid exposure. During any emergency use of pesticides (for example, the eradication of stinging insects that may have appeared unexpectedly) both staff and students should be given time to leave the site of application. Necessary containment of the pesticide is paramount, and after pesticide use, the building should be monitored for problems, and staff and students should be canvassed for complaints related to the application.

TEACHING AND LEARNING PRACTICAL SCIENCES

Participation in the disciplines of the biological sciences is extremely important, because it allows the student to apply information he or she has learned from a printed text through the immediate use of that information in lab work. Applying the information presented throughout a course of study can become an effective means to the lifelong retention of that information. Integrated pest management is a field that allows for the adaptation of a practical science to the solution of problems existing within the confines of the classroom and the school.

Programs that allow students hands-on experience within a discipline can both enhance lessons and aid future scientists toward their adult careers. In such programs teachers can plan lessons in entomology, zoology, chemistry, genetic engineering, bacteriological studies, behavioral sciences, and, of course, environmental sciences. When these studies are offered for credit, they may well enhance the entire learning program, encouraging students to participate in the maintenance of a healthy school.

Several resources are available to foster the practice of IPM as a part of any school science program, and the information necessary to apply this concept is readily available from universities and professional organizations. In field studies students would monitor the structure of various types of organisms, determining the species present within the school building and the extent of the species population. From there, lessons could be planned around identification of given species and how each survives within its particular micro-environment. Studies of habitat modification methods and application of the information learned in classroom study would allow the school to become a laboratory in its own right.

All the ingredients necessary to provide excellent opportunities for students to apply learning in practical programs exist within the confines of their neighborhood school. *Figure 12-1* shows a sample of a lesson-plan outline for environmental science/entomology that can be adapted for any school level.

Classification activities could be incorporated into lab assignments designed to enable students to examine the principles of integrating techniques that would suppress the target organism. Helping the student apply what he or she has learned in the classroom is a practical and immediate way for teachers to extend lessons to real-life experience.

Indeed Jared, and the countless others like him, might be encouraged by such programs to work toward solutions to the chemical problems that have affected all their lives.

RECOMMENDED READING

Abrams, Robert, Attorney General of New York State, March 1993, *Pesticides in Schools: Reducing the Risk*, Albany: Office of the Attorney General.

Buttram, Harold, M.D., "Children and the Dangers of Pesticides," *New Jersey Woman's Journal*, June 1993.

Classification of insects in an urban setting

A) Cockroaches

    1) species identification

    2) digestive characteristics

    3) reproductive characteristics

    4) habitat preference

    e) impact on human beings

B) Urban social insects

    1) Ants

        a) species identification

        b) digestive characteristics

        c) reproductive characteristics

        d) habitat preference

        e) impact on human beings

    2) Wasps and Bees

        a) special identification

        b) digestive characteristics

        c) reproductive characteristics

        d) habitat preference

        e) impact on human beings

Figure 12-1.

A sample lesson plan that may be adapted for any school level

This report sheds light on those issues related to schools and pesticide use. It recommends an IPM approach to managing pests within the confines of public schools.

Leidy, R. B., C. G. Wright, and H. E. Dupree, Jr., "Concentrations and Movement of Diazinon in Air" *Journal of Environmental Science and Health,* B17(4), 1982, pp. 311-319.

This report indicates that the active ingredient in diazinon will move from the original site of application, further indicating that pesticides do not necessarily remain at the site of application.

Morgan, M. Granger, M.D., "Risk Analysis and Management," *Scientific American,* July, 1993, Volume 269, Number 1.

Dr. Morgan looks at the analysis process for determining risks related to a number of toxins. He points out that there are several unknown factors relating to pesticides, and discusses them as risks unknown to science.

13

LEAD POISONING IN SCHOOLS

by Jacqueline A Krohn, M.D.

Lead, the cause of many health problems, is found in soil, air, and water. In this chapter, Dr. Krohn discusses its history, the hazard it represents for children, and treatment for patients suffering from lead exposure. She addresses a number of questions central to the concerns of school health professionals, maintenance staffs, and all others responsible for the health and safety of children in school.

- ☐ *Why is lead exposure so common in areas that may seem safe?*

- ☐ *What are the sources of lead in older schools?*

- ☐ *How can schools be maintained so that lead exposure is minimized?*

- ☐ *How can the water supply in a school be protected from lead content?*

- ☐ *How can diet help protect children and adults from lead poisoning?*

Lead poisoning is thought to have occurred as far back as Roman times, when toxic levels of lead were used for plumbing and as a sweetening agent in wine and foods. (Smith 1986) Because of its extensive use over centuries, lead has been investigated for toxicity more thoroughly than any other metal. Childhood lead poisoning, a preventable disease, is one of the most common health problems in the United States today. (Centers for Disease Control 1991)

Lead has accumulated in the environment not only because of its extensive use, but because of its nature. Once it has been mined, it cannot be disposed of or converted to an inert chemical. (Smith 1986) It is ubiquitous in the environment, and, therefore, all humans now have lead accumulations in their bodies.

There are three sources of lead in the environment: soil, air, and water, each of which is a potential source of lead exposure for children, who tend to have a larger cumulative exposure to lead sources than adults.

Lead levels in the blood of populations of industrialized countries such as the U.S. are directly related to the amount of leaded gasoline in use. The body burden of lead in human bones is five hundred times greater today than it was during prehistoric times, and the present American diet contains one hundred times more lead than did prehistoric diets.

BIOLOGICAL FATE

There are two forms of lead, each of which is metabolized in a different way. One is inorganic (salts and oxides), and the other is alkyl or organic (tetraethyl lead and tetramethyl lead). Alkyl lead has been used as the anti-knock agent in gasoline. (Hammond and Beliles 1980)

The major routes of inorganic lead absorption are ingestion and inhalation of dust and small lead-containing particles. Alkyl lead compounds, on the other hand, can only be absorbed through the skin.

Absorption from the gastrointestinal tract is affected by the amount of calcium, iron, fat, zinc, and protein in the diet. More lead is absorbed when the body is deficient in calcium, zinc, or vitamin C. (Pounds 1985) Iron deficiency increases lead absorption and toxicity, and often occurs with lead poisoning. (Centers for Disease Control 1991) Although fat increases the absorption of lead, protein decreases lead uptake in the body. Large particles of lead are less easily absorbed than small ones. Infants absorb approximately 40% of lead from food, whereas adults absorb only 10%. (Hammond and Beliles 1980) Growing children tend to absorb and retain more of the lead they ingest than adults. More lead is absorbed during fasting periods than at times when more food is ingested. Lead inhaled into the respiratory tract is completely absorbed by the body.

Once absorbed, lead is transported to all the organs and tissues by the blood and is rapidly transferred to bone. After it is absorbed, the rate of excretion decreases, probably because the original dose of lead becomes gradually more deeply embedded in bone and is less accessible to the blood. Autopsy studies show that lead accumulates in the bones throughout life. (Hammond and Beliles 1980)

In persons with long-term exposures, more than 90% of the total body burden of lead is found in the bones as lead phosphate. The remaining 10% is found in the kidneys and liver.

After an adult's single exposure to it, lead has a half-life of 25 days in the blood; in soft tissue, about 40 days; and in the non-labile portions of bones, more than 25 years. (Royce 1990) In bone there is a labile component, which releases lead into the blood readily, and an inert component. Body stress such as pregnancy, breast-feeding, or chronic disease can mobilize inert lead and increase the lead level in the blood. Lead has also been mobilized from the bones in children who were on prolonged bedrest.

Teeth accumulate lead in a dose-related manner. The lead content of children's primary (baby) teeth has been used in many studies linking lead levels and intellectual performance.

Blood lead levels are measured as micrograms per deciliter (mcg/dl), and these values are used as markers of recent lead exposure and dose-response curves, although they do not indicate the total body burden of lead. Ninety-five percent of the lead in blood is associated with red blood cells and the rest with plasma proteins.

A person does not need a major, acute exposure to lead to develop lead poisoning. Because the body accumulates lead over a lifetime and the bones release it slowly, small doses, over a long period of time, can cause poisoning. It is the total body burden of lead that causes symptoms of poisoning. (Royce 1990)

Lead is excreted in stool, urine, skin, and hair. In infants, more is excreted in the stool than in the urine. (Hammond and Beliles 1980)

BIOLOGICAL EFFECTS

Lead impairs the function of multiple organs and systems. The central nervous system, blood, peripheral nervous system, gastrointestinal tract, endocrine system, and kidneys are affected by it.

Lead Affects the Brain

The brain is the organ most sensitive to the toxic effects of lead, which causes symptoms of dullness, fatigue, insomnia, attention problems, depression, restlessness, irritability, headaches, loss of balance, and memory loss. (Royce 1990) The symptoms may progress to coma and death. Permanent damage to the central nervous system is common from chronic or subchronic exposure to high doses of inorganic lead, and this damage can lead to recurrent seizures, hydrocephalus, and mental retardation.

Lead can cause subtle behavioral abnormalities. Children are more sensitive to its effects than are adults. In children up to 36 months of age there is incomplete development of the blood-brain barrier, which allows lead to enter the developing nervous system more easily. Lead poisoning at an early age can result in prolonged, perhaps lifetime, neurobehavioral disorders. Because lead readily crosses the placenta, exposure to it in utero will affect the cognitive and sensory motor functions of the child.

Children under age seven are most sensitive to the toxic effects of lead, and any child with a developmental delay, speech impairment, or behavioral problem should be a candidate for a check of his or her blood lead level. (Royce 1990)

Dr. Herbert Needleman studied lead levels found in the baby teeth of first and second graders. Children with higher lead levels were nearly four times more likely to have IQ scores below 80 and seven times more likely to have learning disabilities. (Weisskopf 1987) There was a mean drop of four to six IQ points for every 10 mcg/dl of lead in the blood. When first-graders were retested five years later, those who originally had higher lead levels had to attend more special education classes and were retained in grade more than children who were virtually unexposed.

In following the progress of children he first examined in the 1970s, Dr. Needleman has discovered that the higher the child's lead level in the initial study, the more likely he or she was to drop out of high school or have a lower class standing and lower reading skills.

Dr. Needleman found that the areas of learning adversely affected by increased blood lead levels were the following: ability to follow simple directions and sequences, ability to organize, tendency to daydream, distractibility, excitability, hyperactivity, impulsiveness, frustration tolerance, reaction time, degree of independent work, persistence with a task, hand-eye coordination, and the ability to function well. (Needleman 1988) This presents a picture similar to attention deficit disorder. Other researchers have corroborated Dr. Needleman's findings. (Baghurst,

McMichael, Wigg, *et al.* 1992; Munoz, Romieu, Palazuelos, *et al.* 1993) Lead can also cause a hearing loss at the higher frequencies, and this can worsen behavioral problems.

Lead also adversely affects the peripheral nervous system. Lead palsy is a weakness of the extensor muscles (muscles that straighten a joint) and can cause wrist drop. Lead poisoning can also cause abnormal sensation, such as numbness or hypersensitivity of the skin. A slowing of the speed of nerve conduction, even when muscle weakness is not apparent, is another result of lead poisoning.

Lead Affects the Blood

Lead causes anemia by decreasing the lifespan of circulating red blood cells, inhibiting synthesis of hemoglobin, and increasing the fragility of the red blood cell membrane. Although lead poisoning in children does not often cause anemia, iron-deficiency anemia is frequently found in children with lead poisoning.

In the gastrointestinal tract, mild lead toxicity causes occasional abdominal pain. Moderate lead toxicity produces diffuse abdominal pain, vomiting, constipation, and poor appetite. Severe lead toxicity causes intermittent severe abdominal cramps. (Royce 1990) Leaded paint chips may be seen on abdominal radiographs.

Kidney damage is common in lead poisoning, because the reabsorption of some essential elements in the body is decreased. These effects can be reversed with chelation therapy.

Lead exposure may also cause high blood pressure.

In the 1920s, lead was added to gasoline, despite warnings by a committee convened by the Surgeon General that lead might result in chronic degenerative diseases. The automotive and oil industry interests won the battle, and no further data were collected. Gasoline producers are now proposing to add manganese, a known neurotoxin, to gasoline. (Urbanowicz 1986)

In 1930, the toxic lead level was considered to be 158 mcg/dl. Now the toxic level of lead is 10 mcg/dl. Dr. Needleman states that 17% of all children have blood lead levels greater than 10 mcg/dl. (Holmes and Breen 1993) Children with blood lead levels between 10 mcg/dl and 19 mcg/dl should be retested every three to four months. Health care workers should take an environmental history of any child with a toxic blood lead level and give educational and nutritional counseling to both child and parents. (Centers for Disease Control 1991).

If a toxic lead level persists for a child, health care workers should perform an environmental investigation (including school and day care) and have as much lead as possible removed from the home. Children with blood lead levels above 20 mcg/dl should be retested and referred for medical evaluation and follow-up. Those with blood lead levels above 25 mcg/dl should be treated with a chelating agent, and those with blood lead levels 20 mcg/dl or above should be tested for iron deficiency. (Centers for Disease Control 1991)

A blood lead level as low as 5 mcg/dl can increase blood pressure. There is no indication of a threshold for lead, and no safe level has yet been found for children. (Royce 1990) In animal studies, lead at picogram levels has been shown to affect nerve transmission. Because of biochemical individuality, a lead level can cause symptoms in one person, while another person can be asymptomatic with the identical lead level.

The test previously used for screening lead in children was erythrocyte protoporphyrin, assayed as zinc protoporphyrin (ZPP). (Royce 1990) This test, however, is not sensitive at the lower levels of lead poisoning, below 35 mcg/dl. It is now recommended that blood lead levels be obtained on patients rather than zinc protoporphyrin levels.

L-X-ray fluorescence has demonstrated elevated bone lead levels in children exposed to lead compared to children not exposed to it. Both groups of children had blood lead levels less than 10 mcg/dl. Since hair concentrates lead levels over 200 times those of blood, it may be a better marker for chronic lead poisoning than blood.

Blood lead levels of 70 mcg/dl and above can cause loss of balance, severe abdominal pain, hyperactivity, apathy, incoordination, paralysis, seizures, and coma. Blood lead levels of 50 mcg/dl or more may cause a flu-like illness, joint pain, headache, tremor, loss of appetite, intermittent vomiting, abdominal pain, and constipation. Blood lead levels greater than or equal to 10 mcg/dl have been associated with decreased intelligence, decreased growth rate, hearing loss, balance problems, behavioral problems, and kidney disease.

SOURCES OF LEAD

Lead in Paint

Children may have lead exposure at school where three potential sources of exposure are lead paint, lead in dust both inside and outside the building, and water that may be contaminated with lead.

Lead has been used in paint because it reduces weathering of the painted surface, and it has also been used for pigmentation of paint and as a drying agent. (Moore 1986) Oil-based paints have typically contained lead, whereas latex water-based paints have usually been lead-free.

The lead content of paint was not regulated until 1977, and lead-based paint produced before 1960 had a higher concentration of lead than paint produced in later years. Lead-based paint in the 1940s often contained up to 50% lead.

Many older buildings, including residential and commercial buildings and schools, have leaded paint that is peeling, flaking, and chipping. Children can ingest loose paint chips because of pica (eating of non-food items), and by mouthing items contaminated with lead from paint, dust, and soil. Lead paint is attractive to children because it tastes sweet.

Even if a room with lead paint is painted over with non-lead paint, those areas with friction, such as windows, will continue to spread lead dust into the air. The new paint is also partially mixed with the lead-based paint, and lead dust will be released when the new paint starts to deteriorate.

Although deleading can be done, it is expensive and in itself can cause lead poisoning. With good clean-up techniques, however, children can return to a school that has been deleaded the next day. (Clark 1993)

If lead-based paint is present in the school, some maintenance activities should be performed carefully and only when children are not in school. Making holes in walls to install electrical outlets or to have access to pipes, tearing out walls, bumping furniture or other objects into painted walls, and closing and opening windows with painted frames and sills can aerosolize lead dust. (National Safety Council 1993)

Sweeping or vacuuming an area of renovation can also cause lead dust to aerosolize. Dust and chips can be cleaned up with a wet cloth soaked in trisodium phosphate (TSP) or powdered dishwasher detergent dissolved in water. Anyone doing such work should wear gloves to prevent skin irritation. (National Safety Council 1993)

There are four methods for dealing with lead paint in a building:

- Encapsulation, in which a substance that bonds with lead paint and prevents it from peeling or becoming dust is applied to the painted surface.

- Scraping or using chemicals to remove the lead paint.

- Removal of paint off-site. If a door has been covered with lead paint, it can be transported from its usual location to another site where the lead paint is removed, and then brought back to the school.

- Enclosing a lead-painted area with paneling or drywall. (Clark 1993).

Since different paints can be used on walls, window frames, doors, and exteriors, each painted surface should be tested, preferably by one of several professional methods. One method uses X-ray fluorescence and can measure lead in all the layers of paint. Another involves removing paint from a two-square-inch surface area and analyzing it in a laboratory. (National Safety Council 1993) Home test kits are available, but their reliability for low levels of lead is unknown.

Lead in the Soil

High volumes of lead have been found in the soil in many cities where contamination results from the deposit of airborne dust that contains lead. Children have a greater risk of exposure to lead in dust from soil because of their shorter stature and poor hygiene. (Moore 1986) In one study, the most important determinant of blood lead concentrations in children was the lead level in soil and dust, both indoors and outdoors. The lead concentration is lower indoors than outdoors, but lead-contaminated soil and dust from outside can be tracked indoors. Lead is harder to remove from carpets than from non-carpeted surfaces. Vacuum cleaning does not remove the smallest particles, but rather, spreads them around.

Soil can be contaminated from lead paint as far as 10 feet from a building. If the soil around a school is lead-contaminated or likely to be lead-contaminated, planting grass or other plants will help. If lead-based exterior paint causes soil contamination, bushes can be planted near the walls. (National Safety Council 1993)

Dust to be tested for lead content should be collected from different surfaces, including floors and windowsills. Samples are collected with a wet wipe, and analyzed by a laboratory for lead content. Soil samples can also be analyzed for lead content.

Lead in the Air

The greatest source of lead in the air is leaded gasoline in automobile exhaust, and the lead level is higher next to busy roads. Such lead may be inhaled directly or deposited in the soil. If it is in the air, it may be absorbed if the particles are less than 5 microns in diameter (about the size of a cell). Children playing near roads and freeways not only breathe the exhaust fumes, but also come into contact with contaminated dirt. (Moore 1986) Since less leaded gasoline is in use now, the blood lead levels of the population have decreased.

Lead can also be found in the air in areas near smelters, where lead is processed, or near battery recycling plants.

Lead in the Water

Water from leaded pipes, soldered plumbing, or water cooling systems may contain lead. Lead levels are high in water that is drawn early in the morning or after vacations and weekends, because the water remaining in the pipes has had longer contact with the lead. In addition, hot water from contaminated plumbing has higher lead levels than cold water.. Approximately 20% of the body burden of lead in children is from water contaminated with lead. (Holmes and Breen 1993)

The Lead Contamination Control Act of 1988, an amendment to the Safe Drinking Water Act, directs that water coolers that are not lead-free be identified; that water coolers with lead-lined tanks be repaired or removed; that water coolers be manufactured lead free; that the drinking water of schools be analyzed for lead; that elevated lead levels be corrected; and that more money be set aside for lead screening programs for children. (EPA 1989)

The Environmental Protection Agency (EPA) is required to help states and localities test for and eliminate lead contamination in drinking water in schools and day care centers. The new law stipulates that drinking water provided by a public water system must have lead levels less than or equal to five parts per billion (ppb) or five micrograms per liter. The Lead Contamination Control Act of 1988 requires schools with their own water supplies to notify parents, teachers, school personnel, and the public that lead test results are available. (EPA 1989)

Lead usually enters drinking water because of corrosion of lead pipes, solder, faucets, or other parts of a plumbing system. Corrosion of lead solder is thought to be the main source of lead in drinking water. The more acidic water is, the more corrosive it is. (Holmes and Breen 1993) Soft water, which causes more soap lather, also causes more corrosion. Less corrosive water will allow a mineral deposit to coat the inside of the pipes, thus preventing the leaching of lead from the pipes. Water can also be contaminated at its source from lead occurring naturally in the ground, from surface water from waste-water treatment plants, or from rain water that has gathered lead particles in the air.

The degree of lead contamination depends upon how corrosive the water is, the amount of lead in the plumbing pipes and fixtures or the water cooler, the age of the plumbing, and whether electrical systems are grounded to the water pipes. If the pipe that carries water from the public water system to the school system contains lead, all the water in the school will be contaminated with lead. If lead solder is used in some of the water outlets in the school but not in others, the lead levels may vary in different parts of the school building. Localized lead contamination can also occur if a water cooler has a lead-lined tank. (EPA 1989) The school official responsible for testing and finding a remedy for lead in school water will have to investigate the type of plumbing used in his or her school system.

Lead plumbing was common until 1930, when copper pipes were introduced for plumbing, though lead solder remained in use for pipe joints. Between 1920 and 1950, galvanized pipes were also used. Today, although a lead ban is being implemented, lead soldering may often be used with copper pipes. (EPA 1989) Lead solder, which was legal through 1988, reacts with copper so that lead is released into the water flowing through the pipes.

Plasticizers in plastic pipes may contain lead. Electric equipment using water pipes as grounding can increase the amount of corrosion in plumbing that contains lead, and if this occurs, an electrician will have to find an alternate grounding system. Faucets, pipes, and pipe fittings labelled "lead free" may contain up to 8% lead. (Holmes and Breen 1993)

Either the local water supplier or the state or local department of health can collect and analyze water samples from a school. The laboratory usually sends a specimen container with instructions regarding sample collection. In a two-step water-sampling procedure, all water outlets can be sampled in the initial step, and then follow-up samples can be collected from those outlets with high lead levels. Samples should be collected before school opens in the morning, before any water has been used. The EPA does not recommend that samples be taken after vacations or weekends, but that all schools flush drinking water outlets after every weekend and vacation.

If the lead levels from all water sources do not exceed 20 ppb, then samples of the water can be taken after weekends and vacations. If lead levels in the water are below 20 ppb after weekends and vacations, then the water system does not need to be flushed after every weekend or break. If lead levels are elevated, flushing the plumbing system is only a temporary measure to be used until permanent solutions can bring lead levels down. The EPA has a standard procedure for flushing water systems. Routine daily flushing of water coolers, however, is not practical because it takes such a long time (15 minutes) and uses a large amount of water. (EPA 1989)

Some permanent solutions to decrease the sources of lead in the water include making the water less corrosive at the local water treatment plant (adding orthophosphates or silicates to make the water harder); installing corrosion control devices for the school system; reducing lead levels at the tap by using reverse osmosis devices and distillation units; removal by a qualified electrician of wires grounded to water pipes; replacing outlets if lead contamination is localized; replacing lead pipe or lead connectors in the water system; repairing and replacing the plumbing system with lead-free solder only; or using time-operated valves that automatically flush the main pipes of the system. If these treatments fail or are not feasible, then bottled water can be drunk by students, teachers, and other school personnel.

Lead in the Art and Food Supplies

Art materials that contain lead should not be used in elementary schools. Non-toxic, unleaded ceramic glazes can be substituted for leaded glazes.

Foods eaten at school could also be contaminated with lead. Food should not be stored in open cans, especially if cans are imported or if they have soldered seams. Nor should foods be stored or served in pottery, especially if it is imported. (CDC 1991) Since plastic food storage bags can have lead in the print, all print should be kept to the outside and should not touch food.

TREATMENT OF LEAD POISONING

Treatment for children with lead poisoning consists of an intravenous infusion of calcium EDTA, either alone or in combination with dimercaptopropanol (BAL), intramuscularly. The combined therapy is more effective than either drug used alone. In four to five days of treatment, 5 mg of lead may be removed from a body burden of 50 to 100 mg or more. When lead is removed, there will be a post-chelation rebound of lead into the blood. (Kosnett 1992) The major source of this mobilized lead is the bones.

DMSA (dimercaptosuccinic acid or Succimer), which is related to BAL, was released as an oral agent for lead chelation in 1991, when it was approved for use in children with blood lead levels greater than 45 mcg/dl. It is given for five days. A recent study shows that six months after chelation with EDTA, children in the population studied had a one-point rise in IQ for every three mcg/dl decrease in blood lead level. (Raff, Bijur, Markowitz, *et al.* 1993)

Adequate protein, zinc, vitamin C, iron, and copper in the diet protect children against lead toxicity. Thiamine (vitamin B1) may also protect against lead toxicity and deposition, as do calcium and chromium. (Shechter 1992) Children should have a well-balanced diet adequate in micronutrients or a multivitamin to ensure protection against the toxic effects of lead.

CONCLUSION

The lead content of dust, soil, paint, and water should be tested in schools located close to highways, or those that were built before 1977, and those that have old plumbing. Since children spend one-third of their day at school, every school building should be investigated as a potential source of lead poisoning.

REFERENCES

Baghurst, Peter A., Anthony J. McMichael, Neil R. Wigg, *et al.*, 1992, "Environmental Exposure to Lead and Children's Intelligence at the Age of Seven Years. The Port Pirie Cohort Study," *New England Journal of Medicine* 327, no. 18: 1279-84.

Centers for Disease Control, 1991, "Preventing Lead Poisoning in Young Children: A Statement by the Centers for Disease Control," Atlanta: CDC.

Clark, Gerry, 1993, "Legal, Economic Webs Tangle Removal Efforts." In *AAP News*, edited by Elizabeth Oplatka. Elk Grove Village, IL: American Academy of Pediatrics.

Doctor's Data, Inc., 1986, "A Summary of Literature Regarding Elements in Human Hair," *Doctor's Data Handout*, pp. 3-6.

Hammond, Paul B., and Robert P. Beliles, 1980, "Metals," In *Casarett and Doull's Toxicology, The Basic Science of Poisons*, edited by John Doull, Curtis D. Klaassen, and Mary D. Amdur, New York: Macmillan Publishing Company.

Holmes, Hannah, and Bill Breen, 1993, "Getting The Lead Out," *Garbage*, pp. 26-31.

Kosnett, Michael J., 1992, "Says Benefit of Chelation for Lead Toxicity Still Unproved," *Pediatric News* 26, no. 7, p. 25.

Lansdown, Richard, 1986, "Lead, Intelligence, Attainment, and Behavior". In *Lead Toxicity, History and Environmental Impact*, edited by Richard Lansdown and William Yule, Baltimore: The Johns Hopkins Press.

Moore, Michael R., 1986, "Lead in Paint," in *Lead Toxicity, History and Environmental Impact*, edited by Richard Lansdown and William Yule, Baltimore: The Johns Hopkins Press.

Moore, Michael R., 1986, "Lead in Soils," in *Lead Toxicity, History and Environmental Impact*, edited by Richard Lansdown and William Yule Baltimore: The Johns Hopkins Press.

Moore, Michael R., 1986, "Lead in the Air," in *Lead Toxicity, History and Environmental Impact,* edited by Richard Lansdown and William Yule, Baltimore: The Johns Hopkins Press.

Munoz, Hilda, Isabelle Romieu, Eduardo Palazuelos, *et al*, 1993, "Blood Lead Level and Neurobehavioral Development Among Children Living in Mexico City," *Archives of Environmental Health* 48, no. 3, pp. 132-139.

National Safety Council, 1993, "National Lead Information Center," Washington, D. C: United States Government Printing Office.

Needleman, Herbert E., 1988, "Why We Should Worry about Lead Poisoning," *Contemporary Pediatrics*, pp. 34-56.

Pounds, Joel G., 1985, "The Toxic Effect of Metals," in *Industrial Toxicology*, edited by Phillip L. Williams and James L. Burson, New York: Van Nostrand Reinhold.

Royce, Sarah E., 1990, "Case Studies in Environmental Medicine. Lead Toxicity," Atlanta: Agency for Toxic Substances and Disease Registry.

Ruff, Holly A., Polly E. Bijur, Morris Markowitz, *et al.*, 1993, "Declining Blood Lead Levels and Cognitive Changes in Moderately Lead-Poisoned Children," *Journal of the American Medical Association* 269, no. 13, pp. 1641-1646.

Schechter, Steve, 1992, "Get The Lead Out," *Let's Live*, p. 80.

Smith, Marjorie, 1986, "Lead in History," in *Lead Toxicity, History and Environmental Impact*, edited by Richard Lansdown and William Yule, Baltimore: The Johns Hopkins Press.

Smith, Marjorie, 1986, "What Is Lead?" in *Lead Toxicity, History and Environmental Impact*, edited by Richard Lansdown and William Yule, Baltimore: The Johns Hopkins Press.

Urbanowicz, Marie Anne, 1986, "The Uses of Lead Today," in *Lead Toxicity, History and Environmental Impact*, edited by Richard Lansdown and William Yule, Baltimore: The Johns Hopkins Press.

United States Environmental Protection Agency, 1989, "Lead in School Drinking Water," Washington, D.C.: The Agency.

Weisskopf, Michael, 1987, "Lead Astray. The Poisoning of America," *Discover*, pp. 68-74.

14

TRACKING MOLD: A Professionally Guided Middle School Science Project

by Richard G. Jaeckle, M.D., Kevin Kuehn, M.S., and Judith Jaeckle

Environmental data gathering sometimes makes an ideal student project. In this chapter, Dr. Jaeckle, Mr. Kuehn, and Ms. Jaeckle describe such a project carried out in four Dallas schools. When a student was able to conduct a two-year study of airborne mycoflora in schools where musty odors suggested the presence of mold, she not only advanced her learning about the environment, but also could present her findings at Regional Science Fairs, as well as at a professional meeting devoted to environmental science. The chapter reveals a number of ways that the relationship of environmental studies to the science curriculum can be explored in other school districts:

☐ *How might a classroom problem such as musty air be used as a starting point for curriculum activities in your school?*

☐ *How might a long-term study of classroom environment be designed for your students' participation?*

☐ *How could students in your school work with environmental-science professionals to design their own environmental-study project?*

☐ *How might a student project in your school district be used to improve conditions in your school buildings?*

☐ *What other school activities can help students become more aware of the need to find cures for all sick buildings?*

Air quality studies from schools are virtually non-existent, so the following airborne mycoflora survey from four elementary schools within the Dallas-Plano Metroplex represents a solid block in the foundation of basic data. The reasons for the lack of studies relate to the financial condition of the school or school district. Numerous other priorities precede concern about air quality, and there is general ignorance of the fact that school buildings could share the same problems as other types of buildings. So the political and economic milieu of schools serves as a bulwark against the intrusions of anyone whose data might suggest increased expenditures that would disturb the delicate balance of budgets and contracts.

The doors in Dallas swung wide open, however, to a student who was performing the annual ritual of a science project during two successive years, seventh and eighth grade. The project used scientific equipment under careful mycologic and medical supervision to guarantee the accuracy of the data and conclusions. The account that follows is drawn from the data collected by the student in her research. Her work not only qualified her for participation in the Regional Science Fair both years, but enabled her to present her findings at the meeting at which the study was first discussed.

METHOD

In the first part of the study, four schools stretching over a 16-mile area within the Dallas-Plano Metroplex were studied on the weekend of February 16 and 17, 1991. At each of the four schools, an outdoor control, the cafeteria, the library, and three classrooms were tested using the Andersen Sampler, which accelerates and impinges mold spores on culture media. Exact spore counts could be determined, since the Andersen is calibrated to a volume of one cubic foot per minute. It was operated for four minutes with a pair of both 2% malt extract and 1.7% cornmeal agar plates at six sites in each of the four schools. After incubation at room temperature for seven days, the colonies were counted and identified.

In the second part of the study, one of the four schools was singled out the following year for an analysis of the effect of air cleaners. Nine classrooms were sampled before and after the addition of air cleaners, on February 16 and 23, 1992, respectively. Three rooms served as controls; four rooms used one filter; and two rooms used two filters.

In addition to the Andersen Sampler with malt extract and cornmeal agars, a Laser Particle Counter and the Burkhart Volumetric Spore Trap were used both before and after one week's operation of air filters. The Burkhart, which was operated for 10 minutes in each of the nine classrooms, is calibrated to sample 10 L/min. (liters per minute) and to impact particles onto a slide coated with an adhesive. The Laser Particle Counter was operated for one minute, sampling one cubic foot. The filters were installed in the classrooms on February 16, and set on medium fan speed. Instructions were given that the filters should not be turned off, but should be left running for a full week. The following Sunday, February 23, 1992, the nine rooms were again tested with the Andersen, the Burkhart, and the Laser Particle Counter. The filters were subsequently removed. Cultures were incubated at room temperature for one week, then counted and identified. The Burkhart slides were also counted and identified. The Laser Particle Counter data, as well as those collected with the Burkhart and Andersen, were converted to counts per cubic meter for standardization.

BUILDING CHARACTERISTICS

The construction of the four schools varied both from building to building and within each building. Since the schools had been constructed in phases, each one had older and newer segments. The heating and air-conditioning systems also differed from hot/cold circulating water to forced air and mixtures thereof.

School #1 had hot/cold circulating water with each room's unit vented to the outside through an exterior wall. Several internal rooms had neither windows nor exterior walls, so the presence or position of a vent in any of these rooms could not be verified.

School #2 had circulating hot water and forced air cooling for an older section, and forced air heating and cooling for a newer section. All classrooms had windows.

School #3 had circulating hot water, with air-conditioning units situated on the roof directly above the classrooms. All rooms had windows.

School #4 had a heating and air-conditioning unit on the roof for every four classrooms. Several internal classrooms were without windows.

School #3 had hard floor covering throughout; the others were carpeted in all areas except the cafeterias. School #3 also had a leaky roof that was completely renovated eighteen months after the completion of this study.

Since Part Two of the study focused on School #1, its building characteristics are elaborated further here. The school, which was built in two stages, was located on a hillside. The older section occupied one level at the top of the hill. The newer section was built on two levels down the slope, with the top floor adjacent to the older section. The lower level of the new section, constructed against the hillside, contained several classrooms without windows. This was particularly important to the study since there was no forced air ventilation, and the rooms without windows had neither exterior walls nor air intakes for the fan units. The odor of the classrooms without windows was especially musty. Hot or cold water circulated to the various rooms for heating and cooling.

All four schools were used daily, Monday through Friday, and portions of the buildings were also used during the evenings and weekends for non-school activities. Some rooms were very heavily used, giving dust and mold spores little time to settle. A detailed activity log would be required for each of these rooms to monitor its traffic.

AMBIENT CONDITIONS

On Saturday, February 17, 1991, the temperature range was 47 to 32 degrees F., and the mold count was 318 spores per cubic meter (mountain cedar 61; elm 128). On Sunday, February 18, 1991, the temperature range was 76 to 46 degrees F. with a mold count of 266 spores per cubic meter (mountain cedar 161; elm 50).

On Sunday, February 16, 1992, the temperature range was 66 to 44 degrees F., and the mold count was 469 spores per cubic meter (mountain cedar 411; elm 328; ash 6; algae 22). The following Sunday, February 23, 1992, the temperature range was 64 to 51 degrees F., and the mold count was 884 spores per cubic meter (elm 27; ash 6; mountain cedar 6).

RESULTS

The survey of the four schools performed in 1991 as Part One of the study are summarized in *Figures 14-1 and 14-2*.

Most notably, the counts in the outdoor controls always exceeded the indoor measurements in every room, because the walls and closed windows of the building formed a barrier to molds from outdoor vegetation. This data is probably the most significant finding in the report. A few rooms with higher than usual mold counts were identified

	Library	Cafeteria	Class #1	Class #	Class #	Outdoor control
School #1	71	62	80	106	53	548
School #2	106	168	62	35	168	1343
School #3	159	282	247	239	239	442
School #4	97	486	292	168	168	530

Figure 14-1.
Four school survey, 1991. Andersen Sampler, malt extract agar.

	Library	Cafeteria	Class #1	Class #	Class #	Outdoor control
School #1	80	88	88	212	106	671
School #2	141	53	88	115	106	2597
School #3	106	168	353	124	256	512
School #4	186	742	283	194	80	830

Figure 14-2.
Four school survey, 1991. Andersen Sampler, cornmeal agar.

as problematic, especially the cafeteria at school #4, which had a characteristically foul odor.

Interestingly enough, the outdoor control was slightly higher, but the scent outdoors was refreshingly pleasant despite the higher count. Moreover, both the cafeteria and the outdoor control had the same predominant species, Cladosporium. So there was no difference in mold count or composition between the foul-smelling cafeteria and the refreshing outdoor control. The most common mold in all rooms was Cladosporium, the same as outdoors. Next came Alternaria, Penicillium, Aspergillus, and lesser known species. The outdoor controls also varied considerably from school to school. The variation in the outdoor controls can be attributed to several factors:

■ the distance between the schools
■ the variation in vegetation near the buildings

- the influence of a cold front which lowered the temperature on the first day of the collection
- the lag period in the effect of temperature on the sporulation of the mold
- the diurnal variation of temperature with the characteristic sporulation of molds in the afternoon and evening

The outdoor control using the Andersen Sampler differed from the mold count in the pollen report, because the latter was performed using the Roto-Rod Collector which produces lower counts than both the Andersen and the Burkhart. The Burkhart counts are actually higher than the Andersen counts, since some of the spores visualized and counted by the Burkhart, would not grow out on the culture media of the Andersen. Finally, some differential in growth of colonies was observed between the malt extract and the cornmeal agars. As can be seen in *Figure 14-2*, however, the colony counts are quite similar and nearly parallel.

Part Two of the study, conducted exactly 12 months after Part One, focused on School #1's mold counts before and after air filtration of one week's duration.

Figure 14-3 illustrates the mold counts of the combined malt extract and cornmeal agars for all nine rooms before and after the week of filtration. The rooms are then grouped by number of filters in *Figure 14-4*, and calculations reveal no significant reduction in mold spores with filtration.

The Burkhart, however, does reveal a significant reduction of mold spores in the rooms with two filters, as shown in *Figures 14-5* and *14-6*.

The Laser Particle Counter was used to monitor total particles, including mold spores, dust, and all other particles. The results are illustrated in *Figures 14-7* and *14-8*.

	7A	8B	5A	6B	4A	3B	4B	7B	CP	OC
Feb 16	119	124	190	123	62	234	176	124	362	936
Feb 23	106	124	428	75	119	150	150	75	132	720

Figure 14-3.
School #1, 1992. Andersen Sampler; malt/cornmeal mean colony count.

	No Filters	One Filter	Two Filters	Outdoor control
Feb 16	141 +/- 28	149 +/- 64	243 +/- 119	936
Feb 23	219 +/-148	124 +/-31	103 +/- 28	720

Figure 14-4.

School #1, 1992. Andersen Sampler; rooms grouped by number of filters.

	7A	8B	5A	6B	4A	3B	4B	7B	CP	OC
Feb 16	493	327	460	428	230	360	360	427	360	4031
Feb 23	426	327	557	393	261	360	229	196	294	1474

Figure 14-5.

School #1, 1992. Burkhart Spore Trap; malt/cornmeal mean colony count.

	No Filters	One Filter	Two Filters	Outdoor control
Feb 16	427 +/- 72	345 +/- 72	394 +/- 33	4031
Feb 23	437 +/- 94	311 +/- 68	245 +/- 49	1474

Figure 14-6.

School #1, 1992. Burkhart Spore Trap; rooms grouped by number of filters.

	7A	8B	5A	6B	4A	3B	4B	7B	CP	OC
Feb 16	9	13	18	15	7	18	32	8	12	16
Feb 23	27	13	9	14	7	39	10	13	4	6

Figure 14-7.

School #1, 1992. Laser Particle Counter (x 1,000).

These results are much more variable, and are more likely to be related to recent activity in the room, since even a few minutes of movement in a room will stir up enough particles to increase the counts. A survey of standard conditions where the amount of activity in a room is controlled

	No Filters	One Filter	Two Filters	Outdoor control
Feb 16	16760 +/- 7846	17976 +/- 9072	9911 +/- 1714	15901
Feb 23	14322 +/- 5097	17685 +/- 12534	8833 +/- 4417	6289

Figure 14-8.
School #1, 1992. Laser Particle Counter; rooms grouped by number of filters.

could not be done within the confines of this study. Nonetheless, no significant reduction was achieved with the Laser Particle Counter.

Other calculations were also performed and are included here. The rooms on the first and second floor were compared, and while there was no significant difference between the two, there was a tendency toward a reduced count on the upper floor. Several of the classrooms also had plants in various numbers, but here again, while a tendency existed toward a lower count with fewer plants, no significant difference was discovered. There was some tampering with the fan speed, but none of the machines was turned off. Three of the filters were still found on the medium setting. Two other filters were turned to high, both in rooms with no windows, as if the occupants hungered for better air. The other three filters located in small rooms where they were very close to students' desks were turned to low, suggesting that the noise they created was a disturbance. The heating/cooling fans were left on in the three rooms with no windows, but in the six rooms with windows, only one fan was left running. This also suggests that leakage from the windows provides some fresh air, whereas the stale air in the windowless rooms motivated someone to keep the fans running.

When we entered one control room for the measurement on the second weekend, a very noticeable odor attracted our attention, and we found a significant elevation in the mold count during the week. The cause was found to be an onion on the teacher's desk which was sprouting. After the colonies were grown out and counted, we realized that in this room not only was the mold count higher, but also that this was the only room where Cladosporium did not predominate. Rather, Penicillium was found in significantly higher concentrations here.

We found the mold count was reduced only 12% in the rooms with windows, compared with 27% in the rooms without windows. Since the windows could not be opened, we surmised that air infiltration around the casements, bringing a higher mold count from outside, actually reduced the efficiency of the filters.

DISCUSSION

This study was prompted by the musty odor in classrooms in several schools, an odor that was frequently described as moldy. The results of the study, including the data from February of two different years, however, failed to document even one room with a mold count higher than that of the outdoor controls. With the exception of some problem rooms, classroom counts were generally considerably lower. School #1 was tested both years, and the indoor counts were remarkably consistent. All four schools are apparently not getting enough fresh air to dilute the body odors, perfumes, volatile solvents from various sources, cleaning solutions, insecticides, etc., brought into the building daily.

The rooms with windows permitted air infiltration, which was apparent when they were compared to the rooms without windows, but even so, the rooms with windows were merely less stale than the others. The odor of the rooms without windows was worse, and a teacher remarked that after physical education, the body odor was almost intolerable and hung in the air for hours. So the odor problem is not due to mold, but rather to stale air.

During the two weeks including the week of filtration in 1992, half of the school was reported absent at one time or another due to colds and influenza. It is impossible to avoid contamination in rooms where the air that is rebreathed is stale from lack of air exchange. So although mold concentration is low indoors compared to outdoors, our findings about molds certainly do not apply to viruses.

Teachers were aware of the stale air, and our air filters were welcomed by teachers and students alike, as a sign that something was finally being done about the stale air problem. The filters were only designed to remove particles, not odors, however. The evidence that the speed of the filter fan had been increased probably indicated the desire for fresher air. Those encouraged by the appearance of the filters must have been disappointed by their removal after one week.

Since only a few plants were kept in the classrooms, there was little apparent contribution from them. In fact, over the period of days or weeks, mold settles out of the air unless replenished quickly. The differential that exists between inside and outside indicates the significant barrier function of a closed building. Obviously, if the windows were kept open, there would be no differential in counts between inside and outside. So the differential indirectly indicates insufficient air exchange.

SUMMARY

The enclosed building with windows shut for year-round heating and air-conditioning effectively keeps out and reduces mold counts indoors. An exception to this probably exists in nearly all buildings, possibly due to conditions specific to certain areas. The efficiency in reducing heating and air-conditioning cost is indisputable, but the cost in air quality and health is substantial. Schools are no exception to that rule, and are perhaps even more vulnerable because of severely restricted budgets and overcrowding.

In other words, schools also suffer from the sick building syndrome, and more commonly than we would think. The solution to this problem is not easy. It starts with increased awareness, and we hope this study, which involved a student in data gathering, will contribute to that goal.

15

FORMALDEHYDE AS A SCHOOL PROBLEM

by David L. Morris, M.D.

Formaldehyde, the simplest of the aldehydes, can cause symptoms of allergy and chemical sensitivity. Because its resin systems are used in so much of the furniture, fabric, glues, and bonding agents found in homes and schools, Dr. Morris points out that it frequently triggers asthma attacks and respiratory discomfort, and in extreme cases, can contribute to severe attention deficit disorder. In this chapter, he addresses the concerns of school health-care providers and others responsible for the health of students. He discusses the desensitization treatment he gives his own patients and answers a number of questions about the prevalence and effects of formaldehyde in the classroom.

☐ *Why does formaldehyde have such a serious effect on the health of some students?*

☐ *What have physicians learned about its pathology over the past 50 years?*

☐ *How can fabrics and other innocent-seeming materials treated with formaldehyde affect otherwise healthy individuals?*

☐ *Why is desensitization a preferred treatment for those suffering the symptoms of formaldehyde exposure?*

☐ *What can a school do to minimize formaldehyde exposure?*

For such a simple compound, formaldehyde is a cause of many complex problems, and these problems are not just toxic. Formaldehyde is an allergen, and it can cause any of the symptoms of allergy *or* chemical sensitivity. Since formaldehyde is ubiquitous, the problems it causes are impossible to avoid.

Formaldehyde is the simplest aldehyde with the organic formula HCHO. The commercial production of formaldehyde involves catalytic oxidation of methyl alcohol in the presence of copper, silver, or iron molybdenum.

It is commercially available as formalin, a water solution of 35%-40% formaldehyde and 0-15% methanol added to prevent polymerization. Physiologically, it is absorbed by all routes, is rapidly oxidized in the body to formic acid, and is excreted in the urine as formate.

FORMALDEHYDE IN THE ENVIRONMENT

Various formaldehyde resin systems (i.e., phenol-formaldehyde resin, resorcinol-formaldehyde, melamine-formaldehyde resin and urea-formaldehyde resin) are produced commercially, and are extensively used in such diverse items as adhesives in plywood glues, and bonding agents in particleboard, plywood, and chipboard; as a foam resin for insulation purposes; and as a glue for carpeting and other floor coverings. All these materials are used in schools.

In the 1960's, I saw a large number of skin problems from formaldehyde in fabrics. I learned from the patients suffering formaldehyde-induced skin conditions that they had symptoms of nasal allergy and asthma, and of chemical sensitivity as well. It also became very evident from observations of other patients, that strange illnesses developed among some occupants of mobile homes. Although such illnesses were initially called toxic problems, most of the patients showed the symptoms and signs of allergy and multiple chemical sensitivity.

Formaldehyde may act as an upper respiratory tract irritant; it has a high solubility in water and is held by the moisture covering the respiratory passages. It interacts with airborne particulates and is carried by them into the alveolar spaces where it may induce inflammation. Formaldehyde is never the only allergen causing symptoms, however, and patients always have other inhalant, food, or chemical allergies.

Evidence currently being accumulated strongly suggests a true sensitizing effect of formaldehyde can culminate in a wide spectrum of clinical disease entities. Formaldehyde is capable of inducing contact dermatitis in both occupational and non-occupational settings (Fisher) and has been reported in rare cases as causing urticarial rashes as well. (Helander 1977; Fabry 1968) Vaughn first reported a case of occupational asthma attributable to formalin sensitivity in 1939 (Vaughan 1939); further reports by Popa, Sakula, Hendrick and Lane have followed. (Popa , Teculescu, Stanescu, and Gavrilescu 1969) Skerfving has incriminated aldehyde pyrolysates from thermal degradation of polyethylene wrap in "meatwrappers' asthma" in Sweden. (Skerfving 1980) Rea has reported cardiovascular and vasculitic reactions occurring in sensitive patients undergoing double-blind challenges to formalin and other environmental chemicals while in environmentally controlled settings. (Rea 1977, 1978) Randolph had earlier reported on the hazards of indoor air pollution from common formaldehyde-containing products. (Randolph 1962)

The true pathogenesis of formaldehyde sensitivity remains poorly understood; many reports attribute symptoms to non-immunological, irritable characteristics of formaldehyde. Attention has been drawn, however, to the fact that common symptoms associated with formaldehyde exposure are, in reality, common allergy symptoms, and it has been emphasized that the problem of formaldehyde toxicity is often a problem of individual susceptibility and "chemical sensitivity." (Morris 1992) It is known that formaldehyde can cause dermatitis on the basis of either irritation or cell-mediated immunity and may induce immediate skin sensitivity. It would seem logical, as Bardana postulates, that "if specific immune hypersensitivity phenomena have been documented on the skin, similar mechanisms may prevail in the upper and lower respiratory tracts." (Bardana 1980) The late-phase asthmatic responses to formalin inhalation challenge found by Popa, Hendrick and others (Hendrick and Lane 1975) is similar to that described in sensitized subjects after the inhalation of other relatively simple reactive chemicals, including toluene di-isocynate (TDI) and platinum salts. The lack of immediate reaction on inhalation challenge argues against a direct irritant effect from the formalin. Also, delayed skin reactivity to a non-irritating intradermal injection of a dilute formalin solution coincided with delayed onset bronchospasm in one of the patients in Popa's study. Indeed, formaldehyde possesses the capability to bind and alter protein constituents. It is not unreasonable to postulate that it may combine with respiratory tract proteins and form an immunoreactive, hapten-protein complex with resultant mediator release. (Morris *et al.* 1971) Alternatively, formaldehyde may directly trigger various complex enzyme systems known to be sensitive to other chemicals (i.e., the kinin/kallikrein system) as described by Bell (Bell 1975) with resultant mediator release and generation of multiple-system functional symptomatology as observed in "chemically sensitive" patients decribed by Randolph and Rea.

We have been able to measure formaldehyde levels accurately in our area. Outside measurements averaged 0.003 parts per million, clothing stores

0.13 parts per million, fabric stores 0.60 parts per million, and there were 1.7 parts per million in a biology wet lab. This correlated with patients' histories, where severely sensitive patients could not even tolerate the level in clothing stores. Although the level of formaldehyde would vary greatly with the degree of ventilation and air exchange, schools could fall into any category. For many of our patients, it is important to be able to open a window and get fresh air into the room. The major problems in schools tend to be new carpets with the gassing out of the glues used for installation and the use of chemicals in the cleaning and disinfecting of the classrooms.

In those exposed to formaldehyde the common symptoms were eye irritation, nasal congestion, and lower respiratory problems, as well as drowsiness, fatigue, dizziness, and "spaciness." The mechanism for these reactions included plain irritation at high levels, but some patients showed definite IgE type reactions with positive skin tests and positive IgE RAST tests on their blood. The patients with skin problems showed positive patch tests and positive delayed intradermal tests usually associated with type 4 reactions. The non-immunologic central nervous system reactions are more likely to be based on the typical reactions involving the central nervous system in multiple chemical sensitivities. The newer theories of direct effect on the limbic system in susceptible individuals help explain these difficult problems.

TOMMY: ATTENTION DEFICIT DISORDER

A typical case is that of Tommy, age 10, who was first seen on September 18, 1992. His history included attention deficit disorder with many outbursts at school of behavior that suggested a possible case of Tourette's disease. He always slept while riding in the family car, was hard to awaken, and was disoriented when the destination was reached. He had a long history of nasal congestion and frequent nosebleeds. The condition had become much worse since the first of September when he started in a new school. New carpeting in that school was emiting a strong odor.

On examination, Tommy exhibited allergic shiners, as well as nasal swelling and post-nasal drainage in the posterior nasal pharynx. His work-up included intradermal testing which was positive for dust and dust mites, alternaria, hormodendrum, and T.C.E. mold mixture. The pollen skin tests were all negative. On radioallergosorbent (RAST) testing of his blood, the antibodies to D. farinae were elevated to 400% of negative control for IgE antibodies, and he showed definite elevation of IgG antibodies to cow's milk at 18 ug/ml. On sublingual challenge testing to formalin, ethanol, and phenol, he showed marked tiredness and headaches on formaldehyde and hyperactive behavior on ethanol. His reaction to phenol also produced drowsiness and spaciness. These symptoms could be relieved by neutralizing doses of chemicals sublingually.

It was suggested that Tommy return to his old school, if at all possible, until the carpet at the new school gassed out. He was also started on sublingual antigens for chemicals and inhalants. Since he was already on Catapres 0.1 mg a.m. and 0.15 mg p.m., Anafranil 5 mg twice daily, and Dexedrine 25 mg 1 1/2 daily, he was not given any additional drugs. In fact, his mother was told to discontinue some of the medications as his condition improved.

When Tommy was seen on October 28, 1992, there had been marked improvement, but it was noted that milk did give him aggressive behavior and that his behavior was "terrible" in art class where there were more chemical odors. He was, however, able to stay in school. By February of 1993, there was again a marked improvement, and he was progressing well at school. Since then, he has been seen approximately every four months and has shown improvement in his intradermal reaction to dust and mites, as well as to some of the molds. He did not require any Dexadrine or other potent central nervous system medications within a month after we first saw him. He continues to do well.

DESENSITIZATION TREATMENT

Over the years, there has been some improvement in the formaldehyde levels in materials such as plywood, carpeting, fabrics, and cosmetics. There are still large exposures from diesel smoke, tobacco smoke, and the materials in new buildings.

Although the preferable main avenue of treatment would be avoidance, in our present society, this is almost impossible. Detoxification by sauna, etc. does not make total sense. While it may be of some help, it is impossible to avoid formaldehyde in the body since it is a product of normal metabolism of amino acids. It is present normally in our bodies in small amounts.

The treatment I use was first published in the *Archives of Clinical Ecology* in the spring of 1982. It involves testing either intradermally or by means of provocative neutralization (intradermally or sublingually), and patients require the same improvements in general health, nutrition, and vitamin and mineral intake that other multiple chemically-sensitive patients require.

Treatment with titrated or neutralizing doses three times daily is safe and effective. The mechanism involved may be that of low dose tolerance, or it may involve the masking effect of small doses of antigens that is seen in other industrial exposures to chemicals. It would be similar to the worker in the nitroglycerine factory licking a stick of dynamite to help avoid the withdrawal and headaches he might have while away from work.

Results of treatment for formalin sensitivity can be shown by decreased skin reaction and by decreased IgE antibodies specific to formalin. *Figure 15-1* shows the formalin skin testing on a patient who was first seen in January of 1990. You will note that a wheal of 14 mm was immediately produced on his skin. The dilution #3 would be five times stronger than dilution #4 and showed a larger skin reaction. By April of 1990, even the stronger dilution #3 produced considerably less skin reaction, a decrease from 14 mm to 7 mm. This was also observable on IgE RAST testing of the patient's serum. *Figure 15-2* shows the initial RAST test of January 1990 with a 2.5 times negative control; by April, the level had decreased to approximately one or equal to the negative control. The dotted line shows that the serum from January was retested on the same RAST run in April and continued to show the much stronger reaction. This gives evidence, both by decreased skin reaction and by decreased IgE specific antibodies in the blood, that this patient did develop tolerance on only four months of sublingual treatment with formalin.

Some people are critical of using formaldehyde sublingually because of possible toxicity. In the 1940's, formaldehyde was given orally (with no adverse effects) in a number of studies in doses of 10,000 to 100,000 times more than the dose we would use in treatment of our patients. Since formaldehyde is impossible to avoid, the use of safe and effective sublingual dosage makes good sense for those patients whose symptoms are difficult to manage.

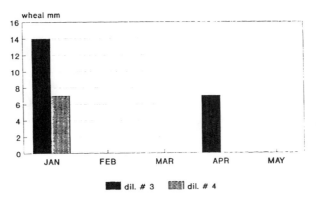

Figure 15-1.
Results of a formalin skin test on the same patient in January and April, 1990.

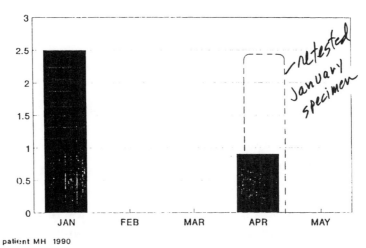

Figure 15-2.
RAST test results for the same patient in January and April, 1990.

SUMMARY

Formaldehyde is a very significant cause of chemical sensitivity. It is probably the most abundant and difficult chemical to deal with in the school, and it is very important that we make efforts to increase ventilation and decrease formaldehyde and outgassing products to prevent problems. Where children suffer from formaldehyde sensitivity, they should be carefully managed by physicians who can use some of the newer methods such as sublingual desensitization to chemicals, molds, foods, inhalants, and other irritants.

REFERENCES

Bardana, E. J., 1980, "Formaldehyde: hypersensitivy and irritant reactions at work and in the home," *Immunology and Allergy Practice*, 2:60-72.

Bell, I., 1975, "A kinin model of mediation for food and chemical sensitivities," *Annals of Allergy*, 35:206-215.

Fabry, H., 1968, "Formaldehyde sensitivity---two interesting cases," *Contact Dermatitis Newsletter*, 3:51.

Fisher, A. A., 1973, *Contact Dermatitis*, 2nd Ed., Philadelphia: Lea & Febiger, pp. 273-277.

Helander, I., 1977, "Contact urticaria from leather containing formaldehyde," *Arch Dermatology*, 113:1443.

Hendrick, D. J., and D. J. Lane, 1975, "Formalin asthma in hospital staff," *British Medical Journal*, 1:607-608.

Morin, N. C., P. E. Zeldrin, Z. Kubinski, P. K. Battacharya, and H. Kubinski, 1977, "Macromolecular complexes produced by chemical carcinogens and ultraviolet radiation," *Cancer Research*, 37:3802.

Morris, D. L., 1992, "Recognition and treatment of formaldehyde sensitivity," *Archives of Clinical Ecology*, 1:1 27-30.

Popa, A., C. Teculescu, D. Stanescu, and N. Gavrilescu, 1969, "Bronchial asthma and asthmatic bronchitis determined by simple chemicals," *Dis Chest*, 56: 395-404.

Randolph, T. G., 1962, *Human Ecology and Susceptibility to the Chemical Environment*, Springfield, IL: Charles C. Thomas.

Rea, W. J., 1978, "Environmentally triggered cardiac disease," *Annals of Allergy*, 40:243-251.

Rea, W. J., 1977, "Environmentally triggered small vessel vasculitis," *Annals of Allergy,* 38: 245-251.

Skerfving, S., B. Akesson, and B. G. Simonsson, 1980, "'Meat-wrappers' asthma' caused by thermaldegradation products of polyethylene," *Lancet*, 1:211.

Vaughn, W. T., 1939, *The Practice of Allergy*, St. Louis: C. V. Mosby, p. 677.

Part Three

Taking Action

16

CHILDREN NEED ALL THE HELP THEY CAN GET!
The Multidisciplinary Team Approach to Treating Environmentally Triggered Illnesses in School-Age Children

Gary Oberg, M.D., F.A.A.P., F.A.A.E.M.

> *The causes and symptoms of any Environmentally Triggered Illness (ETI) are complex. In this chapter, Dr. Oberg discusses the diagnosis and treatment of ETI in school-age children and advocates a multi-disciplinary team approach for consistently successful and cost-effective results. In outlining a team strategy, discussing the possible composition of the team, and setting forth the responsibilities of each of its members, he answers questions that concern all those who work with ETI patients in the school and community.*
>
> ☐ *Why is the team approach desirable for the treatment of school children with ETI?*
>
> ☐ *Who should be part of the multi-disciplinary team?*
>
> ☐ *What are the qualifications of a team member?*
>
> ☐ *What are the responsibilities of a team member?*
>
> ☐ *What should teachers and educational support personnel know and do to be most effective as team members helping to treat children with ETI?*

This chapter presents an overview of the diagnosis and treatment of Environmentally Triggered Illness (ETI), and provides a comprehensive perspective of the ETI complex that will enable the reader to use other information in this book most effectively.

A team strategy is recommended for the treatment of ETI, with close cooperation and communication among all the team members. The success of the treatment is directly related to the knowledge each team member has in his or her area of responsibility. It is critical that the knowledge be shared and applied flexibly and creatively to the unique needs of each ETI case.

To be most effective and responsive to each student's needs, every team member must always strive to maintain the flexible and open-minded scientific attitude expressed by the English philosopher Thomas Huxley:

> Sit down before Mother Nature as a small child. Be prepared to cast aside all preconceived notions and to follow Her into whatever Abyss Sheleads, or you shall learn nothing.

AN OVERVIEW OF THE NATURE OF THE ETI PROBLEM AND ITS SOLUTION

The potential causes of health, learning, and behavioral problems in any particular school-age child may range from quite simple to very complex. Obviously, the possible causes of ETI covered in this book comprise only a partial list of the total causes that may exist. There are many other medical and non-medical causes for problems that may occur in any particular case, but whatever those causes, the more that is known about the nature of each one, the more easily it can be corrected or minimized. For that reason, it is most important that all who deal with children who might have ETI be able to recognize when it, rather than some other medical problem, is present.

ETI is *recognizable, treatable, reversible,* and *preventable.* Indeed, it is most gratifying to the physician to discover that a particular patient has not been doing well because his or her condition involves a previously undiagnosed case of ETI. When the cause is finally recognized as the missing piece in the puzzle, numerous new options for successful intervention are opened up at several different levels.

What is ETI?

The concept of ETI is based on the growing appreciation that a human being is a marvelous, adaptable----but not *infinitely* adaptable---animal, struggling to survive in an often hostile environment by means of a number of inherited, built-in, complexly interacting, and usually reversible biological mechanisms and systems. These systems are designed to maintain homeostasis, to repair injury, and to insure self-preservation. Their ability to function effectively is clearly related to their inherited genetic quality and the status of the nutrients required for their function.

The nature of the interactions between each person and his or her environment changes dynamically over time and seems to be individually specific.

Optimal health requires that all parts of the body be well-nourished and in homeostasis with each other and with the environment. *Homeostasis* is a fundamental mechanism of life itself. It is the inborn propensity of the body to adapt its own operation to maintain the stability of its biological functions. For homeostasis to be achieved, stability must be maintained even in the face of dynamically varying and unpredictable exposures to external and internal environmental stressors that may tend to destabilize and disrupt it.

An *environmental stressor* is any substance or situation that has the capacity to destabilize homeostasis in a *susceptible* individual. Examples of stressors might include biological substances such as dusts, molds, pollens, danders, venoms, foods, and infectious organisms. In addition, inorganic and organic chemicals of all types, nutritional excesses or deficiencies, trauma, psychological stresses, and physical phenomena such as heat, cold, humidity, barometric pressure, vibration, noise, ionizing and non-ionizing radiation, and electromagnetic fields may disturb homeostasis.

Many forms of illness may result when homeostasis between any part of the body and the environment is disrupted. These forms of illness may be collectively called ETI. The form that an ETI takes is the product of each individual's genetic nature and acquired nutritional status as they interact with his or her particular environmental exposures over a period of time. Each individual is genetically and nutritionally unique, and, therefore, the manifestations, progress, and duration of the individual's ETI will be unique to that person.

Effects of ETI

The number of students who have some form of ETI affecting their health, learning, or behavior is likely to be far greater than suspected by most professionals who deal with school problems. There are two main ways ETI may adversely affect a student's ability to perform up to his or her potential. First, the specific symptoms of a student's ETI may sabotage the ability to do school work effectively. A few common examples would include recurrent asthma, nasal congestion, headaches, stomach aches, muscle and joint aches, itchy rashes, and brain function symptoms such as chronic irritability, fatigue, spaciness, attention span dysfunction, and other conditions that inhibit learning. Second, almost any chronic or recurrent ETI can also result in the nonspecific symptoms of just not feeling well, overall achiness, lack of enthusiasm, and apathy about performing tasks. These sensations are also commonly experienced in many acute disorders such as flu and other infections where there is inflammation.

Recognizing ETI

Recognition of an ETI is achieved by the development of a sufficiently detailed, environmentally-focused chronologic history designed to detect various clinical patterns generated by adverse interactions between a student's specific stressors and his or her biological systems. Once a history showing evidence of ETI is established, it should be corroborated by a physician trained in the concepts of ETI, using an appropriate physical examination, laboratory testing, medical imaging, and various other diagnostic testing techniques. Further psychological, social, and/or educational histories and testing should also be performed as indicated by the initial history.

Management and Prevention of ETI

The most important part of management of an ETI is to educate the child and his or her family about the nature of the child's illness and the rationale behind the proposed treatment. The insights gained from appropriate education will help parents and child more effectively comply with and carry out a pro-active, cause-oriented treatment strategy to:

- avoid identified stressors,
- correct nutritional and metabolic dysfunctions,
- and endure an immunotherapy program, when appropriate.

While dealing with specific causes and mechanisms must be the major long term strategy, periodic symptomatic drugs and surgery are an appropriate short term treatment for the amelioration of ongoing symptoms, when and where needed, as long as such symptomatic treatments are effective and without significant side effects.

Prevention of ETl is accomplished by the skillful prophylactic application of the principles and practices of Environmental Medicine. This will result in the adoption of appropriate life styles:

■ that specifically minimize exposures to identified stressors

■ that generally ensure less contaminated air, water, and food, and

■ that pro-actively promote ongoing optimal nutrition and metabolic functioning.

Appropriate treatment plans for each case should result in effective and cost-efficient procedures that can be monitored actively and constantly. Any unsuccess regimens should be adjusted or avoided altogether. The *ultimate long-term goals* of an effective diagnosis and treatment plan should include:

■ Significant reduction or elimination of acute and/or chronic symptoms in any organ or system.

■ Improvement of measured functions in any organ or system.

■ Increased ability to carry out the tasks of daily living.

■ Increased psychological well-being.

■ Reasonable limitation or elimination of exposures to recognized environmental stressors.

■ Increased tolerance of environmental stressors that have previously caused symptoms.

■ Improved ability to prevent the development of new illnesses through pro-active education and the adoption of appropriate life-styles.

Ultimately, the most effective management of ETI will be achieved when all components of society appreciate the profound impact that human interactions with the environment have upon the health not only of our species, but also of our entire biosphere. Knowledge of how humans are vulnerable to the consequences of what they do to their environment will enhance the desire to formulate rational and efficacious policies at all levels that will preserve not only human health, but the health of our whole planet as well. An old Amish saying sets the frame of mind that should be adopted by our society to guide people's interactions with our world: "We have not inherited the land from our fathers. We are borrowing it from our children."

Understanding ETI Can Improve the Health Care System

Comprehensive education in the concepts of ETI, coupled with appropriate training and experience in their application, will result in greatly expanding health professionals' knowledge about the nature of environmental illnesses and increasing the number of effective treatments for them. Augmentation of other current medical models by means of the knowledge gained through the Environmental Medicine model will improve the efficacy and cost-effectiveness of our health-care system. Ongoing research in the field of Environmental Medicine must be encouraged so that the new knowledge discovered thereby will further enhance the ability to prevent and conquer disease and increase the appreciation of the reasons for maintaining a healthy ecosystem.

A widened comprehension of the concepts of ETI will greatly expand public knowledge about the nature of many illnesses, and will allow people to participate more fully in making effective decisions about their own health. Such an understanding will be most appreciated by people who wish to have as much control over their own lives as possible. It will also provide people with greater opportunities to choose effective lifestyles that may help prevent ETIs from occurring. If such illnesses should occur anyway, knowledge about their nature offers patients significantly expanded options for dealing with them effectively at several different levels.

Among government, industry, and health insurance officials, a comprehension of the concepts of ETI will give greater insights into and clearer perspectives on the dynamics of human interaction with the environment and the results of that interaction on health and disease. These insights and perspectives will allow much more informed, rational, and cost-effective approaches to be formulated in the areas of public and private policy designed to deal with health and the environment.

WHY SUCCESSFUL MANAGEMENT REQUIRES A MULTI-DISCIPLINARY TEAM APPROACH

There are three main reasons why the successful management of ETI in school-age children requires a multi-disciplinary team approach:

1. No profession has all the training and skills required to deal with all aspects of a case of ETI.

The range of possible needs in any particular case may require the services of professionals in many different fields. For example, take a typical case of a student with dyslexia, visual perception problems, and ETI manifestations including various allergies that cause chronic sinus headaches, asthma, attention deficit, impulsivity, irritability, and fatigue.

An accurate diagnosis and an effective treatment regimen will require management in several different areas. A *psychologist* or other appropriately-trained diagnostic specialist must assess the student's educational strengths, weaknesses, and coping skills through appropriate testing. The student's *teachers* must carry out an Individual Education Plan (IEP) to deal with these findings. A *physician* must make a diagnosis, determining that the student's particular medical symptoms are due to allergies that cause the sinus, chest, and nervous system symptoms. If it is found that the sinus problems are due to dust, mold, and formaldehyde, better dust and mold control in the child's classroom is required, thus involving the school's *maintenance personnel*.

The jars of formaldehyde-preserved frogs kept on the classroom science shelf next to the student's desk must be removed by the teacher. If the asthma is triggered by heavy exercise, the *coach* or physical education teacher must exempt the student from the mile runs in gym class. If the nervous system symptoms are aggravated by the chocolate milk and donuts the student has for a mid-afternoon classroom snack each day, the teacher is again involved, this time to see that other snacks are substituted.

Since the child may also occasionally need symptomatic medication for attention-span problems, asthma, or headaches, the *family physician* must prescribe them. He or she must also oversee the family's environmental-control education and the immunotherapy regimen of injections that helps control the student's symptoms and builds up eventual desensitization to his or her allergy triggers. When they must be administered in school, the medications are controlled by the *school nurse*. And finally, because both the child and his or her family experience frustration and anger at the inconvenience caused by the student's chronic problems, a *social worker* must provide appropriate counseling to deal with the psychodynamic results of a chronic illness. Since these needs cut across so many traditional professional boundaries, the most efficacious and cost-effective way to achieve all the long-term goals for this and every other case is to have an ongoing, dynamic, cooperative, coordinated, and flexible partnership between a student and family well educated in all aspects of ETI and a multi-disciplinary team consisting of professionals whose areas of expertise are relevant to the case.

2. Management of ETI also often involves important sociological, economic, legal, and political ramifications that must be accommodated appropriately.

In the modernized words of the 17th-century English poet, John Donne, "No man is an island unto himself." Similarly, no case of ETI affects only the individual who suffers from it. Because of the complex nature of ETI, its causes and treatment can be expected to impact in one way or another on other people. This fact may be appreciated best if one stands back and takes a global and anthropological view of the potential relationships between human beings and their environment and how these relationships affect illness and health. Relationships between people and their surroundings do not exist in a stable, static, and isolated state, but rather are a dynamic, concurrent, inter-related, and ongoing process. Under the umbrella concept of humans interacting with their environment, there is a hierarchy of complexity and involvement, starting most simply with the individual in his or her immediate physical or social environment, and expanding upward and outward through several diverse levels to the global society of the species: *Homo sapiens*, interacting with earth, the biosphere on which it lives. In this grand overview, there are five vertical levels of involvement that may influence the management of any particular case of ETI. Expanding from most simple to most complex, the levels are:

- the individual patient and his or her family
- the school
- the medical community
- the student's neighborhood
- the county, state, federal, and international communities and the governments and agencies that manage them

Each of these different levels, through its actions or inactions with the ETI patient, has the capacity either to cause or aggravate illness, or to encourage optimal health. Indeed, all of these levels are inextricably interconnected, so that activity in any one of them has the potential to reverberate up and down through the other levels, with varying degrees of consequences, which in turn may have any combination of sociological, economic, legal, or political ramifications. That is the true nature of the world in which we live. Therefore, these dynamic interactions and their different consequences must be accommodated when they impact on any particular case of ETI. The skills, experiences, and perspectives of a range of professional team members who appreciate and can accommodate these ramifications enhance the possibility for comprehensive and effective solutions in any case of ETI.

3. In the field of education, the framework for the multidisciplinary team approach is already in place----in fact, mandated by federal law----in most, if not all, school districts.

The values of a multi-disciplinary team approach have been appreciated for many years and have resulted in the professional team being mandated by some of the federal laws intended to provide educational programs for children with special needs. The major applicable federal statutes are listed in the RECOMMENDED READING section at the end of this chapter, and are noted in other chapters. In addition, each state, county, city, and local district has laws, regulations, and policies that augment or respond to the federal laws. These different laws and policies provide a framework to guide the interactions between the various team members and the levels of society mentioned above. Hence, it is important that all team members be aware of how the laws may affect their areas of responsibility and how best to comply with them.

THE OVERALL TEAM STRATEGY FOR SUCCESS

Since the framework for a multi-disciplinary team network is already in place in most school districts, a reasonable strategy would be simply to add ETI as a possible cause for problems in students, and adjust all current policies to accommodate this new dimension. Most members of the team probably already have at least an intellectual appreciation of the concept that the environment can affect health and learning. They may, however, need a deeper appreciation of the true scope and importance of the environment as a potential cause of problems in students, and the knowledge that will enable them to deal with ETI as it relates to each of their areas of responsibility.

It is common for someone not experienced with ETI to be discouraged by the daunting complexity of the more difficult cases. It is helpful, therefore, to keep in mind that, regardless of the complexity in each case, if various presenting patterns are observed, an aspect of the environment or diet may be suspected of causing the symptoms. Early recognition of these patterns, which are usually easy to perceive, will enable the team to plan a potentially effective course of action. Although there is no need for any one person to have all the skills and knowledge necessary to deal effectively with all aspects of a given case, each professional should keep in mind that ETI is a potential source of specific symptoms, should know how it may be recognized, how it may impact upon his or her area of responsibility, and how to obtain further help in solving problems outside of his or her area of expertise. All the potential complexities can be handled through the multi-disciplinary team approach.

While evaluating a case, it is important for the professional to keep in mind that it is quite common in many cases of ETI for contributing causes to exist both inside and outside the school environment. Though operating mainly within the context of the school, team members should never lose sight of the complexity of the sources of ETI.

Finally, each team will function most effectively if it meets the following requirements:

- *Visibility and accessibility.* Its existence must be widely known, and access to it should be readily available at all levels of possible intervention.

- *Flexibility.* Its intervention must be based upon the needs of each case, with each team member becoming involved as required.

- *Training and experience.* Each member must have adequate training and experience in his or her particular area of expertise.

- *Knowledge of the ETI concept.* Each member must have an overview of the fundamental concepts of ETI, and how ETI might affect his or her area of responsibility.

- *Protocols.* Each member must have a specific protocol for his or her area of responsibility to rule ETI in or out as the source of a problem.

- *Practical knowledge of ETI.* Each member must know how to treat those aspects of his or her area of responsibility that may be due to ETI.

- *Referrals within the team.* Each member must know when to make appropriate referrals of the case to other members of the team for further evaluation.

- *Monitoring.* Each member must monitor over time the efficacy of the treatment plan in his or her area of responsibility .

- *Adaptibility.* Each member must be willing and able to adjust his or her approach to each case, as required over time, in order to attain the maximum achievement of as many goals as possible.

- *Communication.* Each member must maintain continuous, open, and honest communication with all other members of the team as evaluation and treatment unfold.

- *Cooperation and mutual respect.* Each member must support the recommendations of the other team members and show respect for the others' experiences and perspectives.

- *Documentary evidence.* Dissenting opinions must be put in writing and must include the reasons for the disagreement, along with alternative diagnoses and treatment plans and the reasons for suggesting them. Differences of opinion must be resolved in a professional manner, with the shared understanding that the purpose of all this is to do what is best for the welfare of the student experiencing the symptoms.

- *Time.* Administrators must allow adequate time in the master schedule for each school professional to participate effectively in the team effort.

MEMBERS OF THE MULTI-DISCIPLINARY TEAM

There are two levels of involvement on a team. The primary level includes those members who might be directly concerned with a particular case—patient, family, and friends; school personnel; medical personnel; and community resource staffers. The secondary level includes those who are indirectly concerned in the county, state, federal, or international areas, where policies are set that impact upon all cases. Each team might include any combination of the following:

I. The student and his or her family (parents, siblings, and other relatives) and friends

II. School personnel:

- Board of education/superintendent
- School district's attorney
- District and school building administrators
- Teachers
- Psychologists/social workers
- Other special education diagnosticians, including therapists----physical, occupational, speech and language, vision and hearing, et al.
- School nurse
- Educational support personnel (cafeteria workers; custodial personnel; secretaries, et al.)

III. Medical personnel

IV. Community resources

V. County, state, federal, and international governments and agencies

The responsibilities of each team member in the diagnosis and treatment of ETI is discussed in the following sections.

STUDENT, FAMILY, FRIENDS

All individuals in this group must:

- Acknowledge the presence of the problem(s) as appropriate to the patient's age.
- Be willing to look at the problem(s) objectively as appropriate to the patient's age.
- Want to make things better.
- Give an adequate and sincere trial to all potentially helpful treatment modalities.

Parents

The parents must:

- Provide appropriate positive psychological support to the patient ("psychological vitamins").

- Be the child's advocates and see that all school and other professional personnel provide adequate feedback to each other to monitor accurately the academic, behavioral, and/or medical response to the overall regimen, and to ensure that the ultimate long-term goals are being met over time.

- Visit the appropriate school personnel each spring. Together with school staff, they must review the successes and failures of the current school year and plan the most effective educational strategy for the following school year, carefully choosing teachers, classroom locations, etc.

- Be aware of local, county, state, and federal laws and regulations that might pertain to their child's case, especially those involving the responsibilities of schools for the education of students with special needs.

SCHOOL PERSONNEL, BOARD OF EDUCATION, AND SUPERINTENDENT OF SCHOOLS

All involved in policy-making for the school system should:

- Appreciate the relation between the school environment and the health, learning, and behavior of susceptible students and school personnel.

- Be aware of applicable local, county, state, and federal laws and regulations pertaining to the responsibilities of schools in the education of students with special needs—including those with ETI.

- Accept responsibility for correcting any current situation in their schools that is proved to be contributing to significant ETI in any of their students or school personnel.

- Support a pro-active program in their district to recognize, treat, and prevent future ETI resulting from their district's school environments.

- Appreciate the cost-effectiveness of a pro-active school environmental control program, and ensure that this appreciation is passed down to all levels of school personnel.

The Superintendent and All School Board Members

The superintendent and all school board members should:

- When remodeling or building new schools, hire only those architects and contractors appropriately trained in environmentally safe building and remodeling techniques.

- Acknowledge that they have the responsibility to see that all of their students are taught the importance of the concepts of ETI. They must make sure that an appropriate appreciation of the role the environment plays in health and illness is incorporated into the district's curriculum, in all courses in which this concept has potential impact. Education in this concept at an early age will maximize the opportunity for all children to gain knowledge that will enable them to choose lifestyles in which good health can be maintained, morbidity decreased, and the cost of illness minimized throughout the society.

- Be advocates for the pro-active prevention and treatment of ETI in the rest of the community.

The School District's Attorney

Any legal representative of or advisor to the schools should:

- Have a comprehensive current knowledge of all local, county, regional, state, federal, and international laws and regulations that might impact upon the many possible options available for managing cases of ETI.

- Be able to help the multi-disciplinary team choose the most effective options for managing ETI that comply with appropriate laws and regulations. In advising the school district, the attorney must be guided by the principle of doing what is best for the affected student or school personnel.

District and School Building Administrators

Administrators at the district level or within a school should:

- Establish master schedules that allow the time needed by teachers and other school personnel to participate in the multi-disciplinary team's activities.

- Create job descriptions for all school personnel that incorporate the skills needed to recognize and deal with ETI in the school setting. They must then be sure that all new personnel they hire have adequate knowledge about ETI or can make arrangements to obtain it.

■ Hire personnel who embrace the district's pro-active ETI management program.

■ Note when evaluating staff members how effectively each one deals with ETI issues.

■ Provide appropriate inservice instruction for all staff, to initiate and update periodically the skills needed for each staff member to participate effectively in the district's pro-active ETI program.

■ Be aware of applicable local, county, state, and federal laws and regulations that pertain to the responsibilities of schools in the education of students with special needs, including those with ETI. They must ensure that all other school personnel know and comply with these laws.

Teachers

Teachers, who work with ETI patients on a daily basis and, consequently, need an appreciation for the concept and causes of ETI, should:

■ Be able to recognize presenting manifestations associated with ETI in school-age children and have an overview of possible contributing causes that might pertain to the school setting.

■ Know how to initiate appropriate referrals for further evaluation when a student is having any problems that might be caused by ETI.

■ Choose substances and materials required by certain courses (such as art, chemistry, and home economics) that are as safe as possible, and maintain good ventilation where these substances and materials are used.

■ Appreciate the uniqueness of each child and be aware of how this uniqueness results in the diverse possible presentations of ETI in their students.

■ Help formulate and carry out an educational and environmental control program that minimizes the school's contribution to a student's symptoms of ETI.

■ Work with physicians to ensure the success of the medical component of the treatment regimen; *e.g.*, when medications are required during school hours, send the student to the school nurse at the correct time; provide feedback to the physician about the efficacy of any medical regimen applied in the classroom, and provide adequate control over snacks for students with specific food allergies.

- Exercise environmental controls as required in the classroom; for example, not wearing excessive perfume or other scented products around susceptible students, not smoking around students, keeping classrooms as free as possible of dust, molds, chemical odors, chalk dust, etc.

- Acquire a knowledge of the ways in which the concepts of ETI might impact upon the subject matter they teach, and include that knowledge in course curricula.

- Encourage the school district to offer teacher-training programs incorporating ETI concepts and to include their diverse ramifications in regular curriculum planning for all courses.

- Make known to textbook writers and publishers that ETI concepts should be included in printed instructional materials.

- Be aware of applicable local, county, state, and federal laws and regulations that pertain to their specific areas of responsibility in the diagnosis and management of cases of ETI.

Psychologists and Social Workers

All mental health care professionals should:

- Have a good working knowledge of how ETI can impact on their areas of responsibility, and how to deal with it effectively.

- Be able to perform appropriate diagnostic testing to determine the strengths and weaknesses of each student's learning capacity and style.

- Know how to use appropriate neuropsychological testing to differentiate organic from psychologically caused symptoms.

- Assess each student's emotional status, as well as coping styles and abilities.

- Assess accurately the adequacy of each student's available support groups (family, relatives, friends, school, community, etc.).

- Assist teachers in fashioning effective customized educational prescriptions for each student's needs.

- Recognize and treat effectively the potentially maladaptive psychodynamics that occur between the student, his or her family, and his or her community, as they all attempt to deal with the chronic health, learning, and behavioral problems so often associated with ETI.

■ Have a good working knowledge of all available community support structures and how to utilize them effectively.

■ Be aware of applicable local, county, state, and federal laws and regulations pertaining to their specific areas of responsibility in the diagnosis and management of ETI cases.

Other Special Education Diagnosticians----Physical, Occupational, Speech, Language, Vision, and Hearing Therapists, Et Al.

All special education personnel should:

■ Have a good working knowledge of how ETI can impact upon their areas of responsibility, and how to deal with it effectively.

■ Assist teachers in fashioning effective customized educational prescriptions for each student's needs in their areas of responsibility.

■ Have a good working knowledge of all available community support facilities related to their areas of responsibility, and of how to utilize them effectively.

■ Be aware of local, county, state, and federal laws and regulations pertaining to their specific areas of responsibility in the diagnosis and management of ETI cases.

School Nurses

The school nurse, who is the natural liaison between the physician and other members of the interdisciplinary team and between the team members and outside medical sources, should be:

■ Well trained in the medical aspects of ETI that can occur in school-age children.

■ The first medical contact when a student is having symptoms of any kind at school.

■ The dispenser of medications when necessary at school.

■ A good source of information about how to develop lifestyles that can eliminate or prevent many problems from ETI. Such information should be part of each school's health science curriculum.

- Aware of applicable local, county, state, and federal laws and regulations pertaining to his or her specific areas of responsibility in the diagnosis and management of ETI cases.

Educational Support Personnel

All support personnel, including maintenance staff, cafeteria workers, secretarial staff, paraprofessionals, and others, should:

- Appreciate that many items they use both indoors and outdoors may cause adverse health effects in susceptible students and school personnel; (*e.g.*, many new building materials, new carpeting, types of maintenance materials and cleaning supplies, art supplies, photography supplies, science lab chemicals, gas stoves in the cafeteria and home economics classrooms, pesticides, etc.).

- Have access to information about the manifestations of the common forms of ETI that may be caused by any natural or chemical substances.

- Participate as much as is practical in the district's pro-active program to prevent ETI; *e.g.*, not smoking on school grounds, choosing the safest types of building and maintenance materials possible; using potentially toxic substances only when students and other school personnel are at minimal risk of exposure (at night, on weekends, or during the summer vacation), and maintaining an efficient heating/-ventilating/air conditioning plant with adequate fresh-air exchange.

- Clearly appreciate the cost effectiveness and health benefits of using such a preventive program routinely.

- Be aware of applicable local, county, state, and federal laws and regulations pertaining to their specific areas of responsibility in the diagnosis and management of a case of ETI.

Cafeteria workers should:

- Appreciate that having good sound nutrition is one of the most powerful tools for treating and preventing ETI.

- Provide good nutritious food and clean water in a clean environment for those students who eat at school.

- Be able to provide reasonable alternative foods for those students who are highly sensitive to any of the foods being served on any particular day.

Secretaries, clerks, and other office personnel should:

■ Be aware of those policies that pertain to ETI in their areas of responsibility.

■ Know how to refer any questions about ETI that come into their departments.

MEDICAL PERSONNEL

Whatever their specialty, physicians should:

■ Be appropriately trained in the concepts of ETI so that they are able to take an accurate comprehensive history that will adequately reveal the possible presence of any contributing medical causes for each student's presentating symptoms. If a physician does not have such training, he or she should obtain it or refer the patient to someone who has it.

■ Be able to evaluate properly any suspected medical causes of ETI and know how to refer to other members of the team for further non-medical evaluation.

■ Know how to treat and monitor effectively any medical cause (*e.g.*, detoxification of heavy metals poisoning, correction of nutritional dysfunctions, avoidance education, and immunotherapy for diet and environmental sensitivities, adjustment of medications causing side effects, etc.).

■ Know how to use symptomatic medications, such as the stimulants, anti-depressants, decongestants, antihistamines, bronchodilators, etc., that specifically alleviate symptoms of ETI or symptoms of other common concomitant medical problems for which specific causes cannot be found or adequately addressed in other ways.

■ Act as the patient's advocate with the other members of the multi-disciplinary team who may not appreciate the potentially complicated nature and ramifications of the various medical problems that may occur in a case of ETI. The other team members also need to understand that their cooperation is required to make the medical management a success.

■ Be aware of applicable local, county, state, and federal laws and regulations that pertain to his or her specific areas of responsibility in the diagnosis and management of a case of ETI.

COMMUNITY RESOURCES

Because ETI is *recognizable, treatable, reversible,* and *preventable,* community leaders must encourage community awareness and support for the appropriate recognition and management of this type of problem, not only for the community's students, but also for all of its citizens. There is a need for a general overview of the concepts of ETI, how to use them to maintain optimal health, and how to recognize and treat disease when it occurs. The community should:

- Provide adequate diagnostic and treatment programs for the medical, psychological, social, and legal aspects of ETI within the realm of its responsibilities and capabilities. Information about locating appropriate services and the current status of fees and reimbursement for them must also be provided.

- Provide through one of its agencies specific information about chemical substances, how they might adversely affect various susceptible populations, and the rights of susceptible people who are exposed to these substances.

- Encourage parent support organizations to offer accurate information and responsible support for the various needs associated with ETI.

COUNTY, STATE, FEDERAL, AND INTERNATIONAL GOVERNMENTS

Governing bodies have the obligation to understand and appreciate the nature of the interactions between humans and their environments, and how these interactions can impact, for better or worse, upon the health of the entire population.

Government agencies should formulate rational and efficacious policies at all levels to govern all levels of human interaction with the elements of the environment that can be hazardous. Such policies should preserve and enhance not only humanity's health, but also the health of our whole planet. As part of national policy, local governments could assure that their school districts have adequate funding to correct the causes of ETI and to carry out effective pro-active programs to prevent it.

CONCLUSION

Individuals from all sectors of society who appreciate the implications of ETI must seek each other out and form coalitions dedicated to the formulation of rational policies that will result in an overall decrease in morbidity and a simultaneous reduction of the cost of treating ETI throughout society. More appropriate research is still needed to elucidate the full nature of the mechanisms that govern the interactions between humans and their environment. New knowledge will further enhance humanity's ability to prevent and conquer disease and will increase the appreciation for maintaining a healthy ecosystem.

RECOMMENDED READING

Major Applicable Federal Statutes

The Americans With Disabilities Act

Public Law 89-313 (Title I, State-operated Programs For Handicapped Children)

Public Law 99-372 (the Handicapped Children's Protection Act)

Public Law 101-476 (the Individuals With Disabilities Education Act (IDEA), formerly P.L. 94-142)

Section 504 of the Rehabilitation Act of 1973

The U.S. Family Educational Rights and Privacy Act of 1974

The U.S. Constitution (the 14th Amendment)

Recommended Books & Articles

Beasley, Joseph D., M.D., and Jerry Swift, 1989, *The Kellogg Report: The Impact of Nutrition, Environment, and Lifestyle on the Health of Americans.* Annandale-on-Hudson, New York: The Institute of Health Policy and Practice, The Bard College Center.

Oberg, Gary R., M.D., ed., 1995, *The Core Curriculum Outline and Philosophy Overview of the Field of Environmental Medicine*, Prarie Village, KS: The American Academy of Environmental Medicine.

Randolph, Theron G., M.D., 1987, *Environmental Medicine----Beginnings and Bibliographies of Clinical Ecology,* Fort Collins, Colorado: Clinical Ecology Publications, Inc.

Rapp, Doris, M.D., 1991, *Is This Your Child? Discovering and Treating Unrecognized Allergies In Children and Adults,* New York: Quill/William Morrow.

Rea, William J., M.D, 1992, 1994, 1995, *Chemical Sensitivity (*Volumes I, II, III, and IV), Boca Raton: CRC Publishers,

Thousand, J. S., and R. A. Villa, 1990, "Strategies For Educating Learners With Severe Disabilities Within Their Local Home Schools and Communities," *Focus On Exceptional Children,* 23(3), 1-24.

Werbach, Melvyn R., M.D., 1992, *Nutritional Influences on Illness: A Sourcebook of Clinical Research* (Second Edition), Tarzana, CA: Third Line Press, Inc.

17

PSYCHOLOGICAL EVALUATION AND INTERVENTION FOR THE ENVIRONMENTALLY SENSITIVE CHILD

by Susan F. Franks, Ph.D.; Joel R. Butler, Ph.D.; and Nancy A. Didriksen,Ph.D.

This chapter discusses the role of the psychologist and the reasons why psychological assessment is so important in the treatment of a child with environmental illness. Explaining that the patient's physiological and psychological processes interact to make diagnosis difficult, authors Franks, Butler, and Didriksen give answers to questions educators, school health professionals, and parents ask about psychological aspects of environmental illness:

☐ *Why is the detection of environmental illness difficult?*

☐ *What symptoms of environmental illness might a child display in the classroom?*

☐ *Why is it important that mental health professionals be familiar with the behavioral manifestations of environmental illness?*

☐ *Why are the emotional symptoms associated with environmental illness often confused with those of psychological disorders?*

☐ *How does psychological testing help identify an environmental source of a behavioral problem?*

☐ *What is the role of the environmental psychologist in the treatment of environmental illness?*

Environmental illness results from adverse reactivity after exposure to environmental toxins—heavy metals, solvents, pesticides, and various other poisons. Susceptibility and reaction patterns may be highly unusual even though a commonality of cause or origin exists. The issue of whether the symptoms represented by environmental illness are of organic or psychological origin has been at the core of the controversy over the very existence of the disease and has led professionals who dared to recognize and treat the illness to search for validation of its organic nature——or organicity. But even though EI/MCS will have a biological base rather than being psychogenic, it is not either/or in manifestation. Instead, the reaction pattern will be expressed in a body-mind unity.

Psychological and neuropsychological tests, often necessitated in cases of environmental illness, can be an effective tool in addressing the issue if they are appropriately used. Indeed a competent evaluation by a qualified examiner can be a valuable resource in helping health-care professionals understand the patient, and it can provide information that will contribute to the diagnostic picture. It has been particularly frustrating and disillusioning, however, to witness the use of psychological tests as an attempt to discredit and invalidate the suffering of a growing number of people. Although discrediting may not be the intention, that is what *can* be the result from testing, because the difficulty in interpreting data without an understanding of the illness and its manifestations invariably leads to misdiagnoses. When such misattributions are made, inappropriate intervention follows, and the illness continues at the expense of both the patient and society.

The organic nature of environmental illness is often difficult to detect, because of the subtlety of many of the problems associated with it. Emotional and behavioral signs contribute to the cluster of symptoms, further confusing the diagnosis. In order to demonstrate organic etiology, changes in key areas of a patient's neurocognitive functioning must be present along with an absence of signs that would normally be indicative of a precipitating psychological disturbance. In the absence of a complete psychological evaluation by someone familiar with psychopathology, neuropsychology, and environmental illness it is difficult to delineate adequately the source of observable symptoms. Emotional problems, as well as neurological conditions, can often produce changes in cognitive status that, to the untrained eye, may seem to mimic those characteristic of environmental illness and symptoms produced by adverse reactions to environmental toxins may seem, again to the untrained eye, to be psychological in origin. The environmental health psychologist is typically familiar with psychological, neurocognitive, physiological, and environmental illness symptom patterns that are presented in a variety of contexts and is, consequently, the preferred referral source when environmental illness is suspected.

ASSESSING EMOTIONAL AND BEHAVIORAL CHANGES

An equally important task in any chronic illness is the determination of the extent and influence of psychological problems, both as direct and as secondary factors. There are numerous illnesses that produce emotional and behavioral changes as a direct result of neurological involvement. Such disturbances may range from relatively minor changes in mood, motivation, and activity to severe states of mania, agitation, anger, deep depression, withdrawal, suicidality, and psychosis. Changes in mood and affect can also accompany long-term illnesses as a result of the patient's having to contend with changes in social, work, and academic functioning. The stability of family and peer relationships is often disrupted and the disruption contributes further to negative mood states. Since the emotional consequences for the patient of having to contend day after day with the uncertainty of functional status typically associated with a chronic condition, psychologists can be an invaluable resource in assessing these types of emotional problems and providing support for the chronically ill child.

The task of assessment is somewhat more complex with the environmentally ill child, in that emotional symptoms often comprise both direct and indirect influences of the syndrome. Indirect----or secondary----influences can be anticipated on the basis of the chronic nature of the illness. Emotional fluctuations occur, however, as a direct result of exposure to environmental incitants in the school or home and thus are often rapid and unexpected, even though symptoms may develop slowly as a result of repeated low-dosage exposures to environmental irritants.

These symptoms generally fall within two broad categories; stimulatory reactions and withdrawal reactions. The nature and severity of these reactions are identifiable by integrating information regarding observed behavior and inferred or reported psychological states. Mild stimulatory reactions, often the sign of initial exposure or development of sensitivities, include subjective feelings of motivation, energy, enthusiasm, and well-being that manifest in increased activity and talkativeness. Hyperactivity, attentional problems, tension, and irritability begin to develop as the child becomes more sensitive and the exposure continues.

Higher stimulatory levels produce aggression, anxiety, extreme talkativeness, and even inappropriate laughter. It is at and beyond this point that the affected child is likely to be *misclassified* as having a primary psychological/emotional disorder. The most probable misdiagnoses include anxiety disorders, bipolar disorder, schizophrenia, oppositional-defiant disorder, or conduct disorder. Even when organicity is considered as the basis for disorders, they are likely to be limited to attention-deficit hyperactivity disorder, and the underlying etiology is unlikely to be investigated.

Withdrawal reactions typically include subjective feelings of sadness and depression accompanied by a number of symptoms that vary with the level of severity of the reaction. These may include fatigue, drowsiness, moodiness, indecisiveness, confusion, impaired attention and concentration, poor comprehension, and obvious withdrawal from previous activities. At advanced levels withdrawal, to some extent, may be from reality and reactions can include: lethargy, disorientation, delusions, and hallucinations may be experienced. It is during withdrawal reactions that the child is apt to be referred for a psychological or psychiatric evaluation. General and vague physical complaints often accompany the withdrawal phase, so that the child is likely to be misdiagnosed as having a depressive, somatoform, or bipolar disorder.

At this point, too, a well-intentioned but uninformed search may begin in an attempt to uncover the source of emotional or interpersonal conflict that is assumed to underlie such symptoms. Thus begins the unfortunate, misdiagnosed child's journey through the mental-health system, a journey that invariably includes years of psychotherapy, numerous medication trials, and possible psychiatric hospitalizations, all to no avail. For the appropriately referred and evaluated child, however, a journey toward a healthy and productive life can begin with proper diagnosis and intervention.

The task of the environmental health psychologist in the diagnostic process is to utilize observational and objective data derived from an assessment battery to relate the psychological profile to symptom progression, as well as to recognize signs of neurocognitive involvement. Understanding such information within the context of the disease requires a knowledgeable interpretation of standard test data. The child's performance on measures of attention, concentration, and freedom from distractibility is likely to be diminished, and problems with both immediate and short-term memory will be evident. Reduced speed and efficiency of mental processing results in poor integration of incoming material, effortful or impaired problem-solving, and slowed transition from thought to movement. Interference in perceptual-motor processes may cause rotations or other misperceptions of letters, numbers, or designs. Other commonly noted symptoms include reduced perception of sensations by touch, various articulation difficulties, and balance and coordination problems.

Diagnostic differentiation can be quite complex without a clear understanding of the disease and how it manifests in observable and measurable behavior. The presence of neuropsychological symptoms in association with psychological disturbances is not unusual. For example, problems with attention, concentration, distractibility, and memory can be among the ancillary signs of mood and thought disorders. Behavioral disturbances typical of environmental illness can easily be mistaken as evidence of conduct disorder or oppositional-defiant disorder. Many vague physical complaints are common as well and are usually attended to by the family physician, or if prolonged and in excess, will be presumed incorrectly to be a manifestation of a somatoform disorder, thus denying the biological basis (toxins, chemicals, etc.) of the illness and further denying the need for a treatment program involving both psychological and physiological aspects. An appreciation of the interplay of these body-mind dimensions with environmental factors, in combination with an understanding of psychophysiological processes, allows the environmental health psychologist to contribute to both diagnostic differentiation and treatment planning.

THE INTERACTION BETWEEN PHYSIOLOGICAL AND PSYCHOLOGICAL PROCESSES

The importance of recognizing the interaction between physiological and psychological processes cannot be underscored enough when dealing with the environmentally ill individual. Environmental incitants impact the whole of the individual, directly producing detrimental changes within the immune system, the endocrine system, and the nervous system. The nervous system is made up of various structures and pathways that allow for and coordinate communication between all three systems, including the interaction between thoughts, emotions, and bodily processes. Research has consistently demonstrated the adverse impact of negative emotions such as depression and anger on immune system functioning. Thus, psychological factors can significantly contribute to the total stress load of the individual and can subsequently play a critical role in maintaining and heightening reactivity to the environment. Effective treatment of the environmentally ill must necessarily be comprehensive, taking into account the psychophysiological nature of the disease process.

In order to determine the efficacy of a treatment regimen, baseline data is of primary importance. Optimally, a baseline evaluation should be undertaken prior to initiation of any type of intervention. Subsequent evaluations should be administered at regularly scheduled intervals throughout the course of treatment. Retesting at the completion of a given treatment program or at six-month to one-year intervals is typically sufficient to monitor overall treatment gains or losses effectively. Under special circumstances however, abbreviated testing protocols are utilized to assist in evaluating specific sensitivities, response to various toxic exposures, and reactions to treatment. The use of repeated testing will not only serve to determine the effectiveness of intervention and treatment progress, but will also provide an objective measure of the safety of the school environment.

THE ROLE OF THE ENVIRONMENTAL HEALTH PSYCHOLOGIST

Environmental health psychologists provide services within the field of environmental medicine at a number of levels. As consultants their role is limited to evaluation and assessment for the purposes of diagnostic clarification, recommendations for treatment planning, and monitoring of treatment progress.

Another level of service places the psychologist in the role of providing psychotherapeutic intervention and working directly with the environmentally ill patient.

The primary goal of psychological treatment is to reduce the total stress load of the individual. A cognitive-behavioral approach that emphasizes relaxation, coping, and stress-management skills is the recommended format for psychotherapy. This type of intervention is necessary to address the psychophysiological dimensions of the illness, and biofeedback training is often used as an adjunct to therapy. Other issues secondarily associated with the chronicity and unpredictability of the illness are to be anticipated and should be dealt with accordingly.

Interpersonal and family conflicts often arise as patients tend to adopt a "survival" mode, becoming self-focused on physical functioning and anxious about their possible reactions to the environment. Secondary gain issues may surface if well-meaning family members and friends become overly protective and try to compensate for the patient's weaknesses, rather than encouraging the patient toward independent functioning. Supportive family therapy is helpful, that is, involving the whole family as a treatment team through education; reassurance; positive reinforcement; and relief of tension, anxiety, and depression. Family therapy can provide structure for interactions to occur and it offers hope, direction, and much affection.

Another issue that commonly arises throughout the course of therapy is difficulty with treatment compliance and this is an issue that must be successfully addressed by the psychologist and the whole treatment team if the treatment is to be successful and chronicity thwarted. Restrictions on diet and activity are often not well received by the patient, and it is particularly difficult for children to adhere to instructions that separate them from their peers. Involvement of the family, either through conferences or actual therapy is likely to become necessary as the child and his or her parents try to adjust to the illness and its effects on the family unit.

Traditional psychotherapy (psychoanalytic, neoanalytic-dynamic, nondirective self-theories and behavioristic when used in the established manner) has often been utilized with environmentally ill patients with only a bare modicum of success. However, a part of any of these modalites may be useful, such as counter-conditioning, stress management, behavioral logs, behavioral modification, etc. Although the simple support and encouragement received from an understanding individual within the context of any therapy will help reduce the patient's total stress load and may result in some improvement, it is of critical importance that therapy address the psychophysiological dimensions of environmental illness for long-term success.

SUMMARY

The environmental health psychologist has the knowledge base and training necessary to evaluate emotional and cognitive disturbances resulting from environmental illness, to determine the extent and influence of psychological problems, and to provide appropriate psychotherapeutic intervention. Alternate intervention sources may often be necessary depending upon the availability of a professional familiar with the disease. In such cases, care should be taken to ensure that the person providing such treatment is aware of the body-mind interactive issues involved or is willing to learn about them and that he or she have a background in psychophysiological causation and treatment techniques. Only then may treatment be adequate and/or comprehensive enough to achieve the goals of improved health and well-being for the child.

SUGGESTED READING

Bertschler, J. J. R. Butler, G. F. Lawlis, W. J. Rea, and A. R. Johnson, 1986, "Psychological components of environmental illness: Factor analysis of changes during treatment," Clinical Ecology, 3, 85-94.

Fein, G. G., P. M. Schwartz, S. W. Jacobson, and J. L. Jacobson, 1983, "Environmental toxins and behavioral development. A new role for psychological research," American Psychologist, November 1983.

Franks, S. F., and J. R. Butler, 1993, Biopsychological interactionism: Implications for diagnosis and treatment of environmental patients, Unpublished manuscript.

Hartman, D. E., 1991, Neuropsychological Toxicology: Identification and Assessment of Human Neurotoxic Syndromes, New York: Pergamon Press.

National Research Council, 1992, Multiple Chemical Sensitivities—Addendum to Biologic Markers in Immunotoxicology, Washington, D.C.: National Academy Press.

Parker, R. S., 1990, Environmental Neurotoxins in Traumatic Brain Injury and Neuropsychological Impairment, New York: Springer-Verlag, pp. 258-269.

Rapp, D., 1991, Is This Your Child? New York: William Morrow.

Rea, W. J., 1992, Chemical Sensitivities, Vol. I. Boca Raton: Lewis Publishing.

Rea, W. J., J. R. Butler, J. L. Laseter, and J. R. DeLeon, 1984, "Pesticides and brain function changes in a controlled environment," Clinical Ecology, 2(3), 145-150.

18

CREATING AN ALLERGY-FREE CLASSROOM

by Albert F. Robbins, D.O., M.S.P.H.

In this chapter, Dr. Robbins describes the impact of sick building syndrome on students, teachers, and other school staff. He surveys sensitizing and toxic chemicals, allergens, and toxic building conditions that may be found in schools, and discusses ways of controlling these hazards to promote the good health of students and staff. Suggesting a walk-through of the school building and indicating trouble spots to look for, he answers many questions about the relation between the classroom environment and health.

☐ *What are the most common school-building sources of children's and adults' allergic reactions?*

☐ *What are the chemicals and chemical products most apt to cause sensitizing reactions?*

☐ *How might learning materials such as books and printed papers and learning projects involving pets have negative effects on the health of children and teachers?*

☐ *How can school staff manage allergy sources more effectively in school buildings?*

Among the various health issues facing American schools today, the problem of allergies to the indoor environment is one of the most serious. The proportion of existing commercial buildings in which occupants are exposed to environmental conditions that result in complaints of symptoms or illness has been estimated to be 20% to 30%. (Institute of Medicine 1993) Problem school buildings may be higher according to some sources.

SICK BUILDING SYNDROME AND BUILDING-RELATED ILLNESS

Buildings in which the indoor environment is unhealthy can cause two general types of problems: *sick building syndrome* and *building-related illness.* (Institute of Medicine 1993)

Sick Building Syndrome is suspected when occupants complain of symptoms associated with acute discomfort that persist for more than two weeks at frequencies significantly greater than 20%. The symptoms include eye, nose, and throat irritation, sore throat, headache, fatigue, skin irritation, mild neurotoxic symptoms, nausea, achiness, and odor sensitivity. A substantial percentage of the complainants report almost immediate relief upon leaving the building.

Building-Related Illness is suspected when exposure to indoor pollutants results in clinical signs of a recognized disease that is clearly associated with building occupancy, including some kinds of infections, building-related asthma, humidifier fever, and hypersensitivity pneumonitis. (Institute of Medicine 1993) The percentage of the population that is exposed to either the sick building syndrome or building-related illness is unknown.

The most frequently reported characteristics in problem building investigations include inadequate quantity or quality of outdoor air provided by heating, ventilating, and air conditioning (HVAC) systems, and inadequate distribution of air to and from occupied spaces. (Institute of Medicine 1993)

Environmentally-oriented physicians are concerned that hidden environmental causes of illness are not being appropriately recognized and addressed. Pollutants of indoor air, including dust mites, fungi and their toxins, bacteria, viruses, and toxic chemicals are being implicated in a wide variety of health complaints.

THE IMPACT OF AN ALLERGIC CLASSROOM ON TEACHER AND STUDENT HEALTH

American school children and teachers spend the majority of their waking hours indoors, in classrooms that are mechanically ventilated and, often, windowless, where they inhale little fresh air and are exposed to indoor air contaminants. An increased incidence of asthma, chemical sensitivities, and other allergic diseases is associated with these kinds of indoor exposures.

The knowledge and techniques for elimination of this public health problem, and, thus, for prevention of health risks from indoor air pollutants are now available. (Holma 1994) Putting this information to use in our educational communities should be a national health priority. Every school district throughout America should utilize the known strategies for creating allergy-free classrooms.

Aside from contributing to well-recognized allergic diseases, poorly designed and inadequately ventilated classrooms can impact the learning process negatively. When the indoor air does not contain adequate oxygen content, carbon monoxide levels may increase, leading to headaches, fatigue, and irritability.

In warm, humid climates moisture-laden ventilation systems cause increased mold contamination with resultant sensitization of the occupants of the buildings being ventilated.

Gas heating in schools may expose occupants to increased nitrogen-containing gases that affect nervous system functioning and the respiratory tissues of sensitive individuals.

Chemical pesticide spraying in poorly ventilated areas can result in severe neurobehavioral, allergic, and respiratory problems. Aerosol sprays, cigarette smoke, fragranced products, new building materials and glues, new carpeting, floor waxes, particleboard furniture, paint, chemical cleaning products, and solvents can affect human health adversely.

The illnesses may begin with mild reactions and eventually progress over time (with continued chronic exposure) to severely incapacitating and debilitating allergic illnesses. *Once an individual becomes sensitized to indoor allergens, the sensitization may become irreversible.* The individual may never be able to work in that school again. (National Research Council 1992)

The educational process should ideally include a health goal to create an indoor classroom environment so safe that children are not at risk while they learn. An environment with clean allergy-free air will enhance the positive impact of the teaching and learning experience.

RISK OF SENSITIZATION:

Understanding allergic sensitization is essential for the prevention and control of allergic disease. Complaints of allergic reactions in the indoor environment have received much attention in the media. At first "tight building syndrome" was the term commonly utilized for nonspecific building-related complaints resulting from inadequate ventilation. When many specific causes were identified, the term "sick building syndrome" came into more frequent use. (Holma 1994)

An *allergen* is a biological or chemical substance that causes an allergic reaction. An *allergy* is the state of hypersensitivity that results from exposure to an allergen. After an initial exposure to a particular allergen, an individual who develops an allergy becomes *sensitized* to that allergen, and remains *sensitive* in subsequent exposures, with resulting symptoms. The most common *allergic reactions* are the result of immune system changes and are mediated by Immunoglobulin E (IgE); these classic *allergic reactions* commonly affect the respiratory tract, skin, eyes, nose, and throat. (Institute of Medicine 1993)

Allergic diseases caused by *chemical sensitization* may differ in terms of the symptoms, the mechanisms of action, the biological systems affected, and the treatment necessary. Chemical sensitization may be both immunologic and nonimmunologically mediated. The roles of many chemicals in triggering allergic reactions are currently being studied, and the mechanisms of some chemically-induced allergic reactions remain unclear. Chemical hypersensitivity reactions commonly affect the nervous system, and they may play a major role in behavioral, addictive, and learning disorders. (National Research Council 1992)

RECOGNITION OF THE PROBLEM

The risks posed by indoor pollutants are in fact comparable in magnitude to those associated with exposure to chemicals or radiation in industrial settings. (Nero 1988)

Awareness on the part of school personnel, teachers, parents, and children, as well as other individuals, allergic and nonallergic, who enter the school building, can prevent many of the problems associated with indoor allergens and can alleviate those that remain. Intelligent strategies to coordinate healthy architectural engineering and building design, materials, and construction will optimize health benefits and minimize allergic problems. (Institute of Medicine 1993)

BUILDING-RELATED ILLNESS/SICK BUILDING SYNDROME CATEGORIES (TOXIC, ALLERGIC, INFECTIOUS, INADEQUATE VENTILATION)

The quality of indoor air is a function of the source of pollutants, access to fresh outdoor air, and general ventilation. (Institute of Medicine 1993) Pollutants include toxic chemicals, allergens, and infectious agents or microorganisms. Among the sources of pollution to the indoor environment are poor building design, certain materials for building or furnishing, some human activities, and some consumer products. (Holma 1994)

Toxic or Sensitizing Chemicals

These include fumes outgassing from odorous, highly chemicalized products. Newer buildings have higher concentrations of volatile organic compounds (VOCs) than older buildings do. The majority of VOCs come from texture glue on walls, sealing compounds, floor varnish, paints, and adhesives. (Holma 1994)

Formaldehyde is found in new carpets, carpet backings and adhesive bindings, formaldehyde foam (UFFI) insulation, and formaldehyde wood (particleboard and plywood) cabinets, desks, and other furnishings. Formaldehyde is also present in ceiling tiles, fabric room dividers, chemicalized cleaning supplies, aerosol sprays, and air fragrances that volatilize chemicals into the air.

Gas heat and gas stoves contribute nitrogen compounds to the indoor air.

Carbon monoxide results from poor ventilation. Carbon monoxide gas, though odorless, causes headaches and fatigue in occupants of poorly ventilated buildings. If carbon monoxide, combines with hemoglobin, it produces a serious health risk to the developing fetus of a pregnant woman.

Mycotoxins originate from fungal contamination of air conditioning systems and can readily sensitize the nervous and respiratory systems.

Odorous exhaust fumes from vehicles powered by gasoline or diesel fuel, and sulfur dioxide from air pollution can enter a classroom from a door or window or ventilation system downwind of a highway or school bus stop.

Carpet glues, roofing tars, and paint fumes are emitters of chemicals that can cause sick-building-syndrome asthma. (Holma 1994)

Chemical insecticides, regularly sprayed, are significant toxic offenders. Organophosphates and carbamates are acetylcholinesterase inhibitors that affect and interfere with nervous system functioning. Safer nontoxic pest control methods utilizing integrated pest management are preferable. (Blume 1976)

Chronic exposure to sensitizing chemicals or mycotoxins may lead to multiple chemical sensitivities. (Ashford and Miller 1991; National Research Council 1992)

Lead, which is often underestimated and neglected, is a serious toxic problem in older buildings where leaded paints have been used, or where the school water supply is contaminated. (Tarcher 1992)

Radon gas, which may enter a building through water pipes coming from the ground or through cracks and crevices in the foundation, may also be a serious problem in some localities. The EPA recommends that every school be checked for radon. (Tarcher 1992)

Cigarette smoking, another significant source of indoor air pollution, should be restricted to areas remote from classrooms and other rooms used by sizable numbers of individuals. Smoke enters and contaminates the ventilation system, and the odor of tobacco lingers on furniture and in building materials. (Institute of Medicine 1993)

Figure 18-1 shows those chemicals and chemical products most likely to contaminate the air in a school building.

Allergens

Exposure to airborne particulates and allergens has the potential to sensitize occupants of a building. Allergic rhinitis, asthma, humidifier fever, and hypersensitivity pneumonitis have all been identified as building related illnesses. (Holma 1994; Institute of Medicine 1993)

Dust mites and dust are major problems and accumulate in poorly maintained air conditioning duct systems, as well as on floors, walls, furniture, and other surfaces.

- ☐ Adhesives
- ☐ Aerosol Sprays
- ☐ Air Fragrances
- ☐ Arts and Crafts Materials
- ☐ Carbon Monoxide
- ☐ Ceiling Tiles
- ☐ Cleaning Products
- ☐ Floor Varnish
- ☐ Formaldehyde
- ☐ Gas Heat
- ☐ Gas Stoves
- ☐ Glues on Walls
- ☐ Insulation
- ☐ Lead
- ☐ Outdoor Pollution
- ☐ Mycotoxins
- ☐ Paints
- ☐ Particleboard
- ☐ Perfumes
- ☐ Pesticides
- ☐ Radon
- ☐ Room Dividers
- ☐ Roofing Tars
- ☐ Science Lab Chemicals
- ☐ Sealers
- ☐ Smoke

Figure 18-1.
A Checklist of Chemicals and Chemical Products

Moisture is a major problem contributing to the growth of the microbial population, including mites, molds, fungi, and viral and bacterial agents. When temperature (70 degrees Fahrenheit) and humidity (less than 45%) are properly controlled, mites and mold growth are prevented.

Danders can be a problem if animals are allowed in classrooms. Pollens can enter from the outside air.

Figure 18-2 shows the most common sources of allergens in the classroom.

Infections

Improperly maintained HVAC systems can harbor bacterial, viral, fungal, and mite microorganisms, giving rise to serious respiratory and flu-like episodes, as well as other allergic phenomena.

Inadequate Ventilation

This condition is cited most frequently in building investigations as a factor contributing to allergic, toxic, and infectious air-quality problems.

HOW TO CREATE AN ALLERGY-FREE CLASSROOM WITH ENVIRONMENTAL CONTROLS

The major principles involved in creating an allergy-free classroom include:

1. *Making the proper diagnosis* of the problem building or classroom (i.e., identifying the causes of the problems).

2. *Treating the problems* identified, usually by:

■ *source control*, avoidance or removal by thorough clean-up of as many allergens or pollutants as possible, which can eliminate occupant exposure, or

■ *exposure control*, which can minimize but not eliminate occupant exposures by methods of dilution or air cleaning. (Institute of Medicine 1993)

MAKING THE PROPER DIAGNOSIS

To make a diagnosis of a problem building, begin by doing a walk-through of classrooms and other school areas, paying attention to:

☐   Pets

☐   Chalk dust/erasers

☐   Food odors

☐   Particleboard furniture

☐   Fragrance emitters

☐   Cosmetics, hairspray, nail polish, perfume

☐   Fabric softeners

☐   Magic markers

☐   Paints, glues, solvents, science chemicals

☐   Insecticides

☐   Floor wax

☐   Ammonia-, phenol-, and chlorine-containing cleaning products

☐   Carpeting

☐   Gas Heat

☐   Ozone emitters

☐   Outdoor contaminants: pollens, auto exhaust, sewage, bus-stop odors

☐   Ceiling tiles

☐   Tobacco smoke

☐   Mold growth and dust on books

☐   Flowering plants

Figure 18-2.
Common Classroom Sources of Allergens

Location

What is the school near? Is it in close proximity to a highway, bus stop, industrial polluter, gas station, garbage dump, parking garage, incinerator, etc?

Odors

Take note of any odors coming from any areas of the school, i.e., odors from bathrooms, cafeteria, arts and crafts rooms, carpeted areas, and new construction, as well as those from cleaning materials, pesticides, dust, or gases; musty smells; and aerosol-spray fragrances. Find out where all the chemical cleaning agents, glues, paints, and other remodeling and repairing supplies are stored, and make certain they are not contaminating classroom air.

Windows and exhaust fans

Are there windows or exhaust fans in the rooms, or is the school a tight building? Are there exhaust fans for odorous products (arts and crafts materials, science lab chemicals) and equipment (photocopy machines, computers)?

Heating, ventilating, and air conditioning systems

Equipment problems that have been most frequently reported in investigations of polluted buildings include inadequate specification and installation of air filters for removal of inert particulates and bio-aerosols; inadequate specification and installation of drain pans and drain lines for removal of water condensed from cooling coils and humidifiers; inadequate specification and installation of duct work to prevent microbial contamination; and inadequate specification of humidifiers to prevent microbial or chemical contamination in the humidifier and subsequently in the air. (Institute of Medicine 1993)

Look at the windows, the air flow, the ventilation systems. Are the air conditioning duct systems connected together, or is the system in each classroom separate from those of other rooms? Are the A/C systems sealed tight, or do they pull in dust or other particulates from ceiling tiles, dead ceiling space, or other rooms, etc.?

Are the A/C filters, air handlers, vents, ceiling fans, and duct systems properly maintained? Are there moisture buildups in the ventilation system? Check cooling coils, condensing surfaces, drain pans, dehumidifiers, filters, and air ducts for proper maintenance and cleanliness.

Fresh air intakes should be evaluated and adequately maintained. Recirculated indoor air, if not adequately mixed with fresh air ventilation or if not purified sufficiently, can become a serious health threat to occupants. (Holma 1994; Institute of Medicine 1993)

Evaluate temperature and humidity. It is important to determine and define the indoor air, temperature, and relative humidity conditions that will provide for occupant comfort and at the same time suppress the growth of allergen-producing microorganisms and mites. (Institute of Medicine 1993) The development of allergen-containing reservoirs depends on available water in the micro-environment of the allergen-producing organism. The amount of water in such an environment depends on the relationship between the amount of airborne water vapor and the temperature in the environment (which controls condensation); the ability of substrates in the environment to absorb water; and the presence of liquid water sources. Ambient relative humidity is often considered the major controlling factor for indoor allergens. (Institute of Medicine 1993)

Ask if the A/C system is left on or shut off at night? To control dust mite and mold growth, the average temperature should be no higher than 70-72 degrees Fahrenheit with humidity below 45%, especially in warm, humid climates.

Floor Coverings

Carpeting and padding are sources of dust and mold growth, especially if they have accumulated moisture. Some new carpets can outgas multiple chemicals for several months. Carpets cleaned with chemicals or sprayed with chemical cleaners, pesticides, or deodorizers are sources of chemical exposure, and in many instances, the removal of carpeting has dramatically improved indoor air quality and alleviated allergic symptoms. From the standpoint of preventing allergy problems, flooring should be low-odor and nontoxic. (Blume 1976; Holma 1994)

Hard surface flooring (hardwood, marble, linoleum, vinyl, Mexican tile, or terrazzo) is preferred over carpeting.

Ceilings

Ceiling tiles can easily contribute to poor air quality, because they can emit chemical odors and shed particles.

Look above the ceiling tiles. Many times they are loaded with dust and dirt. Roof leaks should be repaired, and damaged ceiling tiles and air conditioning ducts should be repaired or restored. Sheet rock-type ceiling tiles are recommended. Ceilings and walls may be covered with water-based paints or other water-based coatings. (Holma 1994)

Wall Coverings

Walls should be covered with a smooth surface of water-resistant materials. Low odor, nontoxic, water-based paints can be used. Mold can accumulate behind wallpaper, especially if there have been water leaks from the ceiling into the walls. In case of leaks, removal of wallpaper may be necessary. Aluminum foil-type wallpaper is a good non-allergic barrier.

Nontoxic, low-odor, water-based paints and sealers are available. Old paint on walls may be a source of lead exposure; sealing these walls with a fast-drying sealer may be all that is necessary. (Tarcher 1992)

Particleboard in walls, cabinets, desks (and subflooring in trailers) can outgas formaldehyde and create significant allergic problems. Particleboard should be removed or sealed. All edges and sides of cabinets and desks need to be completely sealed.

Other Pollutant Sources

Dust and mold collectors include old books and magazines, stuffed animals, and stuffed furniture. These should be removed or properly stored. Books or furniture that have been water-damaged may have to be destroyed.

Chalk dust, arts and crafts materials, perfumed or fragranced products, and pets can be major allergen sources. Their presence should be minimized or eliminated in the classroom. (Blume 1976)

Smoking should be prohibited in the school, because it is a major source of indoor air pollution.

Cleaning Products

Only low odor nontoxic products should be used for cleaning and maintenance. Cleaning can be done with fragrance-free soap (for example, Rugged Red by Neo-Life), borax, baking soda, and vinegar (to retard mold growth). These products are available from a number of sources. (Blume 1976, Holma 1994) Dehumidifiers should be used to prevent the growth of mold in hot or moist climates.

TREATING THE PROBLEM

Treatment should begin with a study of the principles of environmental control. *Figure 18-3* lists the most important of these principles and shows how they can be applied to various contaminent sources.

Educating School Staff, Students, and Parents

Lectures on allergies, asthma, and environmental control can be developed as an integral part of the educational program for teachers, support personnel, and parents. Children should also be made aware of the importance of environmental factors in their health.

By creating healthy, allergy-controlled classrooms for students and teachers you are setting an excellent educational example.

Professional Investigation of the Problem

For the latest information on the treatment of sick buildings, contact your local health department, NIOSH, the Certified Industrial Hygienists, the American Lung Association, the EPA, the American Academy of Environmental Medicine, and the American College of Occupational and Environmental Medicine.

REFERENCES

Ashford, N., and C. Miller, 1991, *Chemical Exposures,* New York: Van-Nostrand Reinhold.

Blume, Kathleen, 1976, "Air Pollution In The Schools," *Clinical Ecology*, edited by Lawrence Dickey, Springfield: Thomas, pp. 369-378.

Holma, Bo, 1994, "Indoor Air Pollution," *Occupational Medicine*, 3rd Edition, edited by Carl Zenz, St. Louis: Mosby, pp. 1067-7075.

Institute of Medicine, 1993, *Indoor Allergens,* Washington, D. C.: National Academy Press.

National Research Council, 1992, *Multiple Chemical Sensitivities*, Washington, D. C.:National Academy Press, pp. 13-35, 1992.

Nero, Anthony, Jr., May, 1988, "Controlling Indoor Air Pollution," *Scientific American*, Vol. 258, No. 5, pages 42-48.

□ *Cleaning Products, Nontoxic And Low Odor. Keep the classroom odor-free. Avoid aerosol sprays and chemicalized cleaning products.*

□ *HVAC Maintenance. Maintain adequately fresh air intakes, air purification systems, dehumidifiers, filters, and air conditioning and heating ducts.*

□ *Integrated Pest Management. Utilize the least toxic pest control methods. Any spraying should be done when occupants are not present.*

□ *Humidity, Moisture, And Temperature Control. Maintain this control to minimize airborne microbiological contamination.*

□ *Remodeling. Always undertake remodeling when occupants are not present in the building, e.g., over vacations. Proper sealing off of the area being renovated from the rest of the school will prevent contamination of other areas. Utilize exhaust fans and low odor, nontoxic building and construction materials.*

□ *Furniture. Make sure that low odor, nontoxic and nonallergic furniture is used in the building.*

□ *Storage Areas. Locate storage areas away from classroom ventilation systems.*

□ *Windows And Exhaust Fans. Locate and maintain windows and exhaust fans carefully. Proper location and maintenance will solve the majority of minor indoor air problems when quick ventilation is necessary.*

□ *Floors, Walls, And Ceilings. Make sure that these are made of odor free nontoxic materials.*

□ *Smoking And Fragrances. Avoid smoking and the use of fragrances in the classroom and, if possible, in the school.*

Figure 18-3.
A Checklist Of Important Principles For Environmental Controls

Speer, Frederic, 1970, *Allergy of the Nervous System,* Springfield IL: Thomas Publishing.

Tarcher, Alyce, Editor, 1992, *Principles and Practice of Environmental Medicine*, New York: Plenum, pp. 1-39 and 246.

19

NUTRITION, LEARNING, AND THE SCHOOL CAFETERIA

by Beatrice Trum Hunter

In this chapter, Ms. Hunter, the Food Editor of Consumers' Research Magazine, describes adverse reactions to foods and offers suggestions to cafeteria workers, teachers, parents, and administrators about numerous alternative foods and food substances that can be safely ingested by children with intolerances or chemical sensitivities. In discussing children's intolerances to lactose, gluten, galactose, fructose, and sensitivities to some food additives and colorings, she provides answers to these questions frequently asked by those responsible for nutrition in schools:

- ☐ *What specific food substances influence children's learning and behavior patterns?*

- ☐ *How can the school lunch be made more nutritious for all children?*

- ☐ *What bad effects may some "good" foods such as milk and grain products have on some children?*

- ☐ *What alternative foods may be tolerated by a child with a particular food sensitivity?*

- ☐ *How can an alternative product be monitored for its effectiveness?*

Recent attempts to upgrade school food have been well publicized. The United States Department of Agriculture (USDA) has announced its intention to double the amount of fresh fruits and vegetables available for school lunch and breakfast programs, and to reduce fat and sodium contents. These improvements are laudable. School cafeteria offerings, however, must address the additional needs of some school children in order to provide optimal conditions for learning.

337

DIET AND BEHAVIORAL DISORDERS

A 1993 British study adds support to the idea that dietary manipulation may improve a child's learning ability and behavioral pattern. The children who participated in the study were extensively evaluated with assessment tests. All met attention deficit disorder criteria. The children ranged from 3 to 12 years of age, and had an average range of IQ scores.

For several weeks the children were given a diet of basic foods: turkey, lamb, rice, potatoes, bananas, pears, vegetables, bottled water, sunflower oil, and milk-free margarine. Diets for individual children were adapted to avoid suspected food allergies or aversions.

Seventy-eight children completed the first phase of the study. The parents of 59 of the children (76%) reported notable behavioral improvements; 17 (22%), no improvements; and 2 (3%) worsening of behavior.

In the second phase, the 59 children who responded favorably were challenged with manufactured foods, food additives, and various basic foods that are common allergens. The additives consisted of a blend of 10 food colors (only four of which are allowed in the United States) and two commonly used preservatives, benzoic acid and metabisulfite. Although the levels of the additives were quite low, the adverse reactions they elicited were severe, 70% of the children reacting unfavorably to foods containing them. Both cow's milk and chocolate provoked adverse reactions in 64% of the children; oranges in 57%; cheese made from cow's milk in 45%; wheat in 45%; other fruits in 36%; tomatoes in 22%, and eggs in 18%.

The researchers concluded that diet can contribute to behavioral disorders in children. They recommended that the observations (anecdotal evidence) by parents and other child caregivers be taken seriously by clinicians. Dietary manipulations deserve consideration for treatment of children with attention deficit disorders, hyperkinesis, and other behavioral patterns that can have adverse effects on learning. They noted:

> The ways in which diet worked remain unclear. Toxic, pharmacological, or allergic mechanisms could be involved, and the physiological effects of different foods might induce changes in brain perfusion similar to those reported in attention deficit disorder. (Carter, Urbanowicz, Hemsley, et al. 1993)

WHAT'S THE DIFFERENCE BETWEEN FOOD ALLERGIES, SENSITIVITIES, AND INTOLERANCES?

Some children react unfavorably to certain foods or food components. Frequently, different terms----*allergy, sensitivity*, or *intolerance*----are used interchangeably to describe adverse food reactions: Yet the meanings of these terms differ.

Allergy

Allergy is a confusing term because it has two components: *symptoms* and *sensitization*. A patient thinks about the symptoms manifested in an *allergic reaction*. "After eating shellfish I broke out in a rash." The doctor thinks about the *antigen-antibody* response: the *antigens* are molecules, usually proteins, that stimulate the immune system to produce a response characterized by symptoms, and the *antibodies* are molecules formed by the body's immune system as a specific response to antigens.

A *true allergic reaction* is a complex immune reaction that involves antibodies in the blood, attached to cells, and. on various body surfaces. Medical tests can detect the presence of antibodies and confirm an allergic reaction. When antibodies are present, the person is considered to be *sensitized* to a food or other substance.

Food Sensitivity

A diagnosis of food *sensitivity* can be confirmed with double-blind studies that show an antigen-antibody response. Repeatedly, after a specific food----the suspected antigen----is ingested, a specific antibody to the food will be found. This provides the immunologic basis for true allergy. Because of the confusion resulting from the term *allergy* being applied both to symptoms and to reactions, however, the phrase *food allergy* has been abandoned by the majority of medical professionals and replaced with *food sensitivity*.

The tendency for a child to be food-sensitive is thought to be genetic in origin. Although the incidence of food sensitivity in a child is increased if the parents have allergies---- especially if *both* parents are affected---the child does not inherit a sensitivity to specific food substances. For example, the parent(s) may be sensitive to pollen, but the child may be sensitive to some unrelated grains.

Food Intolerance

In contrast, food *intolerances* may cover a wide range of adverse reactions resulting from a variety of mechanisms, including enzyme deficiencies (example: lactose intolerance); metabolic diseases (example: gluten intolerance); adventitious contaminants (example: aflatoxin molds in food); toxic residues (example: lead, mercury, or cadmium); or neuro-excitors (example: aspartame or monosodium glutamate).

STRATEGIES FOR MANAGING FOOD SENSITIVITY

The basic program for preventing food sensitivity is avoidance of the known or suspected offending food or food component. If a child is known to have certain food sensitivities, there needs to be a cooperative effort between parents and school cafeteria personnel to make certain that the child is not served the offending food or food component. Sometimes a dietitian can help to suggest alternative foods or offer guidance in planning nutritionally adequate meals for the child with special needs.

Cow's Milk Allergy

Common nutritious foods, usually tolerated by children, may be unsuited for a child who is truly allergic. Cow's milk allergy (not to be confused with lactose intolerance) is the most common offender, especially in children. Other common allergens include beef, eggs, citrus fruit, tree nuts, corn, soybeans, and wheat. Hence, label reading is essential for parents and school cafeteria personnel.

Coping with milk allergy serves as an illustration of the strategies necessary to manage all food allergies. Dietary choices should be limited, insofar as possible, to basic foods, and factory-processed foods should be minimized. Many foods may contain milk or non-fat dry milk, including au gratin foods, baked goods, butter, cheeses, chocolates, creamed or scalloped vegetables and soups, cream sauces, gravies, ice cream, luncheon meats, malted milk, margarine, non-dairy creamers with caseinates, pancake and biscuit mixes, puddings, salad dressings, sherbets, and white sauces.

A child on a milk-free diet must be supplied with many of the essential nutrients commonly supplied by milk. For example, alternative foods that contribute calcium include clams, sardines and salmon with bones, oysters, broccoli, almonds, and dark molasses. A calcium supplement may be prescribed by a pediatrician or dietitian.

Stewed fruit or fruit juice may be used as substitutes for milk over cereal. Fruit ices and popsicles can replace ice cream, and milk-free frozen desserts are available.

Lactose Intolerance

If a child avoids milk in the school cafeteria, it may not necessarily be due to poor eating habits. The child may have learned to shun milk after having experienced discomfort such as abdominal pain, bloating, flatulence, and diarrhea. These symptoms suggest *lactose intolerance* (also termed *lactose malabsorption*).

Lactose intolerance (distinctly different from milk allergy) is a common problem, and can range from mild to severe. Various epidemiological studies estimate that from 70% to 90% of the world's population to some degree cannot digest lactose, the main carbohydrate present in milk and other dairy products. Those individuals who tolerate lactose beyond weaning are actually a minority. After weaning, humans experience a decline in lactase, the enzyme needed to digest the lactose. Lactose intolerance is especially high among African-Americans, Native Americans, and Asians.

Two diagnostic tests are available to confirm that a child is lactose intolerant. One is oral, based on routine laboratory procedures. The other is a breath hydrogen test, which is considered more reliable to evaluate lactose digestion. Both tests are available in most hospitals.

If lactose intolerance is confirmed, and the degree of intolerance is determined, a number of different techniques are available to cope with this condition. For the extreme case, all dairy products that contain lactose may need to be avoided. At times, soy milk is available and may be tolerated. Labels on all pre-prepared foods used at school and at home must be read carefully before the foods are served to a lactose-intolerant child. Casein and caseinates, which are derived from milk, can be tolerated because they contain no lactose.. Skim milk and nonfat milk, added to numerous food products, however, should be avoided.

For the child who can tolerate lactose to some degree, there are some coping techniques. The more slowly lactose is presented in the intestine, the more readily it is digested and absorbed. Milk, consumed along with solid foods, delays the gastric emptying, and therefore favors lactose absorption. Thus, some dairy-containing foods in the school cafeteria may be tolerated in the context of an entire meal.

Another strategy is to offer only a small amount of milk to the child over time, rather than the entire container at one sitting. This arrangement would be important as applied to a mid-morning or mid-afternoon snack at school.

Gastric emptying is delayed by the presence of fats and amino acids, the building blocks of protein. For this reason, whole milk, with its full butterfat content is tolerated better than fat-reduced or skim milk. The trend in school food offerings is to serve fat-reduced milk as part of the effort of total fat reduction. An option should be available for the lactose-intolerant child. Likewise, chocolate-flavored milk may be tolerated better than unflavored milk. Though nutritionists may frown upon the use of such products to which sweeteners have been added, there is a beneficial trade-off for the lactose-intolerant child.

Fermented dairy products undergo reduced lactose levels and may be tolerated. Some fermented dairy products, however, are tolerated better than others. Aged cheeses, such as Cheddar or Swiss, are significantly reduced in lactose because the discarded whey contains most of the lactose, whereas the curd contains little. Soft cheeses, such as cottage cheese may have whey added to them. Hence, such cheeses may be less easily tolerated than aged ones.

The lactose level of other fermented dairy products such as yogurt, cultured buttermilk, and sweet acidophilus milk may be just as high as that of whole fresh milk. Their lactose content varies according to the processing technique. Whole-fat fermented products may be tolerated better than low-fat or non-fat ones. Although nonfat milk solids increase the nutritional value and lower the fat contents of any food product to which they are added, they raise the lactose content of such a product.

Commercial food-grade lactases (Beta-galactosidase enzyme preparations from microbial organisms that digest the lactose) are used to produce lactose-hydrolyzed milk and other reduced-lactose products. They can serve as an alternative to fresh fluid milk for the lactose-intolerant child. Such products, which contain from 40% to 90% less lactose, are available from some dairies. School cafeteria personnel and parents should inquire about the availability of such products for school and home use for the lactose-intolerant child.

Another approach is to make regular fluid milk better tolerated by using lactose-reducing products such as Lactaid , Dairy Ease , or Lactogest , produced respectively by Johnson & Johnson, Eastman Kodak, and Thompson Medical. These products are available in liquid or in tablet forms. They add to the cost of the milk, however, and require a 24-hour incubation period in the milk to become fully effective.

An ongoing effort to improve lactose digestion is to add Beta-galactosidase to milk at mealtime. Results of preliminary studies show that adding such lactase enzymes is easy, improves lactose absorption, and decreases the undesirable colonic hydrogen production. Also, when added at mealtimes in appropriate amounts, these lactase enzymes can hydrolyze milk lactose, even when solid foods are eaten at the same time.

Gluten Intolerance

Due to an inborn metabolic disorder, people who suffer from gluten intolerance (also termed celiac sprue, gluten-induced enteropathy, primary malabsorption, and ideopathic steatorrhea) cannot tolerate gluten naturally present in certain grains. Gluten is a water-insoluble complex protein fraction found mainly in wheat and rye, and to a lesser extent in barley and oat.

Children born with this disorder fail to thrive unless they are placed on a gluten-free diet, and follow a lifetime gluten avoidance. Gluten-intolerant individuals who continue to eat gluten-containing grain products, even at very low intake, may experience abdominal distention, diarrhea, nausea, headache, drowsiness, skin rash, anemia, weight loss, and bone or joint pain. In extreme cases, the disorder may contribute to high blood pressure, heartbeat irregularities, and low serum calcium, which can lead to tooth decay.

Frequently, the gluten-intolerant child is also milk-intolerant. Both conditions produce some overlapping symptoms. According to the American Celiac Society, children tend to outgrow celiac-induced milk intolerance within a year or two after adherence to a gluten-free diet.

A gluten-free diet is difficult to achieve in the school cafeteria. Most meals include gluten-containing grains in foods such as bread, pizza crust, pasta, pancake, crouton, flour-thickened soup, stew and gravy, cookies and other bakery products, and ready-to-eat breakfast cereals served in school breakfasts. The introduction of certain ethnic foods such as corn tortillas is a boon for the gluten-intolerant child—provided the tortilla is entirely free of wheat, and that the child tolerates corn.

Gluten offers many technical benefits to food processors, and it is widely used in many food products. Because of gluten's binding qualities, it is used in breadings and coatings, and to bind ground meat, poultry, and fish products. Textured protein products manufactured from blends of wheat gluten and soy have been used extensively as low-cost meat extenders in school cafeterias.

For the child who needs to avoid gluten in the school cafeteria and at home, there are good non-gluten substitutes: potatoes; rice, and corn, and the flours, meals, and starches derived from them; and tapioca, arrowroot, and agar agar as thickeners. Two non-gluten grains, long used in Latin America but relatively recent introductions in the United States, are amaranth and quinoa. Two other ancient grains, Teff and Job's tears, both gluten-free, are currently being introduced. Buckwheat, not a true grain, contains no gluten. Some of these unusual grains can be obtained from special sources.

Other newly introduced grains are spelt and kamut. They actually are forerunners of hybrid wheat. They may be tolerated by some, but not by all gluten-intolerant children. If introduced experimentally, they should be offered sparingly, under the supervision of a health professional who can watch for any untoward reaction. Triticale, a grain combining wheat and rye developed through plant breeding, contains gluten and needs to be avoided. Millet, an ancient grain, may contain some gluten, albeit at a very low level. It may be tolerated by some, but not by all gluten-intolerant children.

In addition to avoidance of gluten-containing grains, school cafeteria personnel and parents need to be aware of other food products that contain fractions of wheat, rye, barley, or oat, found in malt and malted milk powders; hydrolyzed vegetable protein and plant protein; and processed foods containing modified food starch.

According to one processor, wheat germ is gluten-free. The processor cautions, however, that because the germ is separated mechanically, it might be contaminated by a small amount of gluten. Because even a small amount can result in acute illness in gluten-intolerant individuals, it is prudent to add wheat germ to the avoidance list.

The case of gluten intolerance serves as a reminder that foods, regardless of how basic, natural, or nutritious, may not be tolerated by all children. It has been found that other disparate health problems may be associated with gluten intolerance. Cases of dermatitis herpetiformis, psoriasis, eczema, Sjögren's syndrome, rheumatoid arthritis, systemic lupus erythematosis, and schizophrenia have all responded favorably, or the disorders have been ameliorated in patients placed on a gluten-free diet.

Galactose Intolerance

Galactose, a sugar component of lactose and the major component of the main carbohydrate in both human and cow's milk, may also create intolerance problems for children who lack the enzyme needed for its digestion. Galactosemia is a genetic disorder of carbohydrate metabolism. At present, understandings about this disorder are at a stage similar to that of lactose intolerance several decades ago----largely unrecognized and unexplored.

Galactose must be avoided by the galactosemic child. Galactose intolerance may be far less common than lactose intolerance, but it is far more severe for those who do experience it. Such children require a totally dairy-free diet. Otherwise, they fail to thrive, have stunted growth, develop cataracts and liver disorders, and usually die prematurely.

Galactosemia affects one in every 30,000 to 60,000 infants. The acute symptoms occur a few days after birth in an apparently healthy infant. The baby begins to vomit and lose weight, and becomes lethargic. Usually, the symptoms subside when breast milk or cow's milk-based formula are replaced by a non-milk formula. Because the galactosemic infant responds favorably to the same diet as the milk-allergic infant, galactosemia may be unsuspected at an early stage and wrongly attributed to milk allergy. These two disorders are distinctly different entities, which may become apparent during the next stage of growth. The milk-allergic child may continue to thrive when fruits, vegetables, and cereals are added to the diet, whereas the galactosemic child may begin to show poor growth, mental retardation, and speech difficulties.

Recent galactose research may help to explain this puzzle. A joint study, conducted by the Agricultural Research Service (ARS) of the U.S. Department of Agriculture (USDA) and Ross Laboratories, revealed that many common fruits and vegetables, and possibly some grains, contain galactose.

As a follow-up, various amounts of galactose were identified in 12 fruit and vegetable products intended for infant feeding. High levels were present in applesauce, banana, and squash. The researchers examined 45 commonly consumed fresh fruits and vegetables and identified high galactose levels present in tomato, watermelon, papaya, and persimmon, and moderately high levels in banana, apple, date, kiwi, pumpkin, bell pepper, and brussels sprout. Unfortunately, the foods identified as galactose-free are not ones likely to be used in baby food products or to form major contributions to school menus: artichoke, mushroom, olive, and peanut. At present there is a lack of information about whether galactose is present in cereals commonly fed to infants, from grains such as rice, oat, or barley.

Based on this new information, 115 galactosemic children, ranging from infants to teenagers, are being studied. Parents are keeping food diaries for the children. The ARS will make laboratory.analyses of the foods eaten to determine galactose intake levels. The goal is to learn whether the low galactose levels present in non-dairy foods also need to be avoided by galactosemics. A school cafeteria administrator faced with the problem of feeding a galactosemic child needs to consult closely with the parents of the child as well as the health professional who is monitoring a specialized diet.

Fructose Intolerance

Fructose, a natural sugar present in many foods, is problematic for some children. Most can convert fructose to glucose and burn it for energy. Fructose-intolerant individuals cannot make this conversion, because they are unable to absorb fructose into the bloodstream. Instead, the fructose remains in the bowel, where bacterial fermentation produces carbon dioxide, hydrogen, methane, water, alcohol, and lactic acid. Both the alcohol and lactic acid can irritate the bowel lining. The gas, bloating, and abdominal distention, if chronic, can lead to hiatal hernia, or a blow-out of the thin weak-walled portion of the colon.

Fructose intolerance may be a previously unrecognized factor associated with gluten intolerance. Also, it may be a missing piece in the puzzle of irritable bowel syndrome. Symptoms of fructose intolerance are surprisingly similar to those of lactose intolerance. As with galactosemics, a school cafeteria administrator is challenged to feed a fructose-intolerant child appropriately.

Fructose is present in fruits and in honey. Corn that is treated enzymatically, however, can be converted to fructose. Corn-derived sweeteners and syrups have become increasingly important in the American food supply as high-fructose corn syrup (HFCS) which now partially or totally replaces sucrose (table sugar) in many processed foods and beverages. Therefore, label reading of all processed foods is essential to identify the presence of HFCS.

FOOD ADDITIVES

Of approximately 3,000 direct food additives intentionally used in foods in the United States, some are capable of inducing adverse effects in some individuals, though all the mechanisms are not well understood. Food additives represent a category of food components that should be suspected if a child demonstrates any inappropriate symptoms after a specific food or drink is consumed. Some symptoms attributed to certain food additives include headache, numbness, drowsiness, dizziness, mental confusion, severe anxiety or depression, mood swing, impaired cognition, dyslexia, slurred speech, deterioration of handwriting, behavioral change, restlessness, hyperactivity, and aggressiveness. All are relevant to a learning environment.

Among the host of food additives, the sulfiting agents and the food color tartrazine, are prominent as universally-acknowledged inducers of adverse effects. Others include the preservative sodium nitrite; a range of synthetic colors, flavors, and antioxidants; the high-intensity sweetener aspartame; and the flavor enhancers monosodium glutamate (MSG) and hydrolyzed vegetable protein (HVP) which forms some MSG.

Offending food additives can produce a range of reactions, including allergic manifestations, neurologic overstimulation, toxicity, and other untoward effects.

Sulfiting Compounds

If, after eating, a child experiences shortness of breath, labored breathing, tightness in the chest, airway constriction, coughing and wheezing, an asthmatic attack from sulfiting agents used with food may be suspected. Other symptoms might include a rapid pulse, faintness, weakness, sudden generalized flushing, lightheadedness, cold clammy skin, hives, itching, severe abdominal distress, diarrhea, swelling of the tongue, and difficulty in swallowing. Severe reactions could result in the loss of consciousness, anaphylactic shock, cyanosis (blue discoloration of the skin caused by insufficient oxygen in the blood), coma, and death.

The number of children experiencing asthma, the severity of the illness, and the incidence of mortality associated with it have increased dramatically in recent years. More than three million American children under the age of 18 are asthmatic. Sulfiting agents used to preserve the freshness and natural appearance of some foods are among the environmental factors that can trigger asthmatic attacks. As little as 7.5 milligrams (mg) of sulfites taken orally can trigger a reaction in a person who is sensitive to sulfiting compounds. Non-asthmatics, as well as asthmatics, can be affected.

Since 1985, more than a thousand cases of adverse reactions from sulfiting compounds have been reported to the Food and Drug Administration (FDA). As a result of the deaths of some individuals—including children—who went into anaphylactic shock, the FDA took several curbing actions. Now the presence of sulfiting agents at levels of 10 parts per million (ppm) or more must be declared on food labels.

Many convenience foods containing sulfiting agents at levels higher than 10 ppm are used in school cafeterias. According to FDA, foods with sulfiting levels above 10 ppm commonly include baked goods and grain products; dairy products; seafoods; processed seafood products other than dried or frozen; fresh or frozen shrimp; frozen lobster; nut products; plant protein isolates; dried fruits and fruit juices; glace fruit and maraschino cherries; dehydrated and canned vegetables and vegetable juices; dehydrated and frozen potatoes; gravies and sauces; soup mixes; gelatin; jams and jellies; filled crackers; and sweet sauces, syrups, sugar, and molasses.

Physicians who have treated sulfite-sensitive individuals have reported that vitamin B12 is a metabisulfite blocker. They recommend that sensitive individuals should ingest 1,000 to 2,000 micrograms of vitamin B12 before eating any factory-prepared foods.

Parents of an asthmatic child should avoid serving the child any sulfited foods and should make school cafeteria personnel aware of the health problem. Label reading by both the parents and the cafeteria personnel will help to identify those products that need to be avoided by the asthmatic child. There are six sulfiting agents permitted for use with foods: sulfur dioxide, sodium sulfite, sodium or potassium bisulfite, and sodium or potassium metabisulfite.

Tartrazine

The most widely used color additive, FD&C Yellow No. 5, tartrazine, is well recognized as a cause of asthmatic reactions, as well as acute or chronic urticaria (hives), angioedema (abnormal amount of fluid in the heart and blood vessels), rhinitis (runny nose), and purpura (skin discoloration caused by hemorrhage into the tissues), among other effects.

According to the FDA, tens of thousands of Americans are tartrazine-sensitive. In recognition of this fact, the agency required that tartrazine's presence be declared specifically on labels of foods, drugs, and cosmetics long before more recent legislation mandated similar disclosure for other food colors.

Tartrazine is added to numerous food products that are likely to be found in school cafeterias where any convenience food products are used. Although tartrazine is yellow, it is not used merely to color foods that appear yellowish. Tartrazine is used also to adjust hues in products that are brown, green, orange, or other colors. Tartrazine is present in numerous food products including pasta and cheese dishes such as macaroni and cheese; salad dressings; ice cream and sherbets; gelatin desserts; instant puddings and pie fillings; cake mixes and icings; imitation flavorings; and fruit drinks.

The orange drink Tang is used as a screening test for tartrazine reactions in individuals suspected of being tartrazine-sensitive. Following the consumption of an average serving size of this drink, the person is observed for adverse reactions, especially exacerbation of asthma.

Some individuals who are tartrazine-sensitive also react adversely to aspirin (salicylic acid) and to the common food preservative, benzoate of soda (sodium benzoate).

As with sulfiting agents and other sensitizing food additives, parents and school cafeteria personnel need to read food labels carefully to ensure that tartrazine-containing food and beverage products are not served to a tartrazine-sensitive child. The parents need to check medications and toiletries, as well.

SCHOOL CAFETERIAS AND PARENTS' LEGAL RIGHTS

Up to the present, many parents of children with special dietary needs have felt frustrated. They have been told by school officials that the cafeteria is ill-equipped to meet the children's needs. Frequently, they have been advised to send food from home. This arrangement often burdens the children with a psychological stigma in addition to the health problem.

This situation is changing. Ellie Goldberg, M.Ed. an educational rights specialist, insists that new laws and regulations can provide parents with a better alternative. The school is *obligated* to provide alternative choices for children with special food needs.

Goldberg's interest in this issue arose from her daughter's asthmatic condition, and her experience with school cafeterias unable to meet her child's need. Finding legal support in the Rehabilitation Act of 1973, Goldberg has developed expertise to the point that she consults for school administrators throughout the country. She offers them assistance for complying with the regulations, and guidance in developing individual meal plans for children with special needs.

According to Goldberg, Section 504 of the Rehabilitation Act "prohibits discrimination in education or employment on the basis of handicap in any program or institution receiving federal funds. By definition, handicap is any physical or mental disorder or condition affecting one or more body systems that substantially limits one or more major life activities such as walking, speaking, eating, or breathing."

Goldberg explains that "despite the common practice of providing special planning only for students in special education, Section 504 rulings clarify that schools must provide related services and accommodations to 'handicapped students' in regular classrooms." Goldberg interprets this ruling to cover children with food allergies, intolerances, and sensitivities.

The USDA guidelines advise professionals that, "Schools shall make substitutions in foods listed in this section for students who are considered handicapped under 7 CFR part 15b and whose handicap restricts their diet. Schools may also make substitutions for nonhandicapped students who are unable to consume the regular lunch because of medical or other special dietary needs. Substitutions shall be made on a case by case basis only when supported by a statement of the need for substitutions that include recommended alternate foods, unless otherwise exempted by FNS [Food and Nutrition Service]. Such statement shall, in the case of a handicapped student, be signed by a physician or, in the case of a non-handicapped student, by a recognized medical authority."

More recent legislation that encompasses the rights of disabled individuals has wide applications in many areas of concern. Inevitably, the law will have an impact on the school cafeteria and access to appropriate foods for the child with special needs.

The issue of special diets is a relative newcomer in child nutrition programs. The USDA's Food and Nutrition Service Instruction 783-2 Rev. 1, specifically states that "generally, children with food allergies or intolerances are NOT handicapped." Evaluation is made on a case by case basis.

In view of this policy, Professor Cecilia Rokusek at the University of South Dakota's, School of Medicine, has offered parental advice, "When a parent or someone else requests a special diet for a child, there are certain requirements to assure the needs of the child are being met and to protect the school and the school food service personnel." Rokusek instructs parents to obtain a physician's recommendations and attach them to the submitted request for a special diet for the child. She suggests that the request specify required substitutions, or that the physician mark specific deletions of items on the school menu for which substitutions must be made. Rokusek cautions that some substitutions may involve expenses that school cafeterias cannot underwrite. Above all, she emphasizes the importance of parents working cooperatively with the school board and administration, including the food service director.

SUMMARY

Becoming aware of the special requirements of the child with allergies, intolerances, or sensitivities results in raising our awareness of individual differences, and the value of each human being. Adjusting school cafeteria menus insofar as possible to meet special needs requires flexibility and a broader view. The cafeteria challenge should be regarded as an extension of the classroom challenge, to meet the educational needs of each child by providing a nurturing environment that contributes as much as possible to the child's potential for learning and development.

In addition, when school cafeteria personnel learn to adapt to the special dietary needs of children, the level of nutrition will be raised for *all* children who eat at the school cafeteria. Adaptations will result in the use of a greater variety of fresh foods, simply prepared, and offering more choices. Inevitably, as more food labels are read assiduously, the use of convenience foods will be curtailed sharply. This trend will lead to improved nutrition for all the children.

RECOMENDED READING

Bronson-Adatto, C. ed., 1985, *Food Sensitivity. A Resource Including Recipes*, Chicago, IL: American Dietetic Association.

Bronson-Adatto, C. ed., 1985, *Gluten Intolerance, A Resource Including Recipes*, Chicago, IL: American Dietetic Association.

Bronson-Adatto, C. ed., 1985. *Lactose Intolerance. A Resource Including Recipes*, Chicago, IL: American Dietetic Association.

Carter, C. M., M. Urbanowicz, R. Hemsley, *et al*, 1993, "Effects of a few-foods diet in attention deficit disorder," *Arch Dis Child* 69: 564-568.

Chafee, F. H. and G. A. Settipane, Aug 1967, Asthma Caused by FD&C Approved Dyes. *Journal of Allergy* 40, no.2: 65-72.

Coffey, L., 1986, *Wheatless Cooking*, Berkeley, CA: Ten Speed Press.

Cramer, D. W., July 8, 1989, "Galactose Consumption and Metabolism in Relation to the Risk of Ovarian Cancer, *The Lancet II*, no. 8654: 66-71.

"Diet and Behavior: A Multidisciplinary Evaluation," May 1986, *Nutr Rev* 44: 1-254.

Environmental Neurotoxicology, 1992, Washington, D. C.: National Academy Press.

Fields, M., 1986, "Effects of Fructose or Starch on Copper-67 Absorption and Excretion by the Rat," *J Nutr* 116: 625-632.

Foulke, J. B., October 1993, "A Fresh Look at Food Preservatives," *FDA Consumer* 27, no. 8:23-27.

Galactosemia [Fact Sheet], 1992, Cedar Grove, NJ: American Liver Foundation.

Gallagher, C. R., A. L. Molleson, and J. H. Caldwell, October 1974, "Lactose intolerance and fermented dairy products," *Journal of*

the American Dietetic Association 65, no. 4: 34-35.

Gibbons, D. L., 1992, *The Self-Help Way to Treat Colitis and Other Irritable Bowel Conditions*, New Canaan, CT: Keats Publishing.

Gropper, S. S., K. C. Gross, and S. J. Olds, 1992, *The Galactos Content of Selected Fruit and Vegetable Baby Foods: Implications for Infants on Galactose-Restricted Diets*, Auburn, AL: Auburn University.

Gross, K. C., and P. B. Acosta, 1991, "Fruits and Vegetables Are a Source of Galactose: Implications in Planning the Diets of Patients with Galactosemia," *Journal Inher Metab Dis* 14: 253-258.

Hills, H. C.,1976, *Good Food, Gluten Free*, New Canaan, CT: Keats Publishing.

Hills, H. C., 1980, *Good Food, Milk Free, Grain Free*. New Canaan,CT: Keats Publishing.

Hunter, B. T., 1980, *Additives Book* [rev. ed.], New Canaan, CT: Keats Publishing.

Hunter, B. T., 1987, *Gluten Intolerance*, New Canaan, CT: Keats Publishing.

Hunter, B. T., 1994, *Grain Power*, New Canaan, CT: Keats Publishing.

Hunter, B. T., March 1986, "Lactose Intolerance," *Consumers' Research* 69, no. 3: 8-9.

Hunter, B. T., June 1985, "Sulfites: Preserving, Food at a Price," *Consumers' Research* 68, no. 6: 19-22.

Hunter, B. T., 1975, *The Mirage of Safety: Food Additives &Federal Policy*, New York, NY: Charles Scribners' Sons.

Hunter, B. T., 1982, *Wheat, Millet and Other Grains*, New Canaan, CT. Keats Publishing.

Jamieson, D. M., M. F. Guill, B. B. Wray, *et al*, February 1985, "Metabisulfite Sensitivity: Case Report and Literature Review," *Annals of Allergy* 54: 115-121.

Jones, M. H., 1984, *The Allergy Self-Help Cookbook*, Emmaus, PA: Rodale Press.

Lecos, C., and D. Blumenthal, December 1985-January 1986, "Reacting to Sulfites," *FDA Consumer* 19, no. 10:17-20.

Lockey, S. D. Sr., October 1975, "Reactions to Hidden Agents in Foods and Drugs Can Be Serious," *Annals of Allergy* 35, no. 4: 239-242.

Mandell, H. N. April 1978, "Lactose Intolerance----A Case of Bovine Revenge?" *Medical Times,* 71-77.

Miller, S. A. [ed.], 1981, *Nutrition and Behavior,* Philadelphia, PA: The Franklin Institute Press.

Neurotoxicity, Identifying and Controlling Poisons of the Nervous System, April 1990, Washington, D. C.: Office of Technological Assessment, Congress of the U.S.

"NutraSweet" [aspartame] Health and Safety Concerns. November 3, 1987, Hearings before the Committee on Labor and Human Resources, U.S.Senate, 100th Congress, 1st session.

Papaioannou, R., and C. C. Pfeiffer, 1984,"Sulfite Sensitivity----Unrecognized Threat: Is Molybdenum Deficiency the Cause?" *Journal of Orthomol Psych* 13, no. 2: 614.-616.

Prenner, B. M., and J. H. Stevens, September 1976, "Anaphylaxis After Ingestion of Sodium Bisulfite," *Annals of Allergy* 37, no. 3:180-182.

Schwartz, G. R., 1988, *In Bad Taste, the MSG Syndrome*, Santa Fe, NM: Health Press.

Settipane, G. A., June 1977, "Tartrazine Sensitivity and Aspirin Intolerance," *Comprehensive Therapy* 3, no. 6: 15-20.

Settipane, G. A., November 1986, "The Restaurant Syndrome" [editorial], *Arch of Intern Med* no. 1466: 2129-2130.

Stevenson, D. D., R. A. Simon, W. R. Lumry, *et al*, July 1986, "Adverse Reactions to Tartrazine," *J of Allergy Clin Immun*, 78(l), part 2: 182-191.

"Sulfites in food, drinks trigger anaphylaxis in some asthmatics," Sept 12, 1983, *Med World News* 123-124.

The Health Effects of Nitrate, Nitrite, ancl N-Nitroso Compounds, 1981, Washington, D.C.: National Academy Press.

Tichenor, W. S., October 1985, "Sulfite sensitivity, 'minor problem' proves major hazard for some," *Postgrad Med,* 78 no. 5: 320 - 325.

Welsh, J. D., 1972, "Lactose malabsorption, extent and implications," *Med World News, Gastroenterology.* 57-60.

Wood, M., 1982, *Coping with the Gluten-Free Diet*, Springfield,IL: Charles B. Thomas Publishing.

Wood, M., 1981, *Delicious and Easy Rice Flour Recipes*, Springfield, IL: Charles B. Thomas Publishing.

Wood, M., 1979, *Gourmet Food on a Wheat-Free Diet*, Springfield, IL: Charles B. Thomas Publishing.

Zlotlow, M. J., and G. A. Settipane, July 1977, "Allergic potential of food additives: a report of a case of tartrazine sensitivity without aspirin intolerance," *Am J Clin Nutr,* 30: 1023-1025.

Zukin, J., 1982, *Milk-Free Diet Cookbook, Cooking for the Lactose Intolerant*, New York, NY: Sterling Publishing.

RESOURCES

Food Additives:

FDA Adverse Reaction Monitoring System, HFS-636 200, C Street, SW, Washington, D.C. 20204

NOMSG [No MSG], 540 Frontage Rd., Suite 3105, Northfield, IL 60093 (708) 446-3000

Lists of foods and beverages containing tartrazine:

Tartrazine, and Food Allergies, *Amer Family Practice* 25(6):222 June 1982; also see Food Products Containing Tartrazine, Table I *New Engl J Med* 306(11):681-682, Mar 18, 1982; also see Tartrazine-containing Drugs, M. Lee, A. F. Gentry, R. Schwartz,and J. Bauman, *Drug. Intell Clin Pharm* 15(782):81.

Food Allergies: newsletters

Allergy Recognition and Management Newsletter, Allergy Association, Australian, Box 604F, GPO, Hobart 7001, Tasmania, Australia.

Allergy Alert Newsletter, Diet Design, Box 15191, Seattle WA 98115.

Environmental Allergy Society Newsletter, Plainair Environmental Allergy Society, Box 46711, Station "G," 3760 W. 10 Ave., Vancouver, B.C. V6R. 4K8, Canada.

The Human Ecology Foundation Canada Quarterly, RR 1, Goodwood,Ontario LOC lAO, Canada.

Mastering Food Allergies, Mast Enterprises, Inc., 2615 N Fourth St., #616. Coeur d'Alene, ID 83814.

Food Sensitivities:

Fine Print, a newsletter of the Hyperactivity Helpline, Inc. P.O. Box 10085, Alexandria, VA 22310.

The Human Ecologist, publication of Human Ecology Action League, P.O. Box 49126, Atlanta, Georgia, (404) 248-1898.

Pure Facts, newsletter of the Feingold Association of the U.S., P.O. Box 6550, Alexandria, VA 22306, (703) 768-FAUS

Fructose Intolerance:

National Organization for Rare Diseases, Inc., NORD, Box 8923, New Fairfield, CT 06812, (800) 223-8355

Galactose Intolerance:

National Organization for Rare Diseases, Inc., NORD, Box 8923, New Fairfield, CT 06812, (800) 223-8355

Gluten Intolerance:

American Celiac Society, 45 Gifford Ave., Jersey City, NJ 07304, (201) 432-2986

American Digestive Disease Society, 7720 Wisconsin Ave., Bethesda MD 20814, (301) 652-9293

Celiac/Sprue Association, U.S.A., 2313 Rocklyn Dr., S-1, Des Moines IA 50322, (515) 270-9689

Gluten Intolerance Group, P.O. Box 23053, Seattle, WA 98102, (206) 854-9606

Midwestern Celiac-Sprue Association, P.O. Box 3554, Des Moines IA 50322, (515) 274-3044

For a list of manufacturers who do not use gluten as excipients on pharmaceuticals, write: Dr. W. Thompson, Div. of Gastroenterology, Ottawa Civic Hospital 1053 Carling Ave., Ottawa, Ontario, Canada KlY 4E9

Lactose Intolerance:

Lactaid Lactase Supplementation Therapy, McNeil ConsumerProducts Co., Fort Washington, PA l9034, U.S.: (800) 257-8650. Canada: (800) 387-5711; Toronto: (800) 886-2489

National Digestive Diseases Information Clearinghouse, Box NDDIC 9000, Rockville Pike, Bethesda MD 20892, (301) 468-6344

National Institutes of Health, Building 31, Room 2B33, Bethesda MD 20892: Request lactose intolerance kit.

The Newsletter for People with Lactose Intolerance and Milk Allergy, Jane Zukin, P.O. Box 3074, Iowa City, IA 52244

Parents' Legal Rights:

Ellie Goldberg, M.Ed., 79 Elmore St., Newton, MA 02159, (617) 965-9637

20

BUILDING, REMODELING, AND MAINTAINING SCHOOLS:
Practical and Cost-Effective Approaches

by Bruce M. Small, P.Eng.

In this chapter, Mr. Small, an engineer known internationally for his work in low-pollution structural design, discusses the basic principles for construction, renovation, and maintenance of school buildings to foster a healthy atmosphere for teaching and learning. In describing practical and cost-effective methods for lowering the risk of contaminants in schools, he advocates the involvement of teaching and support staff in all decisions regarding building, remodeling, and maintenance. He also answers a number of questions that might be raised by those responsible for planning, constructing, and maintaining school buildings.

☐ *What are the most important considerations for environmental health in planning new school buildings?*

☐ *How can staff and students work together to design and maintain school buildings that promote the health of all those who occupy them?*

☐ *How can school renovations best be carried out to protect the health of students and staff members?*

☐ *What are the most effective ways to maintain a clean and pest-free school building?*

☐ *How can chemically-sensitive individuals be protected from toxic substances in school without undue cost for building and maintenance?*

Only a few basic principles are needed to produce specific, locally-generated solutions to environmental requirements for school construction, renovation, and maintenance. In many cases, design solutions that lead to the most acceptable indoor environments are also cost-effective in terms of life-cycle costing, energy efficiency, and maintaining building integrity. Simple restructuring of priorities and goals—for example, in maintenance practices—can also reduce costs and improve indoor environments. A shift back to the active involvement of staff and students in the design, monitoring, and adjustment of indoor environments may also yield both educational benefits and better designs.

Some areas of "leverage" where the greatest "ecological return" on investment can be achieved include:

- In new buildings:
  - □ *effective, adjustable ventilation systems, and direct venting of special activities*
  - □ *adequate, segregated, and ventilated storage areas*
  - □ *cleanable, durable, and low-odor interior surfaces*
  - □ *use of low-odor carpeting where carpeting is necessary, and use of hard flooring in special ecological areas (perhaps with natural fabric area rugs only)*
  - □ *integrated pest management design*

- In renovations:
  - □ *segregation and exhaust of all areas being renovated in occupied buildings*
  - □ *careful choice of materials and designs as for new buildings*

- In maintenance:
  - □ *a moratorium on use of high-odor cleaning and repair products*
  - □ *adjustment of goals and practices from "super-gloss" and "antiseptic at all costs" to "clean and nontoxic" (goals should be explicitly stated for maintenance staff responsible for cleaning)*
  - □ *training of staff and students in environmental health and ecological maintenance*
  - □ *integrated pest management practices, rather than pesticide use*
  - □ *ecological grounds-maintenance to avoid use of toxic chemicals*

Practical and cost-effective solutions are more likely to be achieved where indoor ecological considerations are accepted as part of the basic design criteria for activities throughout the school system, rather than as a feature added on only to satisfy the special needs of a small number of hypersensitive students or staff. This approach can yield general cost-saving measures, such as switching to less expensive and less toxic cleaning materials throughout a school, rather than continuing the costly and often unsatisfactory purchase of technology, such as expensive local filtration systems.

Co-operative design involving staff, students, and parents or guardians is both empowering and educational. In this way a great deal of experience and expertise can be marshalled at minimum cost to the school board. Networking and sharing of information among many school boards can reduce total research and design costs and avoid expensive failures. Common environmental specifications can bring significant pressure to bear on manufacturers to respond to the need for less-toxic products.

It will become very easy to institute ecological design, renovation, and maintenance procedures as more school boards recognize the potential savings in terms of special education expenses, improved learning, reduction of illness, and avoidance of very tragic and unnecessary restrictions on staff and young people's abilities and activities as a result of unnecessary chemical exposures.

THE DESIGN POPULATION

In the confusion over design standards, indoor air quality standards, health considerations and aesthetics, it is possible to lose sight of the fundamental purpose of a school building. If a school makes people sick, it has failed to provide even the most basic protection, let alone create a productive educational environment in which we can exercise our highest capabilities, free of the adverse effects of the elements.

Our conceptual design population model can have significant implications for the design and interior finishing of school buildings. Because the approximately 15% of the population who are hypersensitive are widely dispersed, over 40% of households contain at least one hypersensitive individual. Therefore, many families with school-age children may have experience with the problem, as will many teachers. Because of the high incidence of hypersensitivity, virtually every school building will contain an identifiable sub-population whose environmental needs are more stringent than the rest, and who cannot under most circumstances be segregated in any practical way from those who are presently less reactive.

Less sensitive individuals also need healthy environments, but their design requirements are usually less stringent than the hypersensitive individuals with whom they learn and work. The wide range of vulnerability of the general population must be taken fully into account in integrated design of schools, since hypersensitivity is now becoming an accessibility issue and a rights issue for people whose bodies are unable to process high levels of pollutants. New school designs may therefore incorporate greater adaptability and a wider variety of environmental conditions within a single building.

HYPERSENSITIVITY IN THE SCHOOLS

Environmental sensitivity means in the most general sense that human beings respond and adapt to the environmental conditions around them. The term is often used more specifically to describe how some human beings respond involuntarily with physical and/or mental changes, when one or more environmental factors around them change. For example, if someone gets a headache when diesel bus exhaust is sucked into a classroom from the school entrance, that person is sometimes referred to as environmentally sensitive.

By this definition, all human beings can be considered environmentally sensitive, although we know there is a wide variation in the nature and degree of human response to environmental conditions. We also know that there can be a wide variation in response to environmental conditions in any one individual over time. (Calabrese 1978) For example, a woman may be more sensitive to certain odors during pregnancy than she is at other times. A person whose arteries are clogged may be more sensitive to carbon monoxide now than he or she was prior to developing arterial disease. (Griffin 1974)

Environmental conditions that tend to trigger similar, adverse reactions in most of the population are referred to as toxic exposures. Other conditions that may trigger reactions in some individuals, but not in others, are considered nontoxic but may be referred to as irritating or in some cases allergenic. For example, ragweed pollen is not considered to be toxic, but it is most certainly a potent allergen for a segment of the population, and its presence in the air can cause major discomfort for some people.

When an individual reacts adversely to environmental conditions that the majority of the population appears to be able to live with or adapt to without impairment, that individual may be referred to as environmentally hypersensitive. (Thompson 1985). That is, the sensitivity to that particular condition is more acute or pronounced for the individual than it is for the vast majority of the population. Environmental hypersensitivity is a naturally occurring phenomenon, and is merely a description of a condition of people who are at one end of a continuum of sensitivity that ranges from relatively hypersensitive to relatively insensitive. Most of the population lies somewhere in-between.

Environmental sensitivity is not a problem. Rather it is a normal fact of human life, and the variation in environmental sensitivity among members of the population must be taken into account in the design and operation of all school environments, just as much as the variation in human size, strength, and agility.

Environmental hypersensitivity is also a normal fact of human life, but it is sometimes defined as a problem since it may affect a student's or staff member's ability to carry out daily tasks in the school environment. Compared to the ability of the general population to adapt to a broader range of environmental conditions, environmental hypersensitivity does constitute a handicap, which, like other kinds of handicap, may require special provisions in schools in order to allow the affected individual to function well.

Environmental hypersensitivity can in some cases be initiated by dangerous school conditions (e.g., emission of some toxic chemicals, including for example the strong odor of hot tar during re-roofing). It can also be aggravated or prolonged by low-level exposures (e.g., by dust and odors emanating from a nearby space that is being renovated). (Rea 1978)

MOTIVATION FOR ACCOMMODATING ENVIRONMENTAL SENSITIVITY IN SCHOOLS

In general, the fact that there is a wide range of environmental sensitivities (from insensitive to hypersensitive) among any school population is not well understood, and has not yet been put into widespread practical use in the design, construction, and operation of schools, except where certain comfort and aesthetic factors such as temperature, humidity, and decor are concerned. (Small 1990)

Environmental sensitivity deserves our consideration because environmental conditions (including physical, social, and organizational) can have significant effects on health, productivity, and quality of thinking in educational environments. (Small 1985) Effective attention to environmental conditions can enhance our chances of maintaining good health, improving learning and productivity, and ensuring the highest quality of thinking in our schools. Untreated or aggravated environmental hypersensitivity can also lead to further deterioration in teaching or learning performance and health, and sometimes to permanent disability. (Thompson 1985) Although environmental factors have been treated as a side issue, they are directly related to education.

Because environmental conditions may affect both health and the quality of the educational experience, school environments are also a significant determinant of the cost of providing educational services. There can be direct costs to the school board, such as salaries of substitute teachers to replace teachers afflicted with environmentally-related illness. There can be costs to affected teachers and to the families of affected students, such as the fees for consulting with a physician and purchasing medicines to alleviate or cure health complaints triggered by environmental factors. School boards may also be spending a great deal of money on special education programs to deal with poor learning exhibited by students whose difficulties may be caused or aggravated by environmental factors. It is plausible that healthy school conditions might reduce such costs, compared to the present norms, although the extent of such a reduction has not yet been quantified. (EPA 1989)

Some estimates indicate that 90% of the cost of providing services consists of salaries and benefits of employees, with capital and building costs and operating and maintenance costs representing the other 10%. This means that if a 10% increase in operating and maintenance costs yielded a 1.1% or more productivity increase (or decrease in absenteeism costs), it would be worth it on a cost basis alone. And conversely, if a 10% decrease in operating and maintenance costs (for example, by reducing the fresh air intake), caused a 1.1% or more decrease in productivity (and increase in absenteeism cost) it would not be worth it, on a cost basis alone.

Both environmental sensitivity and hypersensitivity are also receiving attention in the school environment because in the past they have been a focus for prejudicial behaviors and attitudes. People who were sensitive to environmental conditions were sometimes labeled as weak. Sensitivity was tagged as a female trait and became the target of sexism. (Small 1987) Many female teachers who have spoken up about adverse environmental conditions have been accused of hysteria. And many employees, both male and female, who have been adversely affected by environmental conditions have not spoken up at all, because they have feared being called troublemakers and targeted for job cutbacks. (Small 1985)

DESIGNING SCHOOLS WITHOUT TRIGGER AGENTS

When exposed to high concentrations of pollution in the air in a classroom, a person's body may process the pollutants well, breaking them down or excreting them in such a way that there are no adverse symptoms and no permanent harm to the body. Another person's body may also process the pollutants, but will simultaneously develop a headache or other unpleasant symptom, and might be less efficient about getting rid of the pollutants, leaving them in the body fluids or tissues to contribute to longer-term problems. (Laseter 1983)

Within a certain range of environmental conditions, most human beings remain relatively stable, both physically and emotionally. Those who have become environmentally hypersensitive are less able to maintain stability, because they react adversely to a wide range of environmental factors at relatively low exposure levels, and often in an unpredictable manner. They often return to their baseline states much more slowly than their less sensitive counterparts (e.g., a headache that lasts all day develops after a short exposure to cleaning-fluid odors).

An environmentally hypersensitive individual is decidedly more trigger-able than most of the population. In some cases, the sensitivity is so broad in nature that there are literally hundreds of different environmental agents and factors that can trigger adverse symptoms. Removing many of the environmental triggers can reduce adverse symptomatology and help a hypersensitive person to function more normally. But reducing the triggering by lowering the environmental load does not always reduce the triggerability. Solving school problems associated with environmental hypersensitivity often requires not only identifying and removing trigger agents, but also assisting the affected person to obtain medical and other treatment to reduce triggerability. (Rogers 1986)

Common trigger agents can be grouped into a number of general categories, including particulate inhalants (such as dust, mold spores, and pollens), gaseous inhalants (such as odors from furnishings, building materials, or automobile exhaust), food (including certain food additives or substitutes), water, contact materials (such as fabrics), and physical factors (such as electromagnetic fields, barometric pressure, humidity, temperature, and light). There may or may not be any evidence of toxicity of these trigger agents when encountered by the general population in quantity or in high concentration. Nevertheless, sensitized individuals may experience a wide variety of adverse reactions to such trigger agents.

Sometimes such agents act as triggers of adverse symptoms only when the total load of trigger agents exceeds some critical minimum. (Calabrese 1986) Within the threshold, a person's body may function normally, and no one trigger agent may cause any obvious problems. Above the threshold, in excess of that individual's critical load, adverse symptoms may occur, and there can be evidence of specific physical response to trigger agents that appear benign when the total load is lower.

The level of exposure to trigger agents necessary to initiate very uncomfortable and sometimes life-threatening symptoms is, with some individuals, extremely low indeed. Someone who has acquired an acute hypersensitivity to tobacco smoke can, for example, develop adverse symptoms by encountering the odor of tobacco from the clothes of a smoker, even if the person is not smoking at the moment. It is not unusual for the odor of perfume, after-shave, or deodorant to trigger adverse symptoms in chemically sensitive individuals. Sometimes the mild odor of paper, especially printed stock, or self-inking carbon paper, is more than sufficient to trigger acute attacks or to maintain uncomfortable chronic symptoms. (Fisher 1983)

Others who are closer to the middle of the scale of sensitivity (from hypersensitive to insensitive) usually require stronger odors or more concentrated particulate exposures before chronic or acute symptoms develop. For example, a person might tolerate the overall collection of odors in a school hallway reasonably well, but then might develop respiratory symptoms if he or she entered a clothing store in which new clothing was being unboxed and put on display. (Rogers 1986)

The nature of trigger agents is such that there are no easy standards or guidelines for a school board that would be guaranteed to produce a uniform, healthy environment that would be tolerated well by all students and staff. Reducing known and suspected trigger agents as much as is practical is the basic design goal. And producing a more varied and flexible school environment that can be adjusted and modified to suit the needs of the day is also a practical way of accommodating the phenomenon of environmental sensitivity.

CHARACTERIZING THE DESIGN POPULATION

Just as there are no overall guidelines that can be counted on to cover 100% of the needs of any given school population, it is difficult to design new schools, renovate existing schools, or maintain existing schools properly without a detailed knowledge of the people who will occupy the schools. In most cases, this will mean that a school will need to identify and characterize those individuals who are more sensitive than most to various environmental exposures.

There are various medical and non-medical procedures that have been reported to be useful in confirming the presence of sensitivity to an environmental factor, and the degree or severity of the response to that factor. These include blind or double-blind exposure-challenge testing, skin prick tests, intradermal titration, sublingual provocation/neutralization, various blood challenge tests, and deduction from oral medical history. (Bell 1982)

The medical profession as a whole does not seem to have reached any solid scientific agreement on the effectiveness of these methods, with the exception of exposure-challenge testing. The patient is subjected to a real, measured exposure to a potential trigger agent, and objective parameters involving the patient's state of health are measured pre-exposure and post-exposure under conditions that are carefully controlled to exclude confounding variables. The challenge tests can be repeated to confirm results, and results for persons suspected to be environmentally hypersensitive can be compared to results of identical tests with control subjects who are known to respond within the range of sensitivity of the bulk of the population.

For practical purposes in a school environment, simple experiments with less rigidly controlled conditions can be used to establish, with a reasonable degree of confidence, the environmental conditions under which a teacher or student performs or feels at his or her best. Medical testing can be used to pinpoint and confirm objectively the existence of hypersensitivity reactions to specific environmental agents, or to suggest by deduction the kind of environment that would be best for the person (e.g., whether the essential component is a mold- and dust-free environment, a less-chemically-contaminated environment, a less stressful environment, etc.).

Since environmental hypersensitivity involves very individually variable responses, field testing is essential to confirm which environments are appropriate for which people. This would suggest that setting up schools so that a variety of different environments are available could make such field testing relatively quick and easy. For example, moving a student temporarily to a different floor on which the activities are different from those in the previous location (e.g., fewer photocopy machines, or more openable windows) could provide useful information in a very informal and economical way. Another method is to supply the student with samples of any odorous materials present in alternative workplaces, and let that student and his or her parents or doctor determine, under more controlled conditions, which material exposures would be better tolerated. (Small 1982b)

Sometimes people develop very firm beliefs concerning the environmental agents which they feel have triggered their hypersensitivity responses (or those of their children), particularly when symptoms coincide with a wide variety of environmental agents. Prior to making equally firm conclusions about the kind of environment that might be helpful to an individual, it is sometimes useful to set up informal field experiments to confirm the details, and to sort out any misapprehensions about the true trigger agents. For example, many people who are sensitive to indoor odors blame their symptoms on fluorescent lights, but they have often not been in a position to set up the simple experiment of turning off the fluorescent tubes and substituting local lighting, to confirm whether their symptoms do indeed vanish under the experimental conditions.

Such informal experiments are often very economical, if not free, and have the added advantage of empowering the affected individual (and/or his or her teacher or parent) in becoming part of the investigative team and contributing directly to the solution of the problem. They also serve to provide reasonably credible evidence for staff who have difficulty sorting out which of the individual's (or his or her parent's or guardian's) conclusions about trigger agents are reliable. Where possible, third party observers with scientific and psychological training could be involved to monitor the logic of the experiment and check for possible placebo effects.

It is also important to remember that the goal in the school is to establish the conditions under which a student or teacher remains healthy, achieves optimum productivity, and thinks clearly. Whether the evidence of field experiments confirms environmental hypersensitivity or not may be irrelevant, as long as conditions are ultimately established which achieve this goal.

EFFECTIVENESS OF PROVIDING LESS-POLLUTED SCHOOL ENVIRONMENTS

There appears to be some consensus that a primary action in the initial treatment of most individuals who exhibit signs of specific hypersensitivity to a trigger agent, is avoidance of that agent, at least for an initial period until some form of desensitization can take effect. When multiple agents are involved, the primary treatment often prescribed as an initial line of defense is to lower exposure to as many of the agents as possible that appear to be precipitating the most adverse or debilitating symptoms.

The highest degree of success and the most long-lasting results have been reported in those cases where the individual carries out consistent changes to more than one aspect of his or her environment or lifestyle (e.g., modified diet, modified home environment or lifestyle, as well as modified school or workplace environment or working procedures).

While modified school environments or procedures may reduce the aggravating trigger agents that may be contributing to a deterioration in an individual's health, productivity, or thinking ability, such changes would not necessarily constitute, by themselves, adequate treatment for the underlying environmental hypersensitivity or for any disorder that may have caused that hypersensitivity condition. It is important that individuals affected by hypersensitivity receive competent support from health professionals familiar with this condition or with the underlying causative disorder. School environmental changes that are not backed up by complementary treatments may turn out to be stopgaps only, and the environment that relieved symptoms initially may be insufficient later if the hypersensitivity condition has been allowed to progress to more critical levels.

STAFF INVOLVEMENT IN DETERMINING ENVIRONMENTAL CONDITIONS

By far the easiest way to achieve an effective environment in a school is to involve the staff in the decisions concerning the school environment, including tradeoffs and budgets. Feedback and negotiation may be required on specific environmental proposals. Environmental standards alone are insufficient to create a physical or organizational environment that works for everyone, and considerable flexibility may be required, since there is a wide range of sensitivity in the school population.

There are a number of administrative actions that can contribute to an effective solution when a situation arises in which an environmental factor appears to be adversely affecting someone in a school:

- Solicit information about the situation immediately and enter into direct discussions and negotiations with individuals who appear to be affected adversely.

- Resist all temptation to blame anyone, especially those affected; focus on solutions.

- Gather as much physical information as possible, including environmental measurements where feasible and economical.

- Set up formal or informal field tests to determine the most suitable conditions for those who appear to be adversely affected.

- Establish a suitable interim environment (even if it is makeshift) to enable the affected persons to remain healthy and productive while long-term solutions are worked out.

- Encourage those affected to seek medical advice to determine the extent and specific nature of their hypersensitivity, and whether other actions could also assist them.

- Initiate remedial action to improve the school environment more permanently (considerable creativity and organizational flexibility may be required to provide a compatible environment in times of severe budgetary restrictions).

- Empower everyone concerned with more information about environmental factors, sensitivity, and hypersensitivity.

- Work on and eliminate preconceived prejudices about hypersensitivity. The easiest method is to encourage frequent and direct contact between hypersensitive people and less sensitive people, so that they can see each other as well-rounded human beings, rather than solely through the narrower issue of hypersensitivity.

TAKING ENVIRONMENT INTO ACCOUNT IN DAILY OPERATIONS

School building managers can incorporate a knowledge of environmental sensitivity into their regular operation and maintenance procedures. For example, the following principles can be adopted and translated into specific actions within regular routines:

- Determine which indoor environment standards and guidelines apply in your jurisdiction and incorporate a periodic check to confirm that standards are being met consistently.

- Establish procedures for minimizing the introduction of gaseous and particulate contaminants into the indoor air of your school building at all possible entrance points (e.g. selection of low-odor cleaning materials, regular inspection and maintenance of air filters, institution of restrictions regarding idling of motors in delivery areas and closures adjacent to loading docks, use of low-odor repair and renovation materials, or special ventilation during repairs and renovations, etc.)

- Establish a regular procedure and schedule for monitoring the effectiveness of the environmental conditions you have provided (e.g., by asking the occupants regularly whether and how the conditions affect them).

TESTING PROCEDURES TO VERIFY AND PINPOINT ENVIRONMENTAL PROBLEMS

On occasion, formal testing of school environments will be required to determine levels of specific air contaminants. This is a more expensive procedure than routine inspection, and ideally should be used sparingly after common sense, good detective work, and detailed visual and sensory inspection have failed to pinpoint an environmental problem adequately.

Measurement involves two steps: (1) air sampling, and (2) analyzing the sample to determine the pollutants and measure their concentrations. There are three types of sampling equipment:

■ *personal*----the monitor may be worn or hand-held;

■ *portable*----the monitor may be hand-carried; and

■ *stationary*----the monitor must be operated from a fixed location.

Within each type, monitors can be classified as either active or passive, depending on whether a power source is required for sample collection. Most active monitors use a pump or a blower to collect the sample by causing absorption of the sample in a liquid medium or onto a solid surface. Active samplers are available for measuring either gaseous or particulate matter. Passive monitors collect the sample by diffusion, either directly into a collection medium or across a permeable membrane into a collecting medium. Passive monitors are used primarily for measuring gaseous pollutants and biological contamination (e.g., fungi and bacteria).

The output of monitors also falls into two categories:

■ *analyzer*----the monitor produces a signal that identifies and quantifies the pollutant concentration that is being measured, usually immediately; and

■ *collector*----the sample is collected by the unit and subsequently analyzed in a laboratory, and results are available after a period of delay.

The selection of appropriate monitoring equipment will depend on such factors as cost, availability, convenience of use, and desired level of accuracy. In general, access to equipment that will test for the presence of respirable particulates, bio-contaminants (bacteria and fungi), and total volatile organic contaminants (VOCs) is useful. Measurements of specific gases such as carbon dioxide, carbon monoxide, and formaldehyde can be helpful in some cases. In difficult situations, gas-chromatography and/or mass-spectrometry measurements may be required to pinpoint specific irritating gases and trace them to likely product or material sources. Tracer gas and other techniques may be required to determine the ventilation effectiveness of the building's heating, ventilating, and air conditioning (HVAC) system.

As discussed in other sections, field testing of affected individuals by attempting experimentally to find alternative conditions in which they feel better, may, in some cases, yield useful information that will complement direct air measurements in the suspect areas. In almost all cases, considerable detective work and deduction is required to piece together the evidence into a plausible explanation of the problem and a prescription for solution. In the absence of readily available testing equipment, a great deal can still be accomplished by assembling information from those affected, and the human nose should also be recognized as one of the most valuable detection agents available.

REMEDIAL MEASURES TO CORRECT ENVIRONMENTAL PROBLEMS

Remedial measures to correct specific environmental problems affecting occupants of your school building may be quite diverse in nature, and no one strategy will solve all the problems you encounter. Particularly where environmental hypersensitivity is involved, the solutions you devise may have to be tailored to the individual and may be very local in nature. They may require going beyond established wisdom for building operation and maintenance or ventilation design. They may require a great deal of creativity. And they may require some form of interim measures, even if those measures are relatively makeshift, to fill the gap in time between the perception of the problem and the authorization, funding, and implementation of effective long-term solutions. Delays may cause further deterioration in health for those people who are affected. Every day that the problem remains untreated may represent lost productivity and may be perceived as a form of devaluation of those who are affected.

The list below represents some of the possible remedial measures that might be used to address situations in which occupants feel unwell in their classrooms or work-stations, and wherein their symptoms have been confirmed to be triggered by physical environmental factors such as indoor air pollution. It is intended only to illustrate the variety of solutions that may be involved, and the wide range of options from quick, no-cost measures to extensive renovations. Each new situation will require one of these solutions tailored to the specific circumstances:

- Remove, relocate, or ventilate at source any offending pollution sources, e.g., photocopy machines. (Miksch 1982)

- Check and, if necessary, adjust the operation of the heating, ventilating, and air condition (HVAC) system to design standards (ASHRAE 1989); check for mixing of exhaust air with intake air (Reible 1985); perform basic maintenance to specifications and on schedule.

- Relocate the individual affected to some other area in the building, after confirming experimentally which areas would be more compatible with the individual's particular sensitivities.

- Increase general fresh air ventilation in the immediate vicinity of the affected person.

- Provide some source of fresher air directly to the individual's workstation (e.g., a small vent-pipe tapped into the main air supply duct, and directed close to the individual at breathing level).

- Rearrange building furnishings (e.g., cloth partitions, desks etc.) to allow better air circulation to and around the affected person, without changing the supply air source itself; experiment with simplifying the furnishing arrangements and removing any unnecessary furnishings (e.g., drapes, extra chairs) as a diagnostic measure.

- Clean the air ducts and fans throughout the system delivering air to the area around the affected individual.

- Check and, if necessary, replace the air filtration media in the air circulation system delivering air to the affected individual; take a sample of the filter and offer it to the affected individual for medical testing to confirm whether odors impregnating the filter could be part of the problem.

- Deliver to the individual some samples of various building and furnishing materials present in the area surrounding him or her, and remove those materials that prove, upon medical testing, to be part of the problem (e.g., remove offensive carpeting in one room and replace it with low-odor carpeting, or ceramic or other tile).

- Use alternative, low-odor cleaning materials, particularly near the affected person's work-station (e.g., wipe desks and other surfaces with a damp cloth without cleaners); if toxic cleaning and maintenance products are used elsewhere in the building, ensure proper storage of these products and ventilation of storage areas.

- Alter the cleaning schedule in the vicinity of the affected person or agree on alterations to the location and type of furnishings to make the vicinity more cleanable (e.g. have the area double-vacuumed regularly in the vicinity of asthmatics, or simplify the furnishings so that they can be dusted more effectively).

■ Cease use of high-odor cleaning products, or ensure that janitorial closets are kept closed during the school day so that volatile air contaminants will not be released into the general school air while the building is occupied.

■ Clean carpeting or other fleecy, adsorptive surfaces in the vicinity of the affected individual with steam, water extraction, and/or low-odor cleaners. Such surfaces can adsorb, hold, and then re-emit volatile and particulate air contaminants, and may have accumulated a significant amount of these, for example, during renovations. (California Dept. of Health Services 1992)

■ Find and offer to the affected person alternative furnishings that would reduce the total load of volatile contaminants in his or her vicinity (e.g., a bare hardwood chair may be better tolerated by an environmentally hypersensitive individual than a plush foam-based chair, or a metal desk may be safer than a laminate and composite desk with exposed particleboard underneath).

■ Provide enclosed and, if possible, ventilated storage cupboards in the vicinity of the affected individual so that volatile objects, stacks of books and papers, etc., can be kept organized but separate from the individual (a small computer muffin fan ventilated through a three-inch duct into the ceiling space or directly into an exhaust duct may provide sufficient ventilation for the cupboard and can be run continuously during working hours).

■ Arrange smoking/non-smoking areas so that tobacco smoke does not get into the general school air. Smoking on all school property can be banned so that entrances do not become hazardous to hypersensitive individuals; totally non-smoking buildings are becoming very common

■ For flicker-sensitive individuals, remove fluorescent tubes over the affected person's desk, and arrange sufficient wiring for a stand-alone or desktop incandescent lamp.

■ For electromagnetically-sensitive individuals, work with teachers on furniture arrangement in the classroom to minimize the person's exposure to stray fields from the backs of computer terminals, etc., or add appropriate metal shielding between the affected individual and electronic equipment that may be producing electromagnetic fields.

■ For particularly hypersensitive individuals, arrange a specially-designed area of the building with its own direct air intake, and renovate it with low-pollution materials such as ceramic tiles.

■ Repair any building leaks immediately, and remove and replace materials that have sustained water damage and that could be harboring mold growth.

■ Investigate, clean, and, if necessary, repair air conditioning equipment drainage so that there is no standing water that could harbor bacterial growth. (Hambraeus 1986)

■ Remove deodorizer blocks from washrooms, and institute adequate cleaning and ventilation instead, to avoid odor accumulation. For stubborn washroom odors, consider using an ozone generator (when the building is unoccupied) to scavenge and oxidize offensive odors that have impregnated grouted surfaces).

■ For new buildings or renovations, institute bake-out procedures to elevate the indoor temperature while occupants have been evacuated, to accelerate and ventilate the gassing-off of new building materials (California Department of Health Services 1992).

■ If other methods do not yield results, or as a diagnostic measure, experiment with local portable or in-duct air filters (Sparks 1988) with high-efficiency filtration media to remove airborne particulate contaminants, or with chemically-absorptive media to remove gaseous contaminants. Chemically absorptive media may also prove helpful as diagnostic measures within smaller, relatively closed spaces, but they are particularly expensive to maintain, difficult to assess as to saturation levels, and often inadequate to keep up with the general building contaminants and, therefore, less desirable than source control or the creation of separate, less contaminated areas for hypersensitive individuals.

WAYS OF RESPONDING TO ENVIRONMENTAL SENSITIVITY ISSUES IN SCHOOLS

School building managers who have educated themselves about environmental sensitivity will not have much difficulty responding to specific issues as they arise. In general, common sense is sufficient to reach adequate solutions, and the building manager with reasonable people-skills will have little difficulty working with staff, students, parents, and doctors to agree on appropriate actions.

The following general pointers might be of help when a specific environmental complaint is encountered:

- Treat all environmental complaints with credulity and launch appropriate investigations without prejudice towards the persons who are affected.

- Keep in touch with principal and staff periodically during the investigation, and work together with everyone involved (including affected persons, local school board officials, the building maintenance staff, the building owner, if other than the school board, union representatives, etc) to analyze the situation from as many viewpoints as are necessary to solve the problem.

- Invent ways of verifying information offered by complainants so that remedial actions are based on satisfactory evidence. Solicit co-operation from staff, students, and parents in setting up appropriate experiments to provide this evidence.

- Document all actions taken and experiments conducted, so that information on the timing of your actions can be correlated with changes experienced by the building occupants.

SCHOOL DESIGN STRATEGIES

There are many options for the future for designing schools which deal with environmental sensitivity. Some of the essential procedures in an effective overall design strategy are:

- To establish more stringent standards for all school environments.

- To design or modify schools to provide some space that has fewer environmental triggers that would affect hypersensitive individuals.

- To design schools in future that contain a variety of conditions available in each school to accommodate the full range of sensitivity.

- To design schools in such a way that local modifications can be made easily on an *ad hoc* basis as sensitivity problems arise.

Ecological design strategies suitable for school environments may not coincide with strategies now being used for home environments, since the occupant populations, activities, goals, and purposes of the spaces are different. For example, a hypersensitive individual and his or her family may choose to exclude certain materials and appliances from the home, and to regulate the activity of the family to avoid the use of perfumes and specific volatile grooming products. Instituting similar tactics in the school environment may not be feasible, particularly if the equipment required in the school has no substitute or cannot be dispensed with (e.g., computers may be excluded from the home, but they are presently considered necessary in the school). Regulating perfume use has been considered in school situations and may be effective, but lower level emissions from grooming products (e.g., the variety of mild scents from dozens of kinds of shampoos) are likely to be beyond any practical form of regulation, except by voluntary agreement and co-ordination in small groups of colleagues who operate in close proximity to affected individuals.

The most important item of information from research into environmental sensitivity over the last several decades is that many people are significantly affected by their immediate environment. The second most important item is that these effects vary in nature and intensity from person to person. The old design model, now outdated, was that standardized school building conditions should satisfy everyone, and that anyone who is uncomfortable or ill has a mental problem or is a chronic complainer. The new model is a more positive one: that creatively tailored physical and organizational environments can play a major role in maintaining and enhancing staff and student health and safety, productivity, and clear thinking.

In the old model, building environments were homogeneous. Design criteria sought to provide satisfactory conditions for 80% of the occupants, and did not address specifically how to attend to the remaining 20% of the occupants, some of whom might be feeling uncomfortable, less productive, sometimes ill, and possibly isolated. In the new model, school environments need not be completely homogeneous. They will seek to satisfy all of the occupants, to be healthy for everyone, to promote productivity and clear thinking throughout the school, and to help everyone feel valued.

It has already been well established that people require relatively consistent comfort conditions related to temperature, humidity, odor, and air quality. (Green 1979; NRC-US 1987) Building managers are referred to various existing and common standards of performance for buildings, to provide a generally acceptable baseline school environment. (ASHRAE 1989)

Efficient delivery of service is also an important goal, and this efficiency must include energy efficiency. Energy efficiency at the expense of health and productivity, however, is counter-productive, and creative school building management will not sacrifice one for the other. Building management solutions must achieve reasonable energy efficiency and adequate ventilation for both optimum human health and optimum human performance. (Being able to breathe but not being able to think or stay awake is not enough.)

Indoor air pollution has proven to be a contributor to illness and lost productivity. (EPA 1989) Minimizing indoor air pollution is a requirement for effective learning. There are at least three primary means of achieving clean air in schools:

- *Source control* is the most direct and dependable option, since you either avoid introducing materials and devices that cause indoor air pollution, or prevent their emissions from entering the general school environment.

- *Adequate outdoor air ventilation* is required as one component of a strategy to minimize indoor air pollution. The air delivery system must be sufficiently competent to reach all the occupants of a school building where they work.

- *Air cleaning* can complement but not replace the need for adequate outdoor ventilation and source control. Air cleaning technology is most readily applied to airborne particulates, and is less economical or effective in removing gaseous contaminants.

Control strategies involving source control, ventilation control, and air cleaning should be integrated into the school building design, operating, and maintenance procedures (EPA 1989). Additional strategies such as reconsideration of occupant densities can also be added at any stage. (NRC-US 1987)

Under the new design model, the school board plant manager becomes part of a co-operative team that monitors school environments comprehensively, provides a baseline of generally acceptable environmental conditions, and responds to individual variations which may be required from time to time, in a flexible and creative manner.

Some individuals may require fresher air than others, to perform at their peak, because of the variation in environmental sensitivity among any school population. Some individuals may require much lower levels of specific contaminants in the air they breathe than others do, for the same reason (e.g., sensitivity to chalk dust). Building managers will therefore be required to understand their school's physical facilities in much more detail than before (for example, becoming acquainted with the variations in air quality on different floors and in different sections, due to different pollutant sources and different locations along the fresh air ventilation paths).

They may also be required to devise minor modifications which could create small variations in environmental conditions (for example, a special routing of a small flow of ventilation air to favor the classroom or even desk space of a hypersensitive teacher; a special routing of exhaust air to collect fumes at the source in a photocopy room; or special low-pollution maintenance procedures or products on one particular floor that is to be used by hypersensitive students, etc.).

Of all the possible features that could be incorporated into a new school building to establish a healthy indoor environment, a few stand out because they offer a great deal of benefit insofar as indoor air quality is concerned.

Ventilation is, of course, a key item. The ventilation system must be adequate to meet all modern ventilation standards (ASHRAE 1989) and adjustable to account for periods in which additional ventilation may be required to clear out odors from some unexpected event or high-odor actitivy (e.g., a spill in the chemistry lab or a special celebration or community event with high attendance). Wherever possible, the ventilation system should be designed to ventilate known pollution sources at the point of emission, and to exhaust directly to the outside any odors that would cause a problem if they were recirculated (e.g., fumes in an automobile shop or an art area).

Storage is also a key item. The more streamlined and bare each classroom is, the easier it is to keep dust-free and well-maintained. Items not being used should be in storage cupboards, and the air from storage cupboards should be treated the same way as washroom air, that is, exhausted directly to the outside. This allows new materials (e.g., fresh supplies) to gas off to the outside, rather than to the inside, of the school. Allowance for heat exchange (either air-to-air or by heat pump extraction of exhaust air) will make such ventilation economical and return exhausted heat to the building.

With the help of staff and students, as well as appropriate architectural and environmental consultants, a school board can choose relatively benign interior surfaces, combining the usual criteria of cleanability and durability with new criteria which require the lowest possible off-gassing. Sample materials can be submitted to a staff/student/parent panel to assess the likelihood of particular materials causing problems for hyper-sensitive individuals. All materials to be introduced in a school building should be evaluated for emissions and potential hypersensitivity effects. If school boards combine forces, more sophisticated emission testing can be done economically. If the budget is limited, even subjective evaluation with adult volunteers will help to eliminate the worst materials. (Small, et al. 1995)

Carpeting has in the past been a significant problem in the school environment. The carpeting industry is presently in the process of responding to the problem of emissions, and it is likely that a genuine low-odor school carpeting alternative will be available very soon. Not-withstanding, the principle of offering multiple environments rather than a single homogeneous environment would suggest providing some areas with hard flooring (and if rugs are necessary, only natural fabric area rugs), as an option for carpet-sensitive individuals.

In a new school, there is also the opportunity of introducing integrated pest management design at little expense. This involves arranging the detailing of construction in such a way that there are no easy accesses for insect and rodent pests into the building from the outside, or from room to room within the hidden spaces in the building structure. If there are no places for pests to hide or to travel within the building, the occasional pest incident can easily be dealt with safely and locally, often by simple mechanical means, without toxic chemicals.

In all school situations, temporary or permanent, it also makes sense to allow for enough ventilation of clothing cupboards and boot areas, to eliminate moisture damage and mold growth. Proper structural and envelope design and attention to foundation sealing and roof construc-tion will also minimize the possibility of longer-term moisture problems.

SUMMARY

It is clear that environmentally safe schools can be created. It is also clear that environmentally safe new construction, renovation, and maintenance of schools can be accomplished in practical, cost-effective ways, provided that sufficient attention is paid to indoor environmental factors from the earliest possible moment in the planning process. Like any other design process, the results will be effective in proportion to the creativity applied to the job. No blanket prescription, guideline, or standard can be followed blindly to produce environmentally safe schools.

At the same time, it is possible to use the most up-to-date environmental guidelines (e.g., EPA), ventilation recommendations (e.g., ASHRAE), and the most advanced low-emission materials available at the time, as the core of the design for both construction and renovation. This will create a general school environment that is less likely than conventional construction to precipitate illness in healthy people. Adding explicit consideration for individuals who are more sensitive than most to environmental factors will increase the chances of providing a truly safe environment for the entire school population. Most of this consideration lies in creative ventilation at the source of potential pollutants, and the reduction or elimination of as many known or suspected trigger agents as can be done practically and economically.

Involving the users in the design process and in day-to-day school environmental issues will yield useful design information, and will bring to bear a great deal of expertise at low cost to the school board. Understanding the design population is essential, because the effectiveness of a school environment will be a function of the adaptability of the basic design and the presence of a variety of indoor environmental conditions. The old model of providing a homogeneously controlled space is not sufficiently flexible to accommodate the true range of environmental sensitivity in a typical school population.

There is a potential for reducing both direct and indirect costs by producing healthier school environments, and for reducing a great deal of unnecessary suffering and disability. School boards that incorporate indoor environmental considerations into their operations can look forward to healthier students and staff, lower absenteeism costs, greater educational productivity, and a higher quality of thinking in our schools.

REFERENCES

American Society of Heating, Refrigerating and Air-Conditioning Engineers, Inc. (ASHRAE), 1989, *Ventilation for Acceptable Indoor Air Quality: Ashrae Standard 62-1989*, ISSN 1041-2336, ASHRAE, 1791 Tullie Circle NE, Atlanta, GA 30329.

American Society of Heating, Refrigerating and Air-Conditioning Engineers, Inc., 1991, *Healthy Buildings: Proceedings of IAQ '91, Sept. 4-8, 1991, Washington DC USA*, ISBN 0-910110-83-2, ASHRAE, 1791 Tullie Circle NE, Atlanta, GA 30329.

Ashford, Nicholas A., and Claudia S. Miller, 1991, *Chemical Exposures: Low Levels and High Stakes*, ISBN 0-442-00499-0, Van Nostrand Reinhold, 115 Fifth Ave., New York, NY 10003.

Axelson, O., M. Hane, and C. Hogstedt, 1976, "A Case-Referent Study on Neuropsychiatric Disorders Among Workers Exposed to Solvents," *Scandinavian Journal of the Work Environment and Health*, Vol. 2, pp. 14-20.

Beall, James R., and A. G. Ulsamer, 1981, "Toxicity of Volatile Organic Compounds Present Indoors," *Bulletin of the New York Academy of Medicine*, Vol 57, No. 10, pp. 978-996, December 1981.

Befekadu, Ferede, 1984, "The Effect of Environmental Strain Upon Students' Comfort and Work Performance, in Buildings, Ventilation and Thermal Climate," edited by Berglund, Lindvall and Sundell, *Indoor Air*, Vol. 5, pp. 349-353, Swedish Council for Building Research, Stockholm, Sweden, 1984.

Bellanti, Joseph A., 1974, "Immunological Responses to Chemical Pollutants," *Pediatrics*, Vo. 53, No. 5, Part 11, pp. 818-819, May 1974.

Bell, Iris R., 1982, *Stress, Immune System, and Illness*, Presented at the 16th Advanced Seminar in Clinical Ecology, Banff, Canada, October 3-8, 1982.

Bell, Iris R., 1982, *Clinical Ecology: A New Medical Approach to Environmental Illness*. Common Knowledge Press, Box 316, Bolinas CA 94924.

Berglund, B., U. Berglund, T. Lindvall, H. Nicander-Bredberg, 1982, "Olfactory and Chemical Characterization of Indoor Air: Towards a Psychophysical Model for Air Quality, from Indoor Air Pollution," John

Spengler, editor, *Environment International,* Vol. 8, No. 1/6, pp. 327-332, Oxford and Toronto:Pergamon Press.

Cain, W. S., and B. P. Leaderer, 1982, "Ventilation Requirements in Occupied Spaces During Smoking and Nonsmoking Occupancy; from Indoor Air Pollution," John Spengler, editor, *Environmental International*, Vol. 8, No. 1/6, pp. 505-514, Oxford and Toronto: Pergamon Press.

Calabrese, Dorothy V., 1986, "Concept of Total Load: Man and His Environment," *Environmental Medicine Newsletter*, Vol. 1, No. 2, p. 1, September 1986.

Calabrese, E. J., 1978, *Pollutants and High-Risk Groups: The Biological Basis of Increased Human Susceptibility to Environmental and Occupational Pollutants*, New York: John Wiley and Sons.

California Department of Health Services, 1992, *Draft Guidelines for Reduction of Exposure to Volatile Organic Compounds (VOC) in Newly Constructed or Remodeled Office Buildings,* California Indoor Air Quality Program, Air and Industrial Hygiene Laboratory, Cal. Dept. of Health Services, 2151 Berkeley Way, Berkeley, CA 94704-1011.

Chester, E. H. *et al*, 1979, "Patterns of Airway Reactivity to Asthma Produced by Exposure to Toluene Di-isocyanate: Supplement." *Chest*, Vol. 75, No. 2, pp. 229-231, February 1979.

Committee on Indoor Air Quality, 1987, *Policies and Procedures for Control of Indoor Air Quality: Final Report,* National Research Council, U.S., July 1987, distributed by National Technical Information Service (NTIS), Springfield VA 22161 as Doct. #PB88-110978.

Damstra, Terri, 1978, "Environmental Chemicals and Nervous System Dysfunction," *The Yale Journal of Biology and Medicine*, No. 51, pp. 457-468.

Ensor, D. S., *et al*, 1988, "Air Cleaner Technologies for Indoor Air Pollution," published in *ASHRAE Journal, Engineering Solutions to Indoor Air Problems*, pp. 111-129 (1988), Proceedings of IAQ 88, Atlanta, GA, 4/11-13/88; by Research Triangle Institute for Environmental Protection Agancey, US, EPA/600/J-88/387, distributed by National Technical Information Service (NTIS), Springfield VA 22161 as Doct. #PB90-103060.

Gammage, Richard B., 1986, *Overview of Trends and Problems in Indoor Air Quality,* Oakridge National Laboratory for U.S. Department of Energy, distributed by National Technical Information Service (NTIS), Springfield VA 22161 as Doct. #CONF/8609248-2.

Green, G. H., 1979, "Field Studies of the Effect of Air Humidity on Respiratory Diseases," from *Indoor Climate: Effects on Human Comfort, Performance and Health in Residential, Commercial and Light-Industry Buildings,* Fanger and Valbjorn, editors, pp. 207-223, (Proceedings of the First International Indoor Climate Symposium, Copenhagen, Aug. 30-Sept. 1, 1978).

Griffin, H. E., 1974, *Clinical Application of Air Pollution Research: The Data Base,* in *Clinical Implications of Air Pollution Research,* Finkel, A. J., and W. C. Duel, AMA Air Pollution Medical Research Conference, Dec. 5-6, 1974, Acton, MA: Publishing Sciences Group.

Grimsrud, David T., Richard F. Szydlowski, and Bradley H. Turk, 1987, *Two Studies on the Effects of Small Exhaust Fans on Indoor Air Quality,* July 1987, by Lawrence Berkeley Laboratory for Bonneville Power Administration, distributed by National Technical Information Service (NTIS), Springfield VA 22161 as Doct. #DOE/BP/13655-1.

Hambraeus, A., 1986, *Microorgansims Related to Buildings,* Institute of Clinical Bacteriology, U. of Uppsala, Sweden, *Indoor Air,* Vol. 6, 1986, Berglund, Lindvall and Sundell, editors, published by Swedish Council for Building Research, Stockholm, Sweden.

Harding, Douglas H., 1982, "Health Effects of Formaldehyde." *Occupational Health in Ontario,* Vol 3, No. 2, pp. 64-80, April 1982.

Health and Welfare Canada, 1990, *Environmental Sensitivities Workshop, Ottawa, Ontario May 24, 1990.* J. W. Davies and K. Wilkins, editors. Organized by the Laboratory for Disease Control, Health Protection Branch, Health and Welfare Canada. *Chronic Diseases in Canada,* January 1991 Supplement.

Health and Welfare Canada, 1991, *Environmental Sensitivities,* Issue Paper by Health Protection Branch, Health and Welfare Canada, Ottawa, December 23, 1991.

Hollowell, Craig D., and Robert R. Miksch, 1981, "Sources and Concentrations of Organic Compounds in Indoor Environments," University of

California, Lawrence Berkeley Laboratory, *Bulletin of the New York Academy of Medicine*, Vol. 57, No. 10, pp. 962-977, December 1981.

King, David S., 1981, "Food and Chemical Sensitivities Can Produce Cognitive-Emotional Symptoms," in *Nutrition and Behaviour*, Sanford A. Miller, editor, Chapter 11, pp. 119-130, Philadelphia: Franklin Institute.

Konopinski, Virgil J., 1983, "Formaldehyde in Office and Commercial Environments," Indiana State Board of Health, *American Industrial Hygiene Association Journal*, No. 44 No. 3, pp. 205-208, March 1983.

Kreiss, K., M. G. Gonzalez, K. L. Conright, and A. R. Scheere, 1982, *Respiratory Irritation Due to Carpet Shampoos*, Colorado Health Dept., Epidemiology Division, and Center for Disease Control, Atlanta, Environment International, Vol. 8, No. 1/6, 1982, Oxford and Toronto: Pergamon Press.

Laseter, John L., *et al*, 1983, "Chlorinated Hydrocarbon Pesticides in Environmentally Sensitive Patients," *Clinical Ecology*, Vol II, No. 1, pp. 3-12, Fall 1983.

Miksch, R. R., C. D. Hollowell, and H. E. Schmidt, 1982, *Trace Organic Chemical Contaminants in Office Spaces*, University of California, Lawrence Berkeley Laboratory, Berkeley, CA.

Mueller Associates, Inc., 1987, *Indoor Air Quality Environmental Information Handbook: Building System Characteristics*, January, 1987 for U.S. Department of Energy, distributed by National Technical Information Service (NTIS), Springfield VA 22161 as Doct. #DOE/EV/10450-H1.

O'Brien, I. M., *et al*, 1979, "Toluene Di-isocyanate-induced Asthma: II. Inhalation Challenge Tests and Bronchial Reactivity Studies," *Clinical Allergy*, Vol. 9, pp. 7-15, Blackwell Scientific Publications.

O'Quinn, Silas E., and C. Barrett Kennedy, 1965, "Contact Dermatitis Due to Formaldehyde in Clothing Textiles," *Journal of the American Medical Association (JAMA)*, Vol. 194, No. 6, Nov 8, 1965.

Randolph, Theron G., 1976, *Human Ecology and Susceptibility to the Chemical Environment*, Charles C. Thomas Publisher, 1976.

Randolph, Theron G., and Ralph W. Moss, 1980, *An Alternative Approach to Allergies: The Environmental Causes of Mental and Physical Ills*, Toronto: Fitzhenry & Whiteside Limited.

Rea, W. J., Iris R. Bell, Charles W. Suits, and Ralph Smiley, 1978, "Food and Chemical Susceptibility After Environmental Chemical Overexposure: Case Histories," *Annals of Allergy*, Vol. 41, No. 2, pp. 101-110, August 1978.

Rea, W. J., 1979, "Diagnosing Food and Chemical Susceptibility," *Continuing Education*, September 1979, pp. 47-48, 52-53, 57-59.

Rea, W. J., J. R. Butler, J. L. Laseter,and I. R.DeLeon, 1984, "Pesticides and Brain-Function Changes in a Controlled Environment," *Clinical Ecology*, Vol. 11, No. 3, pp. 145-150, Summer 1984.

Rea, W.J., and Ollie Dawkins Brown, 1987, "Cardiovascular Disease in Response to Chemicals and Foods," in *Food Allergy and Intolerance, Section G*, Chapter 42, pp. 737-753, Jonathan Brostoff, and Stephen J. Callacombe, editors, Balliere Tindall Publishers.

Reible, Danny D., Paul Yonts, and Fred H. Shair, 1985, *The Effect of the Return of Exhausted Building Air on Indoor Air Quality*, Air Pollution Control Association.

Reid, Lynne M., 1979, *Session on Disease Conditions Predisposing Afflicted Individuals to the Toxic Effects of Pollutants: Introductory Remarks*, Environmental Health Perspectives, Vol. 29, pp. 127-129.

Reinhardt, Charles G., 1978, "Chemical Hypersusceptibility: Original Articles."*Journal of Occupational Medicine*, Vol. 20, No. 5, pp. 319-322, May 1978.

Rogers, Sherry A., 1986, "Indoor Air Quality and Environmentally Induced Illness: A Technique to Evoke Chemically Induced Symptoms in Patients," *Proceedings IAQ '86*, pp. 71-77, American Society of Heating, Refrigerating and Air Conditioning Engineers, Atlanta, GA.

Selikoff, I. J., 1975, *Investigations of Health Hazards in the Painting Trades, by the Environmental Sciences Laboratory, Mount Sinai School of Medicine for U.S. NIOSH*, available from Mt. Sinai School of Medicine, City University of New York, New York City, NY.

Selye, Hans, 1976, "Stress: Its Relationship to Man and His Environment," in *Health Promotion Through Designed Environments*, pp. 107-126, Health and Welfare Canada, Health Programs Branch, Ottawa, October 1976.

Sickles, J. E., *et al,* 1987, *A Summary of Indoor Air Quality Research Through 1984,* Research Triangle Institute for Environmental Protection Agency, August 1987, EPA/600/9-87/020 distributed by National Technical Information Service (NTIS), Springfield VA 22161 as Doct. #PB87-234332.

Small, Bruce M. and Barbara J. Small, 1980, *Sunnyhill—The Health Story of the 80's.* ISBN 0-920858-00-7, Small and Associates, Publishers, #2269 Conc. 4, R.R.#1, Goodwood, Ontario Canada L0C 1A0.

Small, Bruce M., 1982, *Environmental Health Factors in Falling Accidents,* November 1982, by Bruce M. Small and Associates Limited, for the Medical Engineering Section, Division of Electrical Engineering, National Research Council, Ottawa, Ontario. Available from Small and Associates, RR1, Goodwood, Ontario L0C 1A0.

Small, Bruce M., 1982b, *The Susceptibility Report*, Report for National Research Council of Canada on Chemical Susceptibility and Urea-Formaldehyde Foam Insulation, published by DECO and available from Small and Associates, #2269 Conc. 4, R.R.#1, Goodwood, Ontario Canada L0C 1A0.

Small, Bruce M., 1983, *Indoor Air Pollution and Housing Technology,* August 1983, by Bruce M. Small and Associates Limited for Canada Mortgage and Housing Corporation, available from Small and Associates, RR1, Goodwood, Ontario L0C 1A0.

Small, Bruce M., 1985, *Recommendations for Action on Pollution and Education in Toronto,* by Bruce M. Small and Associates Limited, for the Board of Education for the City of Toronto, available from Small and Associates, RR1, Goodwood, Ontario L0C 1A0.

Small, Bruce M., 1987, *Healthier Environments for Canadians*, by Bruce M. Small and Associates Limited and Wendy Priesnitz and Associates, for the Health Promotion Directorate, Health and Welfare Canada, Ottawa, Ontario, Doct. HSPB 88-12

Small, Bruce M., 1990, *Accommodating a Range of Human Sensitivities in Building Design*, presented at the Fifth International Conference on Indoor Air Quality and Climate, Toronto, July 29-August 3, 1990, Proceedings INDOOR AIR '90, Vol. 3, p. 319-324, Intl. Conf. on Indoor Air Quality and Climate, Inc., 2344 Haddington Cr., Ottawa, Ontario K1H 8J4.

Small, Bruce M., et al. 1995, "Practical Emission Screening Protocols for Products that Affect Indoor Air Quality" for Green Workplace Office, Ontario Realty Corporation, Government of Ontario.

Sparks, Leslie E., 1988, "Air Cleaners and Indoor Air Quality," published in *ASHRAE Journal*, July 1988, p. 45 (summarizing material presented at IAQ 88, Atlanta, GA 04/88); for U. S.Environmental Protection Agancey, EPA/600/J-88/286, distributed by National Technical Information Service (NTIS), Springfield VA 22161 as Doct. #PB89-197693.

Thompson, George, *et al,* 1985, *Report of the Ad Hoc Committee on Environmental Hypersensitivity Disorders*, Aug. 1985, for the Ontario Ministry of Health, Toronto, Ont., 2 Vol.

Turiel, Isaac, 1985, *Indoor Air Quality and Human Health*, Stanford, CA: Stanford University Press.

U. S. Environmental Protection Agency, 1987, *Compendium of Methods for the Determination of Air Pollutants in Indoor Air,* Environmental Monitoring Systems Laboratory, EPA, National Technical Information Service (NTIS), Springfield VA 22161.

U.S. Environmental Protection Agency, 1989, *Report to Congress on Indoor Air Quality,* August 1989, EPA/400/1-89/001A-D, National Technical Information Service (NTIS), Springfield, VA 22161, Doct. #PB90-167362, 4-volume set. (Individually: PB90-167370, *Executive Summary and Recommendations*; PB90-167388, *1. Federal Programs Addressing Indoor Air Quality*; PB90-167396, *2. Assessment and Control of Indoor Air Pollution*; PB90-167404, *3. Indoor Air Pollution Research Needs Statement.*)

U. S. National Research Council, 1987, *Policies and Procedures for Control of Indoor Air Quality*, for Department of State, Washington DC, distributed by National Technical Information Service (NTIS), Springfield VA 22161 as Doct. #PB88-110978.

21

LEGAL ASPECTS OF POLLUTION IN SCHOOLS

by Earon S. Davis, J.D., M.P.H.

In this chapter, Mr. Davis, an attorney and environmental health consultant, discusses the potential liabilities of schools with environmental problems and offers school administrators ways to avoid expensive litigation that might result from injuries due to various kinds of building pollution. Advising that all school employees be brought into efforts to conquer sick school building syndrome, he answers these questions that should be of concern to all those responsible for a healthy and safe student body and staff:

- ☐ *Why should compliance with environmental regulations be a priority for school administrators?*

- ☐ *Are sick school buildings limited to certain geographic areas or building types?*

- ☐ *What kinds of legal difficulties can arise from school pollution problems?*

- ☐ *What can administrators do to avoid costly problems that might arise from school pollution?*

Operating a school facility is like owning and operating any other type of building. It involves risks that could result in harm to occupants, economic loss to the school district or other owners, the need for special accommodations for people with disabilities, regulatory compliance problems, and the potential litigation that surrounds each of these issues. These risks exist whether the school is public or private.

PURPOSE AND PERSPECTIVE

This chapter surveys the potential scope of polluted school problems, as well as some ways to address their legal implications in a cooperative manner that will help to maintain the health, well-being, and economic integrity of all concerned. Special emphasis is given to an emerging set of issues which present the greatest challenges to teachers, students, and administrators alike. This includes the growing need to accommodate chemically-sensitive students, teachers, and other school staff members.

In this chapter, the discussion of school pollution problems and solutions frequently appears to be directed at school administrators. The reasons for focusing on administrators are pragmatic. First, there is a dearth of information on this topic currently being presented to school administrators. Second, since the extent of cooperation of school administrators will be critical to the success of most efforts to secure a healthful environment, it is important to present this information in a manner most likely to be understood and accepted by them. This is especially true since efforts involving school pollution cut across many traditional boundaries through which teachers and others frequently do not pass, including public relations, personnel, facility management, risk management, health, student discipline and, of course, legal considerations.

In addition, while this is a "legal" chapter, I have purposefully focused on cooperative efforts rather than litigation. Too often, conflicts intensify and cooperative efforts cease when the discussion focuses on legal "rights" rather than on problem solving. References are provided at the end of the chapter for more information on litigation.

WARNING: WHAT YOU DON'T KNOW *CAN* BE HARMFUL—AND COSTLY

At the outset, it is important to recognize that school pollution is a relatively new issue. As such, those normally charged with protecting a school from liability (and its occupants from harm), such as risk managers, facility managers, maintenance supervisors, and attorneys, may not be familiar with the scope of the risks. Too often, people with only a cursory understanding of the issues will consider themselves experts. Familiarity may also be surprisingly limited among those to whom a school generally turns for advice on health issues, such as school nurses, industrial hygienists, HVAC (heating, ventilation, and air conditioning) companies, consulting firms, and health departments.

Adding to potential fiscal concerns, the insurance programs relied upon by the school may include so-called "pollution exclusion" clauses that deny coverage for chemically-caused injuries. This means that the school may have an even higher financial stake in preventing polluted school problems and resolving school pollution problems amicably when they do arise. It is imperative that full reviews of environmental, legal, and disability rights aspects of school pollution be undertaken periodically to ensure compliance and to prevent problems.

It takes little imagination to see how parents who feel their children's health is endangered can generate a great deal of concern and confusion within the school community. Similar problems are generated when school personnel are affected, whether they be involved with administration, teaching, maintenance, or providing other services. With school pollution issues, confusion and anger are easily generated because solid information is often not readily available to either validate or negate the concerns relevant to the issues.

How, then, is it possible to deal with school pollution in a productive and cooperative manner? The fate of most conflicts is probably determined very early in the process. Considering the concern parents have for the health of their children, it is generally unwise for an administrator to disregard the school pollution or to avoid a specific environmental problem, hoping it will go away on its own. A most productive first step would be to adopt and present a conceptual framework designed to facilitate cooperation rather than conflict.

THE CONCEPT OF *PRUDENT AVOIDANCE*—A REASONABLE APPROACH THAT IS RECEPTIVE, RESPONSIVE, AND REALISTIC

In order to identify and deal effectively with school pollution problems schools will need a conceptual framework that includes all interested parties as problem-solving partners rather than opponents. The framework must recognize both health and learning concerns related to the environment, as well as fiscal priorities and constraints. One of the most useful concepts available is that of *prudent avoidance*.

Briefly, the *prudent avoidance* approach recognizes that we have very little scientific data on the long term and more subtle short-term impacts of pollutants and that there is reason to believe that some of these hazards are significant. Given the large data gaps, it would be irresponsible to ignore these risks, especially where reasonable solutions may exist.

Prudent avoidance also recognizes that, because of the lack of information, it is easy to jump for "solutions" that don't work, that can cause even more serious problems or that are simply out of proportion to the likely hazard. As you can see, *prudent avoidance* policies tend to avoid polarization and conflict. People seeking change feel like their concerns are at least respected and the administration is committed to an open attitude. Likewise, administrators feel that they are being allowed to gather the information they need and that their fiscal concerns are respected.

Whether using *prudent avoidance* or any other framework, good decisions require complete information and open minds. As mentioned above, the personnel to whom a school may turn for advice will often have little to offer in a school pollution situation. More often than not, they will under-emphasize the risks and over-emphasize the costs (and the inconveniences) of responding to a perceived problem.

In order for the school community to build up expertise on indoor pollution, it is suggested that a *chemical use* committee or study group be set up to encourage information exchanges between school personnel and parents, as well as others in the community. This book, and the other books and articles referenced herein, provide a nucleus for your library on school pollution.

DEFINING THE SCOPE OF SCHOOL POLLUTION PROBLEMS

The potential scope of school pollution problems can best be addressed by asking the traditional "who, what, when, where, and why" questions. This is the logical first step to establishing policies and legal accommodations related to school pollution. Without a full appreciation of the possible extent of liability and accommodation issues, it is unlikely that an adequate decision-making framework will be implemented. In the process of answering these five basic questions, many of the "legal" solutions will become apparent.

Who Can Be Affected By School Pollution?

Absolutely anyone coming into contact with the school or schoolgrounds can be affected by school pollution. When dealing with any pollution issue, it is crucial to consider the entire process in assessing whether risks are acceptable. While students and teachers are the general focus of our concerns, one must understand that administrative staff, maintenance personnel, students' parents and siblings, delivery workers, cafeteria workers, security guards, outside contractors, neighbors, school district and state officials, and members of the public are all potentially affected by what happens at school.

The greatest amount of concern is directed at students, of course. Because of many factors, children are more susceptible to the effects of toxic chemicals than adults are. Other high-risk groups, however, include those with respiratory or cardiovascular disorders, pregnant women, and the elderly.

The most complex high-risk group is comprised of people with chemical and allergic sensitivities. Unfortunately, because of limited scientific data on sensitivities, most of those falling into this category are not even aware of their problems until they become ill—and it may take numerous bouts of illness reactions before a person understands this linkage. Nevertheless, people with environmental disabilities, such as chemical sensitivity must be provided reasonable accommodations.

In selecting professionals or consultants to deal with a school pollution problem, one should stay away from people who have no knowledge of chemical sensitivity and from those who feel that the problem is not real. Although such views may appear to coincide with a school district's interests, they will tend to result in poor decisions, increased conflict, and a greater likelihood of non-productive litigation. Like lawyers, consultants will generally make a great deal more money if your situation results in conflict and litigation than if it results in *a prudent avoidance amicably achieved.*

What Is School Pollution?

The scope of environmental problems in the schools is broad indeed, as demonstrated by the other chapters in this book. They range from traditional pollutants posing known risks to everyone (e.g., asbestos, radon, lead, and PCB's) to more exotic pollutants with less known risks (e.g., solvents, electromagnetic fields, and pesticides) to more individualized risks to sensitive people (e.g., mold, pollens, perfumes, foods and food additives in your cafeteria, and many other chemicals). Many of these problem areas will overlap.

When Can People Be Affected?

This question is important because it raises the issue of timing—both on a daily and a seasonal level. Frequently, school pollution problems are caused not just by a hazardous activity, but by the performance of that activity at the wrong time. Even if a pesticide application is necessary, it should not take place when students or others are present. Similarly, roof repairs, painting and re-carpeting may be necessary. Such jobs should be performed, however, during vacations, rather than during the school year.

In all, people can be affected by indoor pollution at any time. The beginning of the heating and/or air conditioning seasons (where seasons are relevant) are especially critical times in which changes are made in air-handling equipment. The failure to provide ample (uncontaminated) fresh air is a major concern that plays a role in the vast majority of sick school situations.

Where Is School Pollution a Problem?

This question can be divided into two parts. First, is school pollution limited to certain geographic areas or building types? The answer is no. School pollution can be a problem anywhere, depending upon the nature of the facilities and the maintenance practices therein. Although special concerns occur in "tight" buildings without openable windows, any school building is at risk.

The second part of the question is: What specific areas of school property are potential sources of pollution problems? As can see from the list of examples in *Figure 21-1*, any school area is a potential problem.

Why Is School Pollution a Problem?

As discussed in other chapters, pollution may cause sensitivity reactions, such as asthma and behavioral or cognitive problems, which severely impair the ability to learn, teach, or administer. They may involve acute or chronic poisoning. They may involve the induction of latent diseases such as cancer, mesothelioma, and leukemia or immediate, less serious (but very important) symptoms such as headache, skin rashes, itchy eyes, or coughing.

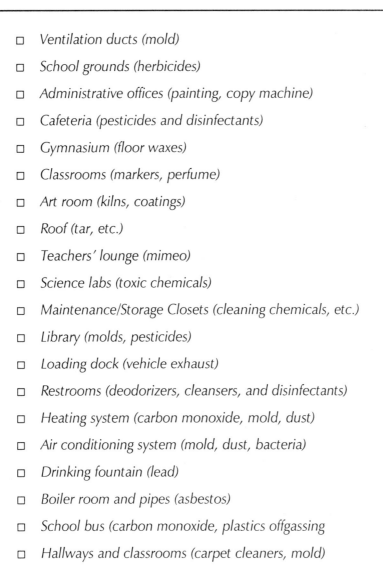

□   *Ventilation ducts (mold)*

□   *School grounds (herbicides)*

□   *Administrative offices (painting, copy machine)*

□   *Cafeteria (pesticides and disinfectants)*

□   *Gymnasium (floor waxes)*

□   *Classrooms (markers, perfume)*

□   *Art room (kilns, coatings)*

□   *Roof (tar, etc.)*

□   *Teachers' lounge (mimeo)*

□   *Science labs (toxic chemicals)*

□   *Maintenance/Storage Closets (cleaning chemicals, etc.)*

□   *Library (molds, pesticides)*

□   *Loading dock (vehicle exhaust)*

□   *Restrooms (deodorizers, cleansers, and disinfectants)*

□   *Heating system (carbon monoxide, mold, dust)*

□   *Air conditioning system (mold, dust, bacteria)*

□   *Drinking fountain (lead)*

□   *Boiler room and pipes (asbestos)*

□   *School bus (carbon monoxide, plastics offgassing*

□   *Hallways and classrooms (carpet cleaners, mold)*

Figure 21-1.
Areas of school property that are potential sources of pollution problems.

WHEN DOES THE LEGAL SYSTEM GET INVOLVED?

Following are four basic legal areas in which school pollution issues may be involved:

- *Disability Rights.* In these issues, a person seeks reasonable accommodations that will allow him or her access to the school facilities as a student, employee, or member of the public. There are numerous state, local, and federal laws protecting the rights of people with disabilities. They may be in the context of equal employment opportunity, educational planning, or community access, and they can range from simple requests to administrative complaints or litigation.

- *Workers' Compensation.* This begins as an informal filing by an employee for work-related injury or disease and/or partial or total, temporary or permanent, disability. If contested by the employer and/or the insurance carrier, litigation can result.

- *Personal Injury Litigation.* Students, employees, and/or others who feel harmed by school pollution may ask a court to award damages for negligent exposure of a student, employee, or other person to harmful conditions or activities on school grounds. If a contractor is involved in work at the school, the contractor may be liable instead of (or in addition to) the school.

- *Environmental Regulation Compliance.* There are a multitude of state, local, and federal regulations relevant to school pollution, including standards regarding asbestos, lead, carbon monoxide, underground storage tanks, radon, pesticide label requirements, waste disposal and hauling, hazardous waste disposal (e.g., old ballasts from fluorescent fixtures), and many others. Non-compliance may result in enforcement actions and possible litigation.

RIGHTS OF PROPLE WITH DISABILITIES TO ACCESS

With the passage of the Americans with Disabilities Act (ADA) and its application to schools, both public and private, the laws regarding access of disabled people to education, employment, and public accommodations have increased in both visibility and stature. The broad language of the ADA clearly extends the right to reasonable accommodations to both students and school employees who have chemical sensitivities such that they are denied access to employment or educational settings and services because they can not fully function in polluted facilities.

Already, the U.S. Department of Housing and Urban Development (HUD) has issued a policy statement and legal memo extending the protection of the law to chemically-sensitive individuals. There is little doubt of its applicability to teachers, students, and others who suffer from illnesses caused by chemical sensitivity.

On the topic of rights, though, it is important to retain the prudent avoidance perspective. *Rights are best understood as representations of the shared values of the community, rather than as absolute entitlements.* The rights of people with disabilities represent the culmination of decades of change in which society has adopted the view that it is in society's interests to stop making it so difficult for people with disabilities to participate in the society's activities.

While the word *rights* is used frequently in this section, it should be understood that the underlying issue is the removal of barriers to participation----not the assertion of some "technical," legalistic concept that places the needs of an individual above those of the larger society. Where barriers are removed cooperatively because it is the logical and decent thing to do, everyone wins.

There are two basic applications of disability-rights laws in school settings. First, students are supposed to get a free, appropriate public education, and they will generally be entitled to accommodations for their sensitivities in public schools. The ADA also provides these same rights to private school students, and they may also be extended to chemically-sensitive parents in both public and private school settings.

Second, teachers and other school personnel who are affected by chemical sensitivities have rights to reasonable accommodation in their employment. Following is a general discussion on accommodations for chemically-sensitive individuals in schools, after which there are more specific discussions of the rights of students and school personnel to accommodations for chemical sensitivity.

Accommodations, Generally

Accommodations for environmental disabilities will frequently include sound indoor pollution practices, including appropriate maintenance with less-toxic substances, integrated pest management indoors and out, appropriate scheduling of remodeling and repairs, and many other activities that will reduce school pollution levels. Such accommodations are likely to be presumed reasonable because of their intrinsic logic as well as the benefits they will present to other school occupants.

Since safer products and practices are readily available, the costs should not generally present a barrier. Therefore, they will not usually be seen as presenting *unreasonable* burdens upon the school that might justify failing to make necessary accommodations.

The Student's Right to Education and Facility Access

There are three basic approaches to accommodating a chemically-sensitive student: at-home programs; separate chemically-safe classrooms; and/or the creation of a school-wide policy to restrict materials, products, and practices so as to provide a reasonably safe environment for the affected student----and everyone else.

Given the psychosocial needs of students and the legal requirements regarding access to the least restrictive environment, some of these options may not be appropriate in a given situation. Because of the great importance of developing peer relations and the full school experience, home schooling and/or home-bound services are a last resort. Where health complications and risks are severe, home schooling and services must be considered, at least as temporary options.

The approach of providing one uncontaminated classroom, which the sensitive student and his or her classmates occupies throughout the school day, may be possible where the curriculum is amenable. Provisions for lunch facilities, specialty classes, rest rooms, assembly halls, etc., may present so many obstacles that this approach will be unworkable. Such dedicated classrooms may be useful on a short-term or transitional basis, however, until broader policies can be implemented for the entire building.

It may appear to be easiest to provide the most stringent environmental controls in one or more specific rooms, rather than apply the same standards to each and every room. Where the problems involve maintenance practices and product selection, however, it will generally be more logical to switch the entire building to less toxic procedures. This is especially reasonable when the additional costs are low and important benefits may inure to the entire school population. Access to specialty classes and extra-curricular activities are special considerations.

Mechanisms for notifying the student in advance of anticipated exposures which create risks of harm and/or learning difficulties must be integrated into any process involving school facilities. Absences due to health hazards should be excused and provisions made for obtaining homework and school materials during periods of hazard (e.g., emergency repairs to the roof). Specific provisions must be made for a safe environment for test taking or other activities when unavoidable exposures will restrict the student's access to parts of the facility.

The School Employee's Right to Reasonable Accommodations

Most of the above discussion on the students' right to reasonable accommodations is applicable to teachers and other school personnel with disabilities involving chemical sensitivity. The mechanisms are different, though, as employees face more complicated employment situations in which retention, promotion, and job assignments may depend upon the administration's perceptions of the employee, rather than the reality of the disability. While children frequently face similar challenges and require substantial advocacy efforts by their parents, school employees may be especially vulnerable to having their disability concerns misinterpreted as uncooperativeness, disrespect for authority, and/or inability to work well with others.

Employees with chemical sensitivities, if they can perform their basic job functions given a *clean* environment, are entitled to reasonable accommodations. Federal laws, such as the Americans with Disabilities Act and the Federal Rehabilitation Act, and state human rights laws are enforced in educational settings by various governmental agencies. The Equal Employment Opportunities Commission, the Department of Education, the Department of Justice, the Department of Labor, and the Department of Health and Human Services all may have relevant information. The degree of relevance depends upon the situation in a given state.

The chief question becomes, *What is reasonable*? Frequently, changes in maintenance practices, an agreement to forego installation of carpeting in a classroom, the prohibition of smoking in the teachers' lounge, the rescheduling of renovation work, and classroom assignment are all issues that may be put "on the table." Given that such accommodations frequently serve to enhance the health and well-being of all building occupants, it is likely that *reasonableness* will be interpreted broadly where administrative agencies are called upon to decide disputed cases.

If a school employee becomes so chemically sensitive that he or she can no longer perform the requirements of a job, even in a clean setting, the employee may have to turn to litigation, workers' compensation claims, disability insurance, and/or social security disability. At that point, the individual's experience and talents are lost to the school----and his or her economic survival is at stake.

To the extent that schools provide safe environments and make accommodations for students and employees who require them, these kinds of lose-lose situations can be minimized. If a school employee is forced to quit his or her job----or is laid off----because he or she cannot work in the school's environment (and cannot secure a transfer to a safer building or classroom), he or she may nevertheless qualify for unemployment compensation if otherwise able to work in a different setting. Obviously, it would be in the interest of a school to assist such an employee in finding gainful employment, even if the school administration does not feel legally responsible for the disabilities.

A Case In Point: When Scents Don't Make Sense

The question of perfumes and scented cosmetics, particularly in junior high or high school settings, raises particular challenges for administrators. If a teacher is severely affected by perfumes, options will include prohibiting fragrances in one or more areas/rooms of the school. One way to make the decision more reasonable would be to frame it as a disciplinary rule prohibiting any use of perfumed or scented products which cause another student or teacher to become ill or unduly distracted from his or her work.

It is not likely that increased ventilation or air filters will solve a problem with perfumes. Increased ventilation may be useful as a moderate step, however, before an administration concludes that more drastic action (e.g., the restriction of perfume use) is needed. In the latter case, the administration should already have made every effort to accommodate those wishing to wear scented products. When balanced against the health of a student or teacher, perfumes (like smoking in many public places) may just have to go.

Given the volatility of adolescent behavior, there may be instances where perfumes are intentionally used by students to make other students or teachers ill or uncomfortable. Such actions should be dealt with immediately as disciplinary problems. If they persist, even after discussions and warnings, they should be treated seriously. For a teacher or student to face intimidation from those using perfumes as a weapon, would be grossly inappropriate.

Where a student's health (or a teacher's ability to work) is placed at risk, few communities would uphold the right to wear perfumes as superior to the right to an education (or the right of a school employee to earn a living.) It has been well documented that fragrances and perfumes----even those called "natural"----generally contain toxic substances that can trigger asthma and allergies as, well as eye and throat irritation, headaches, and discomfort in the general population.

WORKER'S COMPENSATION

Workers' compensation systems vary a great deal from state to state. Federal workers' compensation programs also exist for school personnel on federal lands and in the District of Columbia. In general, workers' compensation programs provide compensation for loss of income and medical costs for illnesses which are related to their work.

While some state systems make distinctions between *pre-existing conditions* and those resulting from exposures peculiar to a particular occupation (e.g., something a worker would not be exposed to at home or in regular office workplaces), most will find sufficient work-relatedness to require compensation for chemical sensitivity induced by or greatly exacerbated in the workplace. Many insurance companies at this time, however, are still actively attempting to discredit chemical sensitivity and will appeal awards to employees, even against the employer's wishes.

This creates a very uncomfortable and potentially adversarial situation between the employee and the school. It is best if early accommodations can be provided to keep the employee from becoming totally disabled in the first place. That way everyone wins. The school administration not only retains an experienced staff person, but also avoids litigation and short circuits the morale problems that frequently result. The employee can continue to work and be productive and can better afford doing things that can improve his or her health.

PERSONAL INJURY LITIGATION

Over the past few years there has been a dramatic increase in litigation associated with indoor pollution in commercial buildings. Schools and school districts have not been frequent defendants in personal injury suits, in part because most of the activities resulting in health damage to school occupants have involved independent contractors, such as roofing companies, exterminators, etc. These contractors can frequently be sued without involving the school itself.

In addition, the novelty of chemical sensitivity disorders has led to some conservatism among many employees, parents, and plaintiff's lawyers. As a result, while the potential for litigation is great, schools have generally faced their legal challenges in other fields, such as disability rights and workers' compensation. As more becomes known about school pollution and chemical sensitivity, however, there is likely to be a significant increase in litigation involving schools.

ENVIRONMENTAL REGULATION COMPLIANCE

Compliance with environmental regulations is addressed in publications by the U.S. Environmental Protection Agency, such as the following:

- *Environmental Hazards In Your School: A Resource Handbook*, Publication #2DT-2001, U.S. Environmental Protection Agency, Washington, D.C., October 1990.

- *The Inside Story: A Guide To Indoor Air Quality*, Publication EPA/400/1-88/004, U.S. Environmental Protection Agency, Washington, D.C., September 1988.

- *Building Air Quality: A Guide For Building Owners And Facility Managers*, Publication EPA/400/1-91/033, U.S. Environmental Protection, and the National Institute for Occupational Safety and Health, Washington, D.C., December, 1991. ($24.00)

  Although this detailed publication has a good deal of relevant information for schools, this initial version tends to downplay subtle health problems and makes only a brief reference to accommodations and sensitivities.

It is important to note that requirements regarding asbestos may be changing and that concerns about lead and hazardous wastes (e.g., PCB's in fluorescent fixture ballasts) are likely to lead to far greater restrictions in the future. The school administration must keep up to date on these fast-changing requirements in order to avoid costly mistakes that might result in litigation, in addition to risking the health of students and school personnel.

CONCLUSION

The information in this chapter is intended to increase awareness and cooperation between administrators, teachers, parents, and students regarding school pollution and chemical sensitivity. As we all learn more about this complicated subject, we will face many decisions. How far should I push my need for a less contaminated environment? How seriously should I take requests for special accommodations that threaten to change the way things are done in my school?

If one views the school as a self-contained community, it is easier to put school pollution in perspective. Your students are involved with environmental issues. You have fire safety programs, as well as visits from school nurses and poison prevention agencies. Classroom projects encourage car pools, the use of public transportation, and activities to help save the rain forests, and end global pollution threats.

Yet, your school may be using toxic herbicides to rid a lawn or playing field of weeds. These chemicals present a significant risk to maintenance personnel, other staff members, and students. Most such chemicals are cosmetics, not necessities. They pollute the groundwater and may be harming migratory birds and interfering with your local ecosystem, regardless of what the producers and distributors who profit from selling or applying them may say.

Your school may be using toxic disinfectants that may be causing learning problems as well as headaches, sinus infections, and irritability. You may be routinely spraying pesticides indoors, unaware that the standard practice has changed in the past few years. These pesticides are toxic and generally unnecessary and ineffective.

In all of these legal contexts, it is important to understand that school pollution is generally preventable. Frequently, sound construction and maintenance practices cost less than more toxic and polluting alternatives. One example is the over-use of carpeting, which is more costly and difficult to maintain properly than are tile floors.

Another example is the unnecessary use of toxic pesticides in lieu of integrated pest management techniques that are less costly and more readily available. Consider the exposures endured by maintenance workers who apply these chemicals and cafeteria workers who must spend hours around toxic pesticides. Further, the use of highly toxic herbicides on school grounds poses so many needless risks (and so few real benefits) as to be entirely unreasonable.

Your school may be the source of many different environmental insults which may separately, or in combination, be affecting your students, your administrative staff, your teachers, and your other employees. They may even be lowering your performance test results.

In reality, we are all in the same boat. Anyone can become chemically sensitive. A school superintendent may be the one seeking reasonable accommodations from his or her school board. A building custodian who appears to be clumsy or irritable may be suffering from low-level poisoning. A teacher who can't seem to keep things straight may be similarly affected by some contaminant in the classroom.

If there is one message in all of this it is that *the environment is not just out there.* The environment is also wherever people are. It is, most certainly, in our schools. Unless we are aware of contaminants in our own schools----our most precious community asset----the lessons about endangered species and rain forests will be doomed to fail. After all, how can we understand and respect the habitat needs of other species and yet turn our backs on our own friends and neighbors? How can we conceptualize a global environment when we can't even recognize hazards in our indoor environment?

Without a doubt, we as a society have a long, long way to go in understanding our environment. With all of our technological and scientific successes, high numbers of sick buildings, and rising incidences of chemical sensitivity, chronic fatigue syndrome, the Gulf War "mystery illness," and other possibly related disorders serve to remind us of our limitations. Indeed, that this book even requires a chapter about legal implications is a sad commentary on our times. Working with these limitations, however, and keeping open minds and cooperative spirits, we can, and must, create healthier schools for everyone's sake.

RECOMMENDED READING

Davis, Earon S. and M. Lamielle, 1992, "Legal Responses Vary to Chemical Illness," *Indoor Pollution Law Report*, New York: Leader Publications December 1991-January 1992.

Ashford, Nicholas A., 1991, and Claudia S. Miller, *Chemical Exposures: Low Levels and High Stakes*, New York: Van Nostrand Reinhold.

Lamielle, Mary, "The Delicate Balance," Newsletter of the National Center for Environmental Health Strategies, Voorhees, NJ.

Davis, Earon S., *et. al.*, 1993, "Can Your School Make People Sick?" Reported by Marleis Lauterjung in *Special Report of the 1992 Joint Annual Conference*, p. 13, Springfield, IL: *Illinois School Board Journal*, Illinois Association of School Boards, April 1993.

Davis, Earon S., 1992 "Multiple Chemical Sensitivity: A New Disease," *TRIALBRIEFS*, Raleigh, NC: *Journal of the North Carolina Academy of Trial Lawyers*, Volume 24, Number 4, 1st Quarter 1992, pp. 24-30.

National Research Council, 1991, *Multiple Chemical Sensitivities*, Washington, D.C.: National Academy Press.

Wilkenfeld, Irene, September 1992, "Sick Schools Pose Certain Risk," *Indoor Pollution Law Report*, New York: Leader Publications.

Rapp, Doris, *Is This Your Child?*, 1991, New York: William Morrow and Co.

Krieger, Roy W., 1994, "On the Line" [regarding electric power lines], Chicago: *American Bar Association Journal*, January 1994.

DeLong, Lynn, 1988, "Roof Repairs Can Endanger the Health of Students and Staff," *The Executive Educator*, February 1988.

Flax, Ellen, 1988, "Pesticides in Schools: Focus Shifting from Indifference to Concern," *Education Week, April 20*.

"Position Statement: The Use of Pesticides in Schools and Child Care Centers," 1992, Chicago: National Parent Teachers Association.

U.S. Department of Housing and Urban Development, Memorandum from George L. Weidenfeller, Deputy General Counsel to All Regional Counsel, April 14, 1992. (Accepting MCS as a disability on a case by case basis.)

22

TAKING ACTION:
What You Can Do If Your School Building Is Sick

by Mary Lamielle

Being a successful advocate for a healthy school requires determination, persistence, a reasonable attitude, and good documentary backup. If you want to improve air quality in your school, Ms. Lamielle tells you how to approach the problem, whether you're a teacher or other school staff member, a parent, or any other community-spirited citizen. Describing how various individuals have assumed the role of advocate, she answers these questions all aspiring environmental advocates face:

☐ *What is my goal for a healthier school?*

☐ *How should I plan the steps to reach that goal?*

☐ *When should I undertake my mission?*

☐ *Where in the school system should I begin my discussions of the problems?*

☐ *Who will make up my advocacy team, and whom will we approach to describe the problem and work toward a solution?*

☐ *How should I feel if the problem isn't solved at once, and what should I do then?*

Healthy indoor air doesn't just happen. It takes an investment of time and energy, a thirst for knowledge, and a commitment to insure a safe school environment. But the payoff is significant---healthy, productive students and staff.

Most schools do not have programs or policies to minimize indoor air contaminants. In many instances the lack of information and expertise have led to indoor air problems that could have been prevented.

These problems don't just go away. A solution-oriented approach is crucial to address potential concerns and to prevent health threats. This approach requires an awareness of the types of health hazards and ways to deal with them in an effective and efficient manner.

To illustrate the range of problems encountered in schools, I will discuss several school pollution incidents, and the efforts taken by concerned people to resolve these situations.

KICKING THE PESTICIDE HABIT

Rachel's mom knew that pesticides were being applied in her daughter's elementary school. She had seen the applicator spraying inside the school during the morning hours just before students entered the building. On other occasions she had smelled the distinctive solvent odors of synthetic pesticides.

Mom knew these toxic chemicals were hazardous to her daughter and her classmates. She knew she had to protect them.

Initially she felt powerless. An educated professional with a background in cardiovascular research, she felt unprepared to tackle the situation due to a lack of specific information on pesticides. She also felt intimidated at the thought of approaching the school system with her serious concerns.

Rachel's mom became an indoor air advocate out of necessity. She educated herself about the threat of pesticides by reviewing scientific papers and government literature. She also received guidance from public health advocates on the approach she might use with the school administrator to present her concerns most effectively.

Mom made an appointment to meet with her daughter's principal and the director of operations for the school district. Her goal was to reduce pesticide usage in the school system. She carefully selected three items to share with these individuals at their meeting. Included were two government publications: *Pest Control in the School Environment: Adopting Integrated Pest Management*, a 43-page booklet issued by the U.S. Environmental Protection Agency (EPA) in August 1993, and *Pesticides in Schools: Reducing the Risks*, a 33-page report issued by the New York State Attorney General's Office in July 1993.

The school officials were very receptive to our Mom's request. They admitted an unfamiliarity with the concept of integrated pest management (IPM) but were eager to learn. Some questions about specific pesticide procedures in place at the school, including the choice of pesticides and the frequency of use, were answered with the aid of a log maintained by the director of operations. Other questions asked by mom were responded to through follow-up correspondence from the school system.

As it turned out, the school had no policy regarding posting and pre-notification for pesticide applications. Following the meeting, the school promptly instituted a pre-notification system. The school district has also contracted with a pest control operator with expertise in IPM. The new program took effect on July 1, 1994.

When Rachel was told that the school system was going to implement IPM, she proudly told her mom, "One person can really make a difference."

AVERTING THE CRISIS

Not all indoor air problems are as easily defined or as successfully addressed. Our second example focuses on teachers' efforts to get the school administration to acknowledge their growing health concerns regarding a sick building, and to act to remedy the complex pollution problems before they reached a crisis situation.

"What stinks down here?" It's what fellow teachers asked when they entered the newest wing of the school building. The "new" wing, now two years old, still reeked of a mix of noxious fumes from construction and construction-related activities, as well as maintenance practices.

The original structure, now five years old, was itself a problem for some faculty members. By the third year many staff members experienced a mix of symptoms which resembled recurrent episodes of flu, colds, and allergies. Headaches, eye irritation, sore throats, dry throats, and loss of voice were common. So too were problems with fatigue, thinking clearly, and mood swings. Some of these symptoms continued to intensify, particularly for faculty members assigned to the new wing. Some students also complained of fatigue and "not feeling well." At least one student in the new wing developed asthma.

Teachers had also become concerned about the incidence of cancer (six faculty members had developed cancer, with one death from brain cancer), miscarriages, and an infant born with birth defects so severe that the child died within two weeks of birth. While it is uncertain if the incidence of cancer and reproductive problems were related to the exposures triggering chemical sensitivity in some occupants, the cancer threat had served to fuel the fears of faculty members.

Rather than administrative action to minimize pollution levels in the new wing, a series of projects and practices further contributed to the seriousness of the health hazards. The doors in the area were varnished while students were in the building. While class was in session, maintenance personnel experimented with various solvents to find the right chemical to remove an odorous, oily film on all of the new chalkboards. Teachers were told not to use the operable windows which might have helped cleanse the indoor air of these various contaminants, could they have been opened.

The individual heating and cooling systems did not work in some classrooms. At least one classroom simmered in spring and fall, which would have caused increased volatilization of off-gassing chemicals from the new furnishings. The fan noise from the heating, ventilating, and air-conditioning (HVAC) system was so loud that students cheered when it broke.

To add to the chemical soup, the grounds around the new construction were hydroseeded. During this process grass seed is mixed with a green dye and water, then sprayed on the dirt. This "green" dirt emits toxic fumes from aldehydes and triphenol methane for weeks after application. These noxious chemicals were applied within a few feet of the fresh air intakes, permitting the entry of hazardous chemicals into the classrooms. Pesticides were also sprayed in the building.

Some faculty members felt "overwhelmed" by the circumstances. Teachers were variously told that the cause was "blackboard dust" or that they were "approaching middle age." Some faculty members may have run interference for the administration by minimizing concerns raised by parents regarding indoor air problems, rather than revealing the school administration's inaction.

The school administration was not responsive to the health complaints. It engaged in a variety of delay tactics, including a proposal to survey the faculty and then to survey faculty members at neighboring schools to compare health complaints. No action has been taken to remedy the situation.

The teachers ultimately contacted the Occupational Safety and Health Administration to request a health hazard evaluation. While discussions are underway to arrange a government look at the indoor air situation, a signature is required to initiate the process. Aware of the lack of support from the administration, teachers wonder, *Do I dare sign my name on the complaint although I'm promised anonymity?*

Sometimes teachers or other faculty members have dared to go on record with pollution problems in a less than supportive atmosphere because they have become unable to work and have found their health continuing to deteriorate. One teacher who reported severe illnesses triggered by chemical exposures in her workplace summarized her experience. "Up until I became ill and voiced my opinion regarding air contaminants in the school environment, my observations and recommendations were sought after and widely accepted. Suddenly my word and fine reputation seemed to hold no weight."

Teachers are faced with the moral, economic, and practical dilemma of balancing their own health and that of their students against possible penalties of intimidation, retaliation, and more subtle forms of harassment and discrimination. Teachers who report problems or file complaints frequently find themselves ostracized by their colleagues and friends. They sometimes become the focal point that further deflects attention from the real problem.

Teachers play a crucial role in protecting our children's health in the school environment. They are the eyes and ears of the parents. But they also bear an undue burden to act in resistant, difficult, or hostile circumstances. They may face employment consequences far beyond anything enumerated in their job descriptions.

While it is good business sense and good public policy to prevent indoor air problems and to act quickly to resolve indoor air complaints, enlightened school districts are still in the minority. Many school systems have resisted acknowledging such difficulties. This reluctance may be due, in part, to the fact that this issue is relatively new, problems can be difficult to pinpoint, and information on sound indoor air practices may not be readily available.

There are few federal regulations that address airborne contaminants in the non-industrial setting. Even industry's minimum ventilation standard known as ASHRAE Standard 62-1989, which serves as a guide for most office environments, is not mandatory in schools. The exception is New

Jersey, where state regulations require compliance with the ASHRAE standard as a minimum ventilation rate in public buildings, including schools.

When an indoor air problem is suspected, the tendency may be either to try to ignore it or to look for a quick fix or a way to deflect complaints. Under certain circumstances indoor air testing may be initiated either by the school administration or by a complaint signed by a staff member in an attempt to identify more serious problems.

Some individuals mistakenly believe that indoor air testing will identify the source of more serious exposures. While there are some tests that may help identify or verify an indoor air problem or the presence of indoor air contaminants, in many instances testing doesn't provide specific answers or remedies. There are no "safe" levels for most indoor exposures. To complicate the situation further many people injured by chemical exposures will find their symptoms are triggered by more and more different substances and products at lower and lower exposure levels.

The testing itself may be compromised when building maintenance personnel make substantial changes in building ventilation prior to scheduled testing to permit maximum fresh air entry and therefore invalidate the testing. In other circumstances testing has been conducted in areas of a building not specifically identified in the complaint, rather than in the problem spots. For example, the front office is tested when complaints have focused on the air quality in the gymnasium.

The lack of regulations and the absence of "safe" levels do not mean that it is necessarily difficult or futile to improve indoor air. Information on known indoor pollution sources and alternative products and practices can help the school community recognize potential problems and address them promptly.

School personnel, parents, and students may have the most opportunity to find occasions to enhance the indoor environment. The school administration and school board must complement these activities by providing support and guidance to facilitate change. In the ideal situation school administrators should be charged with coordinating programs and policies in the quest for safer school environments.

BECOMING AN INDOOR AIR DETECTIVE

If you're concerned about school pollution, become an indoor air detective. It's the first step toward curing a sick school and keeping a good indoor environment healthy. Our indoor air detective must be familiar with basic information on indoor pollution sources. This sleuth must be observant and develop a practical and intuitive awareness of exposures and practices that might compromise the health of students and staff. While faculty members and parents are the most likely choices for this role, students at all grade levels should be taught to recognize problematic products and practices that might contaminate the indoor air, and to call for procedures and policies that are friendly to a healthy school building.

In some schools our indoor air detective might be forced to operate as an individual without the support of the school administration. Ideally, though, our "experts" might come together as part of an Indoor Air Quality Task Force or an Indoor Air Quality Team with the cooperation and approval of the school administration. This team should include representatives from the faculty, support staff, building operators, maintenance personnel, the school board, and the school administration, as well as parents and students. This group should be charged with review of all products, practices, procedures, and policies that may affect a school's air quality.

A team approach is recommended in a guide on school indoor air quality currently nearing completion at the U.S. Environmental Protection Agency. The guide should prove a valuable asset both in motivating schools to take these issues seriously, and to provide basic direction oriented toward addressing and preventing school air quality problems.

In the meantime, let's take a look at products and practices that should be restricted or banned from the school building. We'll also look at problematic exposures and alternatives available to curtail pollutant levels. The examples are taken from problems reported to the National Center for Environmental Health Strategies (NCEHS), a national organization that supplies information to the public on indoor pollution and chemical sensitivities, and tracks those injured by school, workplace, community, and home exposures to chemicals. The Center provides guidance for solving school pollution problems through careful product selection and appropriate programs and policies oriented toward a safe school environment. This includes extensive work with those in need of accommodations in the classroom due to environmental disabilities. To contact the Center, write NCEHS, Attn. Mary Lamielle, 1100 Rural Avenue, Voorhees, New Jersey, 08043, or call (609) 429-5358.

IDENTIFYING PROBLEMATIC EXPOSURES

There are some practices, such as smoking in or near the school building, that most health-oriented faculty members and parents would agree should be prohibited in a safe indoor environment. Just as scientific findings have substantiated the clear danger presented by tobacco, the seriousness of the pesticide threat in the classroom has also been validated by science and the government. Many schools contract for routine pesticide application rather than acting to control a specific pest problem. This method creates ambient levels of toxic chemicals which are hazardous for all building occupants, particularly children. A previously referenced booklet from the U.S. EPA, *Pest Control in the School Environment: Adopting Integrated Pest Management*, endorses the move from synthetic pesticides to IPM, integrated pest management, a technique that requires the use of least toxic products and practices to control pests. The concept of IPM is not new, but its practice on a broad scale is more recent. Instituting IPM in your school system may take the urgings of parents, students, and staff as illustrated in the narrative of Rachel's mom.

To the list of products and practices that should be restricted, add a policy that would limit construction and renovation activities, such as painting, floor covering installation, and roofing, to hours when the building is unoccupied, preferably during summer breaks and vacations. Exposure to the mix of noxious fumes from new construction or remodeling is frequently cited as a cause of sick building syndrome and multiple chemical sensitivities. The area should not be occupied until all work is completed, and the space has had sufficient opportunity to ventilate.

Contract specifications for all construction and remodeling materials should require selection of least toxic products to provide maximum protection for students and staff. A similar policy should be in place for contracting for building furnishings, supplies, and cleaning products. While some less toxic materials may be more expensive, careful choices will improve the indoor environment and ultimately reduce the costs of building operations and maintenance.

If your school has an Indoor Air Quality Task Force/ Indoor Air Quality Team, the group should call for a review of all specifications for products purchased by the school system. Material Safety Data Sheets (MSDS) and label directions should be examined to identify potential hazards. A product which calls for use in a well-ventilated area or warns against breathing vapors during or after use does not belong in the classroom.

The first step toward a less problematic cleaning regimen may be as simple as switching from petroleum-based cleaning products to vegetable-based cleaning products; from chlorinated cleansers to a nonchlorinated cleanser such as Bon Ami; from more toxic disinfectants to borax and hot water.

Maintenance personnel should be aware that more is not necessarily better; that products marketed to freshen indoor air may further contribute to pollution levels; that fragranced and pine-scented cleaning products have no place in the school environment.

Cleaning policies should prohibit the use of pine oil products and air fresheners in light of EPA research findings. EPA's *Total Exposure Assessment Methodology (TEAM) Study,* under the direction of Lance Wallace, found that most indoor levels for select volatile organic compounds were two to three, and up to five times greater than levels found outdoors. The study revealed that both the turpene known as alpha-pinene----a mutagen found in pine-scented products----and limonene----a carcinogen also found in pine-scented products----were ten times more concentrated indoors than out. This 10-to-1 ratio was also found for paradicichorobenzene, the active pesticide ingredient in mothflakes that is present in most air fresheners. These chemicals are serious indoor contaminants.

Many classroom activities from the use of solvent-based markers to freshly copied paper may pose health consequences. Teachers should educate themselves before selecting items for use in their classrooms. They should be alert to student comments and complaints, or changes in behavior. Parents, too, need to be vigilant. If you don't approve, tell someone why.

Our Center has received numerous complaints about classroom practices that may have put students in jeopardy. A sampling of pollution-generating activities are described below. A teacher educated on indoor pollution issues would not have engaged in these practices.

- Students in a fifth grade class were permitted to use individual bottles of solvent-based *White Out* correction fluid to avoid crossing out mistakes.

- Second grade students in an academic enrichment class complained of headaches from breathing noxious fumes from bottles of rubber cement.

- Each student in a class was asked to bring in a model and model glue to use during an extended afternoon recess period.

- A high-school student taking a chemistry test experienced a severe headache and could not concentrate after the proctor used a window cleaning product.

Fragrances and fragranced products are another emerging pollution problem crying out for a solution. From perfumes, shampoo, and hairspray to detergents, fabric softeners, and dryer sheets, personal products are causing illness and controversy. Perfumes, in particular, are a health and safety issue for increasing numbers of students and staff.

Many approaches have been used to try to resolve requests to minimize or eliminate classroom fragrance exposures. Some people in need of a fragrance-free environment have never experienced a challenge to their request. One teacher sends a note home with each student on the first day of school. She explains that she is "allergic" to perfumes and requests that students respect her health problems by refraining from using scents.

In another instance, however, a librarian asked her fifth grade students to refrain from using fragrances for their next class which was to be held in a more confined meeting space than usual. In what may have been a challenge to the teacher's authority, two students brought perfume to school and applied it in homeroom right before library class. The students obviously had no understanding of the request, treated it as a preference rather than a health issue, and chose to defy the teacher without, perhaps, being aware of possible health consequences.

In a different school district, a request made by a mother on behalf of her first grader emphasizes the hidden nature of these disabilities and the very real resistance to modifying behaviors to accommodate the hypersensitive. The mother asked her child's teacher to refrain from the use of perfume because her daughter was ill from the scent. The teacher emphatically refused to change her behavior. The parent took her request to the principal. The principal refused to act. He showed a lack of understanding of the nature of the disability by commenting that he had observed the child in the classroom and had seen no evidence of breathing difficulties or asthma. These were not symptoms identified by the child's physician. With no "evidence" of illness, the principal denied the request.

Many of the indoor air problems discussed in this chapter could also be addressed as an accommodation request under disability laws for students and faculty members with chemical sensitivities. The accommodations may range from simple, inexpensive requests to eliminate solvent-based markers to the complex, more costly request for a sophisticated air purification system for a classroom. Students have rights under federal and state laws for education of the handicapped/disabled. Protections are also afforded under the Americans with Disabilities Act and related state laws.

BECOMING AN INDOOR ADVOCATE

Once you've identified a problem that needs to be addressed, it may be time for the indoor air detective to become an indoor air advocate. If the school system has an Indoor Air Quality Task Force or an Indoor Air Quality Team, bring your concerns or your complaints to that group. The team has likely developed a solution-oriented approach to resolve an indoor air problem in an effective, expeditious, and economical fashion. If there is no procedure in place for addressing complaints, you'll need to determine the most appropriate and receptive contact.

Next, define your goal. Your goal will influence the manner in which you'll pursue this issue. With goal defined, focus your efforts on the next steps: investigation, education, communication, and resolution.

The investigation should include a review of all practices relevant to your concerns. Observation and common sense will play a role in determining the seriousness of the situation.

During the education phase, you should look for information on the products, procedures, and policies related to your situation. Contact the appropriate federal agencies such as the EPA Indoor Air Quality Clearinghouse at (800) 438-4318, or if the issue is pesticides, the National Pesticide Telecommunications Network, at (800) 858-PEST. You should also contact comparable environmental health organizations: the National Center for Environmental Health Strategies at (609) 429-5358 and the National Coalition Against the Misuse of Pesticides at (202) 543-5450.

You may want to consider making your request for modifications to correct a school pollution problem by turning to federal and state disability laws if the affected faculty member or student has environmental disabilities. If this approach is taken, you should have a detailed letter from the physician treating the case that identifies the specific accommodations required to meet medical needs.

As you approach the communication phase, several important decisions must be made. If your child is experiencing symptoms caused by polluted air in the school, who should you talk with first----the teacher or the principal? Except in an emergency situation, work with the person who is closest to the problem and farthest from the top of the hierarchy. Often it is the classroom teacher who can best help you solve the problem. If you are not trying to resolve a problem but are interested in changing policies, you may need to make various contacts and look for strength in numbers.

You should also decide if you should go solo, invite an expert or an advocate, or look for more broad-based support before moving forward.

Carefully select several documents that highlight your concerns. Do not overwhelm the school system representative with information. Prepare a written summary of your position.

Set up an appointment. When you meet, your approach should be knowledgeable and credible. Be confident and goal-oriented; set a tone of reasonableness. Try to resolve the situation in a friendly atmosphere. Don't force a resolution if none is possible immediately. Meanwhile, be flexible and willing to cooperate or compromise if the opportunity presents itself.

Ask for a letter summarizing the meeting, including the agreements reached, the points under consideration, and those issues for which no resolution was achieved. You may also wish to send a follow-up letter summarizing your understanding of the meeting.

DON'T BE DISCOURAGED

Feel good if you've been successful, or if you have made progress toward your goal. If you don't get what you've asked for, don't be discouraged.

But, be sure to ask why. Keep in mind that indoor air quality is a relatively new issue, and change is not always easy. Make sure that the school district representative understands the incentives to resolve indoor air problems as quickly as possible. School districts have a responsibility to provide a safe and healthy environment for learning.

For more information on school pollution issues and classroom accommodations for those with environmental disabilities, contact the National Center for Environmental Health Strategies, 1100 Rural Avenue, Voorhees, New Jersey, 08043, or call (609) 429-5358.

A HEALTHY SCHOOL VOCABULARY

adhesives, materials, often composed of volatile organic compounds, used to secure carpeting to a floor, or fabric to a wall or other surface.

aeration, the process of supplying air to a room or other area in a building.

air change, the substitution of one quality of air for another in a building, generally to upgrade air quality.

allergy relatives, illnesses related to or with symptoms similar to allergies, such as asthma and hay fever.

ammonia, a colorless gaseous alkaline compound of nitrogen and hydrogen often used in cleaning materials; its pungent odor can cause considerable airway irritantation.

asbestos, a group of fibrous minerals that readily separate into microscopic particles; in accumulation, a serious irritant to airway and lungs.

backdraft, an explosion of gas from incomplete combustion in a furnace or other heating appliance.

bakeout, the process of heating a building to disperse volatile organic compounds and other noxious substances.

benzene, a colorless liquid hydrocarbon often used as a solvent in cleaning; flammable and highly toxic.

biocide, a substance such as a pesticide, which is destructive to many different organisms.

breathing zone, that area of a room where occupants' heads are generally located; also *head space.*

cadmium, a bluish-white malleable metallic element used in protective coatings; highly toxic.

capture at source, a method of isolating contaminants at their source, rather than allowing them to permeate the air of a building.

carbon tetrachloride, a colorless nonflammable liquid used in some cleaning materials and as a refrigerant; highly toxic.

chlorine bleach, the derivative of a halogen element used in cleaning materials; in concentration can be a severe airway irritant.

chromium, a blue-white metallic element, found only in combination and used in building and furnishing; can be toxic in concentration.

coal tar, a tar obtained by distillation of bituminous coal, used especially in making dyes and some medicines; can be an airway irritant.

combustion gases, gases resulting from the burning of any fuel.

daylight, natural light produced by the sun; preferable to any artificial lighting for maintaining mental and physical health.

downdraft, a downward current of air or other gas in a heating conduit.

ductwork, any part of the system of passages by which a building is heated, cooled, lighted, or supplied with water.

dust, particles of earth or other matter resulting from disintegration.

dust mites, microscopic organisms found in dust, often causing skin and airway irritation.

electromagnetic field, the area covered by waves or pulses from any electronic source, from high-voltage power lines to household appliances; electromagnetic fields are believed capable of causing cancer and other disease.

ethanol, a colorless flammable liquid used in cleaning materials; highly toxic.

exhaust, gas or vapor escaping from burned fuel which reduces air quality; can cause severe irritation to the airway.

exhaust hood, a canopy with a draft for carrying off noxious fumes, smoke, or dust.

exfiltration, passage of air from a room or other area of a building.

fiberglass, glass in fibrous form used in the construction of buildings and in products such as textiles.

filter, material used to screen out particles or gases that may be injurious to human health.

filtration, the process of passing liquid or air through material to screen out injurious substances.

floor wax, substance for preserving flooring materials, particularly in heavily-traveled areas; ingredients can be injurious to health if inhaled.

floor stripper, appliance or substance used to clear floors of surface buildup; use of strippers requires care to avoid injurious consequences.

flush out, procedure for eliminating lead and other harmful substances from water systems.

formaldehyde, a colorless, odorous chemical substance used as a preservative or disinfectant; its fumes can cause severe nasal and airway irritantation.

formalin, a clear liquid product of formaldehyde; also an airway irritant.

friable, refers to asbestos in a condition that easily crumbles or that can be reduced to powder by hand pressure.

fungicide, a substance used to eliminate fungus.

green materials, those cleaning substances and construction materials that are non-toxic to humans.

head space, the area in a room where occupants' heads are located under routine conditions, also *breathing zone.*

heavy metal, a metal having a high specific gravity relative to size; examples: lead, cadmium, mercury.

hydrocarbon, an organic compound containing only carbon and hydrogen, which occurs in petroleum products.

infiltration, passage of air into a building.

Integrated Cleaning Management, a system for cleaning a building with the least toxic cleaning materials.

Integrated Pest Management, a system of pest control utilizing the least toxic materials.

labile, readily or constantly undergoing chemical physical, or biological change.

lead, a pliable but inelastic bluish-white metallic element generally found in combination with other substances; extremely toxic when accumulated in the body.

lead chromate, a volatile compound found in art materials; example, chrome yellow.

make-up air, fresh air substituted for contaminated air in a building.

mercury, a heavy silver-white metallic element, liquid at room temperatures; highly toxic.

mildewcide, a substance used to eliminate mildew.

mycotoxin, a contaminant or poison emitted by fungus, especially by mold.

naphtha, any of several volatile, frequently flammable liquid hydrocarbons used chiefly in cleaning substances.

natural materials, generally used to describe materials that are nontoxic to humans; the term should be viewed critically as a buzz-phrase, particularly in product advertising.

outgassing, (also offgassing), emission of fumes from building or furnishing materials, cleaning substances, and other products used in residential and public buildings; generally produced by volatile organic compounds, and often leading to poor air quality, if the building is not properly ventilated for an appropriate period of time.

particleboard, a building or furnishing material composed of very small particles of wood bonded together by a synthetic compound; frequently a source of outgassing.

particulates, microscopic forms of substances that contaminate air and water, causing health problems when inhaled or ingested..

pesticide, a substance used to eliminate insects, rodents, and other biological forms found in buildings; often toxic to humans as well as other organisms.

phenol, a caustic crystalline acidic compound present in coal tar and wood tar, and in dilution often used in disinfectants; highly toxic.

power lines, overhead cable systems providing electric power to large areas; a major source of electromagnetic contamination.

radon, a heavy colorless gaseous element formed by the disintegration of radium.

reintrainment, a rechanneling of air through the walls and other conduit systems of a building.

sick building, any structure in which the quality of the air is so poor that the health of occupants is in jeopardy.

silica, silicon dioxide occurring in crystalline form in sand and some semi-precious stones.

solvent, a substance, usually liquid, capable of dissolving or dispersing other substances.

stack, a vertical conduit carrying off bad air, gases, fumes, and other products of combustion.

steam extraction, a method of cleaning carpeting that is preferable to the use of toxic cleaning substances such as shampoos.

toluene, a liquid hydrocarbon produced from petroleum and coal, often used as a solvent, and as an antiknock agent in gasoline.

toxic substance, any material that causes illness to humans; a poison.

toxicologist, a scientist who studies poisons and other injurious sub-stances.

trigger agent, an inhalant, food, water, contact material, or other physical factor that causes syumptoms of discomfort or illness in a building's occupants.

ultraviolet, light waves situated beyond the violet end of the visible spectrum; capable of damaging eyes and skin.

vacuum, a method of cleaning surfaces and air by sucking up particulate matter; often displaces contaminants, rather than eliminates them.

ventilation, the process of circulating air in a building.

ventilation efficiency, air circulation that allows the maintenance of the highest air quality at the lowest cost.

ventilator, any of various types of equipment that circulate air through a building.

volatile organic compound, an easily-vaporizing substance that is a combination of chemical elements, used in various construction and maintenance operations; generally a severe irritant, especially in poorly ventilated areas.

xylene, any of three isometric hydrocarbons in coal tar and wood tar, a mixture of which yields a colorless, flammable liquid used in cleaning products and fabric dyes; a contaminant capable of causing symptoms of discomfort or illness.

ADDITIONAL REFERENCES AND RESOURCES

EPA REGIONAL OFFICES AND STATE CONTACTS

The Environmental Protection Agency's (EPA) Regional Offices and the designated agency within each state can supply schools with considerable information on mitigating radon and managing asbestos. This includes publications, information on training programs, and consultative services.

EPA Regional Offices

Region 1
(CT, ME, MA, NH, RI, VT)
JFK Federal Building
Boston, MA 02203
Radon: 617-565-3231
Asbestos: 617-565-3836

Region 2
(NY)
28 Federal Plaza
New York, NY 10278
Radon:617-565-3231

(NJ)
2890 Woodbridge Ave.
Edison, NJ 08837-3679
Asbestos: 908-321-6671

Region 3
(DE, DC, MD, PA, VA, WV)
841 Chestnut Building
Philadelphia, PA 19107
Radon: 215-597-8326
Asbestos: 215-597-3160

Region 4
(AL, FL, GA, KY, MS,
NC, SC, TN)
345 Courtland Street NE
Atlanta, GA 30365

Radon: 404-347-3907
Asbestos: 404-347-5014

Region 5
(IL, IN, MI, MN, OH, WI)
77 West Jackson Blvd.
Chicago, IL 60604
Radon: 800-621-8431 (except IL)
800-572-2515 (IL only)
Asbestos: 312-353-6901

Region 6
(AR, LA, NM, OK, TX)
1445 Ross Avenue
Dallas, TX 75202
Radon: 214-655-7550
Asbestos: 214-655-7244

Region 7
(IA, KS, MO, NE)
726 Minnesota Avenue
Kansas City, KS 66101
Radon: 913-551-726
Asbestos: 913-551-7391

Region 8
(CO, MT, ND, SD, UT, WY)
999 18th Street
Denver Place, Suite 500

Denver, CO 80202-2405
Radon: 303-293-1440
Asbestos: 303-293-1442

Region 9
(AZ, CA, HI, NV)
75 Hawthorne Street
San Francisco, CA 94105
Radon: 415-744-1046
Asbestos: 415-744-1127

Region 10
(AK, ID, OR, WA)
1200 Sixth Avenue
Seattle, WA 98101
Radon: 206-553-7299
Asbestos: 206-553-1094

State Radon and Asbestos Contacts

Alabama
Radon: James McNees
205-242-5315
800-582-1866
Asbestos: John A. Sikes

Alaska
Radon: Charles Tedford
907-465-3019
800-478-4845
Asbestos: Maggie Hamley
907-465-6002

Arizona
Radon: John Stewart
602-255-4845
Asbestos: Fernando Mendieta
602-542-1654
Norman Petersen
602-230-5858

Arkansas
Radon: Lee Gershner
501-661-2301
Asbestos: Wilson Tolefree
501-562-7444

California
Radon: J. David Quinton
916-324-2208
800-745-7236
Asbestos: James Lim
415-703-5111

Colorado
Radon: Linda Martin
303-692-3057
800-846-3986
Asbestos: David R. Quimette
Thomas M. Tayon
303-692-3150

Connecticut
Radon: Alan J. Siniscalchi
203-566-3122

Asbestos: Richard J. Laiuppa
203-566-1260

Delaware
Radon: Maria Rejai
302-739-3028
800-554-4636
Asbestos: Robert Foster
302-739-3930

District of Columbia
Radon: Robert Davis
202-727-7106
Asbestos: Edgar Kennedy
202-724-4706

Florida
Radon: N. Michael Gilley
904-488-1525
800-543-8279
Asbestos: Roger Loomis
904-922-8955

Georgia
Radon: Richard Schreiber
404-894-6644
800-745-0037
Asbestos: Marvin Bradford
404-363-7020

Hawaii
Radon: Russell Takata
808-586-4700
Asbestos: Kenneth Hall
808-586-4200

Idaho
Radon: Pat McGavarn
208-334-6584
800-445-8647
Asbestos: Gary Barnes
208-334-3896

Illinois
Radon: Richard Allen
217-524-5641

800-325-1245
Asbestos: R. Kent Cook
217-782-3517

Indiana
Radon: Michelle Starkey
317-633-0154
800-272-9723
Asbestos: David K. White
317-232-8219

Iowa
Radon: Donald A. Flater
515-242-5992
Asbestos: C. Milton Wilson
515-281-4743

Kansas
Radon: Harold Spiker
913-296-1561
Asbestos: Gary Miller
913-296-1547

Kentucky
Radon: Jeana Phelps
502-564-3700
Asbestos: Parker Moorer
502-564-2150

Louisiana
Radon: Matt Schlenker
504-925-7042
800-256-2494
Asbestos: Nathan Levy
504-765-0902

Maine
Radon: Bob Stilwell
207-287-5676
800-232-0842
Asbestos: Ed Antz
207-582-8740

Maryland
Radon: Leon J. Rachuba
410-631-3301

800-872-3666
Asbestos: Mardel Knight
410-631-3846

Massachusetts
Radon: William J. Bell
413-586-7525
800-445-1255
Asbestos: Paul Aboody
617-727-3983

Michigan
Radon: Sue Handershott
517-335-8194
Asbestos: Wesley Priem
517-335-9280

Minnesota
Radon: Sheila Brunelee
612-627-5012
800-798-9050
Asbestos: William A. Fetzner
612-627-5097

Mississippi
Radon: Silas Anderson
601-354-6657
800-626-7739
Asbestos: Dwight Wyle
601-961-5171

Missouri
Radon: Gary McNutt
314-751-6083
800-669-7236
Asbestss: Tom Cruise
314-715-4817

Montana
Radon: Adrian C. Howe
406-444-3671
Asbestos: Same as above

Nebraska
Radon: Joseph Milone
402-471-2168
800-334-9491

Asbestos: Kurt F. Bottger
402-471-2541

Nevada
Radon: Stan Marshall
702-687-5394
Asbestos: David Going
702-687-5240

New Hampshire
Radon: David Chase
603-271-4674
800-852-3345, ext. 4674
Asbestos: Joy E. Hanington
603-271-4609

New Jersey
Radon: Tonalee Carlson Key
609-987-6369
800-648-0394
Asbestos: James A.
Brownlee
609-984-2193

New Mexico
Radon: Ron Mitchell
505-827-4300
Asbestos: New Mexico Env.
Dept.
505-827-0062

New York (State Health)
Radon: William J. Condon
518-458-6495
800-458-1158
Asbestos: George R. Estel
518-458-6483

North Carolina
Radon: Felix Fong
919-571-4141
Asbestos: John J. "Pat" Curran
919-733-0820

North Dakota
Radon: Arlen Jacobson

701-221-5188
Asbestos: Ken Wangler
701-221-5188

Ohio
Radon: Marcie Matthews
614-644-2727
800-523-4439
Asbestos: Marty King
614-466-1450

Oklahoma
Radon: Gene Smith
405-271-5221
Asbestos: Charles Sewell
405-528-1500

Oregon
Radon: George Toombs
503-731-4014
Asbestos: Alice Dehner
503-229-6353

Pennsylvania
Radon: Michael Pyles
717-783-3594
800-237-2366
Asbestos: Sharon Lawson
717-772-3396

Puerto Rico
Radon: David Saldana
809-767-3563

Rhode Island
Radon: Edmond Arcand
401-277-2438
Asbestos: Donna L. Sousa
401-277-3601

South Carolina
Radon: Albert Craft
803-734-4631
800-768-0362
Asbestos: Jean Wheeler
803-734-4750

South Dakota
Radon: Mike Pochop
605-773-3351
800-438-3367
Asbestos: Bob McDonald
605-773-3153

Tennessee
Radon: Susie Shimek
615-532-0733
800-232-1139
Asbestos: Bobby Jernigan
615-532-0554

Texas
Radon: Gary Smith
512-834-6688
Asbestos: Athan U. Ogoh
512-834-6600

Utah
Radon: John Hultquist
801-536-4250

Asbestos: F. Burnell Cordner
801-536-4000

Vermont
Radon: Paul Clemons
802-828-2886
800-640-0601
Asbestos: Karen Crampton
802-863-7231

Virginia
Radon: Chris Dixon
804-786-5932
800-468-0133
Asbestos: Nelle P. Hotchkiss
804-367-8595

Washington
Radon: Kate Coleman
206-753-4518
800-323-9727
Asbestos: James Catalano
206-281-5325

West Virginia
Radon: Beattie L. DeBord
304-558-3526
800-922-1255
Asbestos: Richard L. Peggs
304-558-0696

Wisconsin
Radon: Conrad Weiffenbach
608-267-4795
800-798-9050
Asbestos: Regina Cowell
608-267-2289

Wyoming
Radon: Janet Hough
307-777-6015
800-458-5847
Asbestos: F. Gerald Blackwell
307-777-7394

MISCELLANEOUS RESOURCES

American Environmental Health Foundation, William Rea, MD, 8345 Walnut Hill Lane, Suite 225, Dallas, Texas 75231-4262, Phone: 800-225-2343; 214-261-9515; Fax: 214-691-8432.

HealthComm, Inc., Jeffrey Bland, PhD, 5800 Soundview Drive, Gig Harbor, WA 98335. ULTRACLEAR.

National Center for Environmental Health Strategies, *The Delicate Balance*, Mary Lamielle, Director, 1100 Rural Avenue, Voorhees, NJ 08043, Phone: 609-429-5358.

New York Coalition for Alternatives to Pesticides (NYCAP), P.O. Box 6005, Albany, NY 12206-0005, Phone: 518-426-8246; 518-426-9331. Publishes a newsletter about pesticides and other environmental issues.

PACE Chemical Industries, Inc. 710 Woodlawn Drive, Thousand Oaks, CA 91360, Phone: 805-499-2911. Crystal Aire sealant.

Practical Allergy Research Foundation (PARF), P.O. Box 60, Buffalo, NY 14223-0060, Phone: 800-843-3440. General information, books, pamphlets, and videos.

The Bio-Integral Resource Center (BIRC), P.O. Box 7414, Berkeley CA. BIRC is a non-profit institution providing education and research on integrated pest management. Members receive The IPM Practitioner and Common Sense Pest Control quarterly. The BIRC catalogue contains the following resources (please inquire about prices):

1. Common Sense Pest Control: Least Toxic Solutions for your Home, Garden, Pets, and Community, by William Olkowski, Sheila Daar, and Helga Olkowski (Taunton Press, 1991, 715 pages). Virtually every pest found in or around schools is discussed in this book along with practical, least-toxic methods for solving them.

2. Implementing Least-Toxic Pest Control in Schools: A Practical Handbook, by Helga Olkowski, Sheila Daar, and William Olkowski. 1994. Bio-Integral Resource Center. 200 pages.

3. What Is IPM?

4. Directory of Least-Toxic Pest Control Products

5. IPM Policy and Implementation

6. Contracting for IPM Services

7. Delivering Integrated Pest Management Services

8. Videos:

   A. IPM for Turfgrass

   B. Integrated Pest Management

E. L. Foust Co., Box 105, Elmhurst, IL 60126, Phone: 800-225-9549; Fax: 708-834-5341. Vapor barrier. Free catalog.

Environmental Education and Health Serices, Inc., Mary Oetzel, 3202 W. Anderson Lane, No. 208-248, Austin TX 78757, Phone: 512-288-2369. Safe building/design consultant.

Environmental Health Servbices, 3202 West Anderson Lane, #208-249, Austin, TX 78757.

The Guide for Planning Educational Facilities. (1991) Chapter titles include: Project Budget and Cost Control, The School Site, Developing a Master Plan, Educational Specifications, Spaces for Learning, Equipping the Facility, Financing the Capital Program, Renovation, and much more. Available from the Council of Educational Facility Planners,

International, 8687 East Via de Ventura, Suite 311, Scottsdale, AZ 85258, 602-948-2337.

The Healthy House by John Bower (1989). New York: A Lyle Stuart Book. Published by Carol Communications.

The Healthy House Institute, 7471 North Shiloh Road, Unionville, IN 47468. 812-332-5073, publishes the following (please inquire about prices):

1. HH Report 101: The Unhealthy House, 4 pages. Describes the problems associated with poor indoor air quality, including the primary culprits and the health consequences.

2. HH Report 103: Painting, 16 pages. Why you should be concerned about the negative health effects of paints, finishes, and strippers, and how to minimize your risk. Contains a list of sources of healthier painting supplies.

3. Healthy House Building by John Bower. 384 pages softcover, 1993. This book is a detailed guide to healthy house construction with thorough step-by-step instructions as well as tips for alternative techniques and re-modeling projects. This book contains over 200 illustrations and photos.

Personal consultation services are available from John Bower. This could involve questions about a new construction project or about solving an existing problem.

Maryland State Department of Education, Baltimore, Maryland, publishes the following (please inquire about prices):

1. Indoor Air Quality: Maryland Public School s (1987)

2. Indoor Air Quality Management Program (1989)

3. Controlling Environmental Tobacco Smoke in Schools (1991)

4. Controlling Indoor Air Quality Problems Associated with Kilns, Copiers and Welding in Schools (1991)

5. Air Cleaning Devices for HVAC Supply Systems in Schools (1992)

6. Carpet and Indoor Air Quality in Schools 1993

7. Science Laboratories and Indoor Air Quality in Schools (1994)

8. Interior Painting and Indoor Air Quality in Schools (1994)

Order from: Allen Abend, Chief, School Facilities Branch, Maryland State Department of Education, 200 West Baltimore Street, Baltimore, Maryland 21201-2595, 410-333-2534. Bulk purchase discounts are available.

Nontoxic Art Supplies. For a *free* list of nontoxic art supplies contact: Art & Craft Materials Institute, 100 Boylston Street, #1050, Boston, MA 02116. 617-426-6400.

Sick Buildings: Definition, Diagnosis and Mitigation by Thad Godish (1994). Available from Lewis Publishers, Inc., 121 South Main Street, Chelsea, Michigan 48118.

ABOUT THE AUTHORS

Annie Berthold-Bond is the author of the *Clean and Green: The Complete Guide to Nontoxic Housekeeping* and editor of *Green Alternatives Magazine*. (Chapter 7)

Mary Ann Block, D.O., is a physician and Assistant Professor at the Texas College of Osteopathic Medicine. (Chapter 6)

Joel R. Butler, Ph.D., is a clinical psychologist and director for Environmental Health Psychologists in Dewey, Oklahoma. (Chapter 17)

Earon S. Davis, J.D., M.P.H., is an attorney and environmental health consultant in Wilmette, Illinois. (Chapter 21)

Nancy A. Didriksen, Ph.D., is a clinical health psychologist in private practice in Hurst, Texas, and Adjunct Professor of Psychology at the University of North Texas. (Chapter 17)

William Forbes, is a pest management specialist with the Montgomery County Public Schools in Maryland. (Chapter 12)

Susan F. Franks, Ph.D., is a psychologist and Assistant Professor at the University of North Texas Health Science Center. (Chapter 17)

Beatrice Trum Hunter, is the Food Editor of *Consumers' Research Magazine*. (Chapter 19)

Judith Jaeckle, is a middle school teacher in Dallas, Texas. (Chapter 14).

Richard G. Jaeckle, M.D., is a psychiatrist and allergist in private practice in Dallas, Texas. (Chapter 14)

Shirley W. Kaplan, M.A., L.C.S.W., is a psychotherapist and Licensed Clinical Social Worker in private practice in Wilmette, Illinois. (Chapter 3)

Jacqueline A. Krohn, M.D., is a physician at the Los Alamos Pediatric Clinic of the Los Alamos Medical Center. (Chapter 13)

Kevin Kuehn, M.S., is a mycologist who is currently doing doctoral work in mycology at the University of Alabama. (Chapter 14).

Mary Lamielle, is the President of the National Center for Environmental Health Strategies (NCEHS) in Voorhees, New Jersey, and editor of *The Delicate Balance*, the NCEHS newsletter. (Chapter 22)

Joseph Lstiburek, P.Eng., principal of Building Science Corporation, is a widely recognized expert on indoor air quality. (Chapter 5)

Andrew A. Marino, Ph.D., is a biophysicist and Professor in the Department of Orthopaedic Surgery at the Louisiana State University Medical School. (Chapter 11)

Norma Miller, Ed.D., a former art teacher, is an Education and Environmental Consultant in Fort Worth, Texas. (Chapter 4)

David L. Morris, M.D., is a physician specializing in pediatric and adult allergy/environmental medicine in LaCrosse, Wisconsin. (Chapter 15)

Gary Oberg, M.D., F.A.A.P., F.A.A.E.M., is Medical Director of the Crystal Lake Center for Allergy and Environmental Medicine in Crystal Lake, Illinois. (Chapter 16)

Mary Oetzel, is an indoor air quality consultant and president of Environmental Education and Health Services, Inc., in Austin, Texas. (Chapters 8 and 9)

Doris Rapp, M.D., is an internationally recognized authority on environmental medicine and author of, among others, *Is This Your Child?* She is Clinical Assistant Professor of Pediatrics at the State University of New York at Buffalo. Her frequent appearances on the *Donahue* television program have heightened the public's awareness of the impact of environmental hazards on children. (Chapter 1)

William J. Rea, M.D., F.A.C.S., F.A.A.E.M., a pioneer in the field, is the Director of the Environmental Health Center in Dallas, Texas. (Chapter 2)

Albert F. Robbins, D.O., M.S.P.H., is a physician specializing in occupational and environmental medicine in Boca Raton, Florida. (Chapter 18)

Bruce M. Small, P.Eng., is an engineer known internationally for his work in low-pollution structural design, which he does from his home base in Goodwood, Ontario, in Canada. (Chapter 20)

Irene Ruth Wilkenfeld, is an environmental health writer and consultant in Granger, Indiana. She also runs Safe Schools, a research information network and workshop provider. (Chapter 10)

INDEX

A

ADA

   See Americans with Disabilities Act

adhesives, 4, 8, 21, 74, 102--03, 178--80, 185, 188, 271, 280, 325

administration, 4, 6--7, 26, 33, 58, 127, 130, 133, 139, 199, 246, 351, 393--94, 401--03, 405, 411--15

aggressiveness, 243, 347

air conditioning, 63, 81, 85, 88, 101, 121, 158, 308, 322, 325--26, 330--31, 373, 376, 392, 396

allergens, 33, 65, 68, 75, 124, 126--27, 187--89, 279--80, 321, 323--26, 328, 331--32, 338, 340, 363

   fabric softeners, 46, 418

allergy, 8, 12, 15, 21--22, 28--31, 33--34, 75--76, 127--28, 130--31, 134, 279--81, 297, 321, 323--24, 328, 331, 333, 339--41, 345

American Academy of Environmental Medicine, 189, 193, 311, 333

Americans with Disabilities Act, 11, 398, 401, 419

amino acids, 39, 41, 283, 342

antigens, 65, 283--84, 339

antihistamine, 47

asbestos, 65, 106, 109, 153--54, 166--72, 178, 222, 395, 398, 404

asthma, 12, 27, 29, 57, 63, 70, 76, 121--22, 126--27, 182, 197, 279--81, 286--87, 293, 297, 322, 326, 333, 347--50, 354, 375, 396, 403, 411, 419

B

bacteria, 10, 18--19, 43, 65, 90, 100, 121, 138, 141, 187--88, 322, 328, 346, 372, 376

brain damage

   lead exposure, 48

breast-feeding, 41

budgets, 136, 139, 141, 147, 188, 270, 278, 370, 381

bus, 397

bus exhaust, 118

C

carcinogens, 74, 100, 102, 154, 185, 215--16, 286, 417

carpet, 4, 8, 10, 15--16, 19--22, 28, 30, 32--34, 42--43, 68, 74--76, 86,